SECOND CHANCES

CRITICAL GLOBAL HEALTH

EVIDENCE, EFFICACY, ETHNOGRAPHY

Edited by Vincanne Adams *and* João Biehl

SECOND CHANCES

Susan Reynolds Whyte, Editor

SURVIVING AIDS
IN UGANDA

DUKE UNIVERSITY PRESS Durham and London 2014

Library of Congress Cataloging-in-Publication Data
Second chances : surviving aids in Uganda / Susan Reynolds Whyte, ed.
pages cm—(Critical global health : evidence, efficacy, ethnography)
Includes bibliographical references and index.
ISBN 978-0-8223-5795-7 (cloth : alk. paper)
ISBN 978-0-8223-5808-4 (pbk. : alk. paper)
1. AIDS (Disease)—Patients—Uganda. 2. HIV-positive persons—Uganda.
I. Whyte, Susan Reynolds. II. Series: Critical global health.

RC606.54S43 2014
362.19697′920096761—dc23
2014012919]

Cover photo: Sign for the Antiretroviral Therapy Clinic and the Outpatient
Department (O.P.D.) at Kagando Hospital, Kasese District, Uganda
(21 January 2013). Photograph by Susan Reynolds Whyte

Duke University Press gratefully acknowledges the support of
the Danish Ministry of Foreign Affairs, which provided funds
toward the publication of this book.

CONTENTS

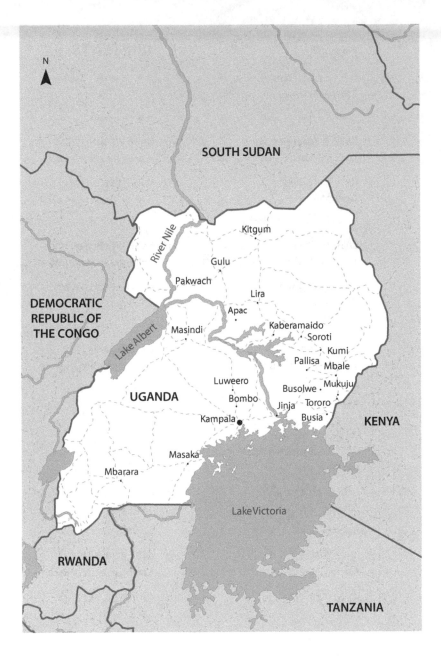

MAP 1

Uganda, showing places
mentioned by our interlocutors.
(Map by Kristian Bothe)

POLYGRAPHY

Second Chances is neither a monograph nor an edited volume in the conventional sense. It is the work of eight people, four from Denmark and four from Uganda, coordinating closely to assemble one common body of material about a unique place and time in African history. Monographs are almost always solo books, written by a single author who disciplines the data to tell one story. In the nature of things, they cannot always fully reflect the contributions of colleagues, field assistants, interpreters, and informants. Edited volumes have multiple authors, each with a set of data and an analysis, often from different countries, intended to illuminate the same overall theme. Our book is a polygraph, written by a set of authors about a collection of people and families who share common circumstances. It is "multi-sighted" in that eight pairs of eyes (and ears) were at work, and it is multisited in that it describes a range of people, locations, treatment programs, and dimensions of concern. Taken together, the stories and chapters form one overarching narrative about the generation of people who knew acquired immunodeficiency syndrome (AIDS) as a fatal disease and experienced the advent of life-prolonging antiretroviral therapy. The polygraphic form suits the task we have set ourselves—to illuminate both the diversity and the historical uniqueness of a generation.

This polygraph does not pretend to be a lie detector, but like those machines, it records changes in the (social) body occurring simultaneously in response to questions—about how to live with the human immunodeficiency virus (HIV). Whereas lie detectors are supposed to assess the validity of people's evidence, our polygraph assembles evidence and gives the reader the opportunity to assess our interpretations of the first generation of AIDS survivors and its second chances.

Our corpus of material comes from long conversations with people about their lives before and after antiretroviral therapy (ART) and from repeated visits to their homes. By listening to their retrospective accounts and following them over time, we came to have a sense of the directions their lives were taking and the concerns to which they returned in conversation after conversation. We wanted to preserve the integrity and situatedness of persons, so we have built our book around eleven personal accounts. They are the main "cases"—biographical versions of our original inspiration from the extended case method of the Manchester School.[1] So often, excerpts from interviews or focus group discussions are used as anecdotes or snapshots to legitimate a point the analyst wants to make. In the process, lives and contexts are chopped up, leaving the reader with little possibility of an alternative interpretation. Even though we have chosen and edited these accounts in relation to certain themes, each provides a surplus of information and ideas relevant to other topics, as well. Our intention is to give readers the opportunity to think in cases, to compare them, and see how they complement one another.[2] Differentiation allows more interesting generalizations.

Each of these stories prefaces an analytical chapter about the primary concerns of members of the first generation. The chapter themes do not directly follow the categorical interests of many global health actors—such as adherence, stigma, disclosure, transmission, and counseling (although all of these are illuminated from our interlocutors' perspectives). They stay closer to the affairs and preoccupations of second-chance life worlds. Roughly, these are about the everyday dramas of treatment (chapters 1–3), family relations (chapters 4–6), and livelihood and daily life on medication (chapters 7–11).

The idea that we were studying a generation took shape gradually; it emerged partly through our interlocutors' accounts, but also through our own experience. We all knew the situation before AIDS treatment was available, and we were working together over the years when the antiretroviral medicines were rolled out. Thus, our own historical location was essential to the bigger story we were trying to grasp. Michael and I, the oldest members of the team, did our first fieldwork in Uganda from 1969 to 1971, not so long after independence, in the pre–Idi Amin period our younger acquaintances sometimes wistfully call the "original Uganda." Returning frequently after

1988 and keeping contact with families we had known, we witnessed the onset of the epidemic and mourned the loss of many friends from our early days as young doctoral students. The rest of our group came of age as researchers in the time of AIDS. Lotte Meinert and Hanne O. Mogensen were closely involved with people who were sick and dying during their fieldwork in eastern Uganda. Godfrey Etyang Siu, Jenipher Twebaze, Phoebe Kajubi, and David Kyaddondo, like all Ugandans, were affected by suffering and death in their own families and among friends and colleagues. Even more than we from Denmark, they could not get away from AIDS. Public talk of the epidemic was constant after 1986; private distress and helplessness over the lack of treatment was just as constant until 2004.

We began working together under an Enhancement of Research Capacity project that ran from late 1994 to 2008. Supported by the Danish International Development Agency, it linked two Danish universities with the Child Health and Development Centre, a small, cross-disciplinary unit at Makerere University. The theme of our cooperation was the changing relation between communities and health systems. We called our project TORCH, for Tororo Community Health, Tororo being the district where our project was anchored and where, by the end, five of us had done long-term ethnographic research for doctoral dissertations. Although our project initially did not address AIDS (many other researchers were flocking to that topic), we did studies with health workers and families seeking treatment for all kinds of problems, which provided a necessary context for our work on second chances toward the end of the TORCH project.

We ourselves formed generations in an academic genealogical sense. Michael and I are the grandparents. Under TORCH, Michael was the supervisor of David, then a lecturer in Social Work and Social Administration at Makerere. I advised the two Danes, now my colleagues, Lotte and Hanne. The next generation of Ugandans, Jenipher, Phoebe, and Godfrey, all went on to earn doctorates in various aspects of AIDS in Uganda after TORCH ended. Hanne supervised Jenipher, who was awarded her degree in Copenhagen. David and I are co-supervising Phoebe, who is registered at Makerere University. After completing a master's at Copenhagen, which I co-supervised, Godfrey went on to earn a doctorate at the University of Glasgow, working with Janet Seeley, whom we met through our research. Academic generations are much shorter than kinship generations; still, by any standards, our engagement with one another has been enduring and fruitful.

When treatment for people with AIDS first became available in Uganda, it was far too expensive for most people. As the price fell, it came almost in reach of families with a modest income, while a few fortunate individuals were able to get the medicines for free. The inequities of this situation drew several of us to do a small pilot study of the diverse ways people were struggling to gain access to the life-saving treatment as a multitude of projects emerged after 2002. We retained an interest in diversity and the "projectification" of treatment when we launched the study that we have come to call Second Chances.

In late 2005, we approached six different sources of ART, three in Kampala and three in southeastern Uganda (Tororo, Mbale, and Butaleja districts), with a request to help us identify people willing to be interviewed about their lives and treatment. From earlier fieldwork, Hanne and Lotte knew people receiving treatment from a seventh source, whom we approached directly as friends and former neighbors. Using these methods, we found forty-eight individuals, whom we interviewed once between December 2005 and March 2006, in a very open format, taking extensive notes but without using a recorder. These were long life-story interviews about how they fell sick and got on treatment, but also very much about their families, partners, work, and daily lives. About half of the conversations were in people's homes, and most of the others took place in a quiet corner of the clinic, under a tree, or even, in one case, in the back of a car.

These forty-eight were by no means representative of people living with HIV or even of those on ART. People who were extremely ill at the time, as well as those whom the health workers considered difficult, and, most of all, those who did not have the economic, social, or cultural capital to get on treatment and stay on it for a while were not among our interlocutors. We tried to encompass variation by choosing both urban and rural sites and by identifying programs that provided only free treatment and others where some clients were paying a fee. We asked the treatment providers to help us find a balance of men and women, with different occupations, and to include people who were paying for treatment. We ended up with informants who were generally somewhat better educated than the average Ugandan in their age range of 30–50. But none were members of the powerful and prosperous elite; those people usually prefer discretion, and many get treatment from private doctors. The people whose lives we heard about, and those we later followed, almost all had financial problems, although there were differences in their livelihood situations. There were teachers, health workers, and soldiers who earned modest monthly salaries, artisans who maneuvered for contracts, and people struggling with small business ventures or farming. Most of these forty-eight people were well settled into their treatment regimes. Thirty had started ART more than a year before we spoke to them; only six had been on the drugs for less than six months. At that time, seventeen of the forty-eight were getting their antiretrovirals on a fee basis (although some were not paying out of their own pockets). The most common drug used was the generic Triomune from Cipla, an Indian pharmaceutical company. The forty-eight were evenly divided between men and women, and twenty-five were married.

Of these forty-eight, we chose twenty-four whom we contacted again to ask whether we might continue to visit them. We selected people from each of the seven treatment sites, men and women, including some who were paying for treatment. We tried to preserve the variety of livelihoods, and, of course, we approached people who had already indicated that they would be open to talking more with us. The ensuing seven visits took place between April 2006 and June 2007. From the first interview to the last visit, we thus cover a period of about eighteen months in the lives of these people. Two seemed uninterested in further visits, and we stopped bothering them, but one, whom we had decided to exclude because she lived so far away, kept looking in whenever she came to Kampala—she included herself in our study. Thus, we ended by following twenty-three people on treatment; in fact, there were more, for many households included several HIV-positive people, and some of these others were also on ART.

By "we," I mean primarily the Ugandan members of the team, who alone did most of the original forty-eight interviews and made the follow-up visits, each having five to seven people to follow. The Danish team members occasionally went along when they were in the country and followed the visits through the written notes. Especially when the Danish researchers had known the family before, it was evident how the quality of the relationship depended on the particular people engaging one another. Sometimes Hanne and Lotte were surprised at the picture that emerged when a Ugandan researcher started a relationship afresh with someone they thought they knew.

In the follow-up visits, we found people in their homes or at their place of work. Talking to people in those places, rather than at treatment sites or nongovernmental organization (NGO) projects, as is often done in health research projects, decentered AIDS. Sometimes people did not even mention their illness and treatment during the several hours that a visit lasted. Family matters and everyday affairs engaged attention and conversation rather than the material needs and donor resources that preoccupy NGO project meetings. This produced evidence that was less influenced by clinic and NGO discourse and practice. It provided insight into how illness and treatment fit into other concerns. Even though the visits were relatively short and intermittent, they gave a social context for the patients who were treated as individuals at the clinics. Our method had something of the rhythm of ordinary social interaction, which involves meeting again, the next day or years later, and updating one another on what has happened in the interim.[3]

Calling our informants "interlocutors" is accurate. There was no real question guide, and the visits took the form of conversations. David, Phoebe, Jenipher, and Godfrey were from three regions of Uganda and spoke different languages, so that some of the conversations could happen in the mother tongues of researcher and interlocutor. Otherwise, they found a common language; in no case was an interpreter necessary. As visitors from the national university, the Ugandan researchers were treated with respect. They always brought a small gift in kind for the household and were often served refreshments. But the particular relationships and the kinds of engagements developed differently. Some people asked for advice; some wanted to borrow money; some phoned or sent SMS messages between visits. Several of the men asked to be given money instead of comestible gifts for the household. Some interlocutors became friends who wanted to share confidences. Others maintained a certain reserve throughout or seemed unforthcoming at some visits and much friendlier at others.

The characteristics of both parties shaped the relationships. Gender played a part in some, as when Jenipher realized that Dominic's wife assumed she was a potential co-wife, and his father called for a piece of charcoal to write her phone number on the wall of the house. David saw that it would be unwise to call on Jackie at home, given the jealous suspicion of her partner. Phoebe visited a soldier who was separated from the mother of his children. When they hung on Phoebe and wanted to go with her, their father explained that they were missing their mother. Friendship and enjoyment of each other's company developed in many cases as the researchers returned again and again. One of Godfrey's interlocutors, from his home area, always expressed admiration for his education and accomplishments and asked his advice on financial matters. David had a background as a trained AIDS counselor and social worker, besides being a full-time university teacher. It was difficult for all four Ugandans to convince interlocutors that they were not health workers or counselors associated with the treatment programs. But it was hardest of all for David, especially because three of "his" people sometimes visited him at his office in the health sciences faculty at Mulago, the national referral hospital.

The challenge for Jenipher, David, Godfrey, and Phoebe was not so much establishing rapport; they are all experienced fieldworkers and friendly, interested people. The difficult part in this type of research is writing up notes immediately and fully to capture the conversation and convey the situation. The Ugandan scholars managed this brilliantly. Theirs was the task of polygraphy in the old sense of copious writing. Their notes filled hundreds of pages and were full of particulars that made people and circumstances come alive for us in Denmark. As individuals, the four visitors were sensitive to different nuances, but all wrote notes that were rich and thoughtful. Their notes were the direct source of the eleven case accounts in this book. To remind readers that this kind of global health "evidence" is produced through intersubjective relationships, we retain in the accounts some details of personal interaction as the researchers recorded them.

After a failed attempt at a computerized thematic analysis, we sat down together at the broad hardwood conference table in our research center in Kampala to brainstorm. On the basis of the interviewers' field notes and headnotes, experiences and reflections, we agreed on the main topical concerns that became the chapters of this book. At further meetings in Kampala and one in Copenhagen, we discussed possible ways to deal with the themes and chose the protagonists whose stories would be presented at greater length. Jenipher organized the notes, and I went through them all and made a kind of index according to our themes. We agreed that the material is ours in common and that any one of us can use it in teaching and writing.

In an attempt to keep everyone involved, we divided the cases and the chapters. Each of the Ugandans wrote about the people they visited, with editorial input from the Danes who followed each "case." Danes and Ugandans drafted the analytical chapters, each working on topics in which they were especially interested. My task differed from the usual responsibilities of editors. The common material was enormous, and I had to decide what would be used where, since the chapters drew on all forty-eight original interviews and twenty-three extended cases. As the overall conceptual themes of generation, sociality, and second chances emerged, I tried to develop them from chapter to chapter to create in our polygraph something of the coherence of a monograph.

Confidentiality was an issue right from the start. Sometimes the visitors were warned not to speak about the reason for their visit when certain others were present. Godfrey became adept at changing the subject whenever one of Matayo's colleagues came into the room where they were talking. Jenipher was quick to hide her notebook when a customer called at Alice's shop. Phoebe visited one family where no one but the mother and one daughter knew why she kept coming. In the notes and in conversations with one another, we used a pseudonym for each interlocutor—so systematically that we hardly remember their real names any longer. In writing, we have sometimes changed details that might make people recognizable.

After the visits ended, Jenipher continued to follow some of the people she had worked with in our study as part of her doctoral project, and a few of the others kept in touch sporadically. Mostly, though, the engagements with our interlocutors ended after the eighth visit. It had to be so. Social life is as much about cutting relationships as about creating and maintaining them. Still, for a few who became friends, the classic fieldworker worries about having exploited friendship remains. Godfrey wrote about John, who admired him so much:

> I worked with John through his grief and joys, and this is perhaps what ensured that we had such a productive connection during the study. However, I feel a great sense of shame and guilt for failing to reach out to John and find out what has happened after fieldwork. My failure to keep his phone number after fieldwork at times haunts me, and I feel I betrayed John. I prioritised my work, my other research, and abandoned the relationship I had built with another human being, a person who had lots of expectations for long-lasting ties. My research colleagues and I know that this is the right thing to do since the research had come to an end; yet looking back, it is obvious to me that this wasn't the best decision.

We from Denmark felt that our engagement with the challenge of AIDS endured through our Ugandan colleagues, who remained at Makerere as a strong resource base for future projects on AIDS. But they ended their relations with the interlocutors whose lives and experiences are the substance of our book. As Godfrey wrote, that sometimes feels wrong. Yet in a broader sense, the Ugandan researchers continue to follow closely the fate of the first generation struggling with second chances. It is their generation, too.

SUSAN REYNOLDS WHYTE

Notes

1. Kapferer, "Situations, Crisis, and the Anthropology of the Concrete."
2. Biehl and Petryna, "Critical Global Health."
3. M. Whyte, "Episodic Fieldwork, Updating, and Sociability."

INTRODUCTION

The First Generation

Susan Reynolds Whyte

I did not know I would live. I knew I would die.
JULIA *(widow, mother of seven, nurse)*

I really thank this government—or whoever brought these drugs.
MOSES *(widower, remarried, construction worker)*

In the space of the first decade of this millennium, thousands of people in Uganda who should have died from AIDS got a second chance at life. Antiretroviral therapy (ART) was the technology that saved them and created a generation of people who learned to live with treatment. They are the first generation: those who benefited from the scaling up of ART, when prices of antiretroviral medicine (ARVs) fell, free drugs became available, and a multitude of programs emerged to offer treatment and support. They had known AIDS as a fatal disease and had seen their loved ones die after terrible suffering. They tested positive for the human immunodeficiency virus (HIV) at a time when death was certain. The increasing availability of ART between 2000 and 2010 was a watershed not only for them, but also for their families, and for the hard-pressed health workers and community supporters who had struggled to help the sick and dying. With the prospect of treatment, hundreds of thousands were willing to be tested, and the enlightened discourse about "living positively" was immensely strengthened. Because ART is not a cure but a lifelong treatment regime, its consequences are far-reaching for society, families, and individuals. To realize the second chances, care must be given and taken continuously.

Three themes intertwine in our understanding of these people and times. One is that of generation. The first generation to live with ART was a biogeneration, defined by the management of an epidemic with medicine and an innovative package of care. Our work starts from there and poses questions about shared historical experience and generational consciousness. The second theme is sociality. We examine the ways that social relations mediated responses to the disease and ask how sociality was changed in the process. The third theme is second chances: what people made of the reprieve that ART gave them. We ask how they reflected on everyday life and future possibilities once these were restored to them. Generations, sociality, and second chances are heuristic concepts that push us to explore the mesh of history, social relations, consciousness, and subjectivity in a particular place and time. They are modes of asking, rather than absolute answers, about a process that is still unfolding.

By inquiring in these ways, we bring to the study of global health a deeper historical perspective and a broader social and existential field of vision. The notion of generation places the epidemic and response in the context of ongoing changes in Ugandan society and political economy. Sociality requires us to look at the everyday forms of interaction that are often beyond the purview of health-policy makers, even though they are essential strands of the web in which health rests. Second chances look beyond medical treatment and biological survival toward well-being—or, at least, the hope of improved being. Taking this broad approach means using ART as an optic for seeing lives and the context in which they are lived, just as it means using lives and context for understanding ART.

ART as a Historical Event

The "event" that defined the first generation was the rollout of ART beginning in 2004. But the event took its significance from the AIDS epidemic and the attempts to deal with it that preceded the rollout. The treatment itself was not new: highly active antiretroviral therapy (HAART, now commonly called ART) had been available in Uganda since 1996. But few people could afford it, and the projects that provided free treatment were grossly insufficient for the need. It was the advent of free medicine at many different treatment sites within the space of a few years that made the vital shift from availability for some to possible accessibility for many.

The expansion of ART happened dramatically. In 2003 the Uganda AIDS Commission reckoned that ten thousand people were receiving antiretroviral medicine. By 2007, the estimate had risen to 115,000. This was only a third of those who were in need of ART.[1] Yet it was a more than tenfold increase in the space of four years. The rapid expansion was possible through resources from many donors and especially two big programs. Money from the multinational Global Fund to Fight AIDS, Tuberculosis, and Malaria, established in 2002, and the US President's Emergency Program for AIDS Relief (PEPFAR), established in 2003, became available in 2004. These programs allowed organizations that were already providing AIDS care to add ART to their services.

The AIDS Support Organization (TASO), born in 1987 and one of the best-known patient organizations in Africa, was finally able to start giving ART to some of its long-standing members by the end of 2004. Even more revolutionary was the establishment of HIV clinics in government hospitals and upper-level health centers. Some of them had already been "pre-adapted" to HIV treatment by donor programs that supported other medical responses to the epidemic. (HIV testing was available in or near health facilities through the US-funded AIDS Information Centre; other donors had provided for the Prevention of Mother-to-Child Transmission of HIV program to be integrated in antenatal services; treatment of opportunistic infections, within some health units was supported by World Vision.) The number of sites where ART was available grew from 175 in 2005 to 286 in 2007.[2]

Since then expansion has continued. By 2011, the number of people on ART was being estimated at 291,000,[3] more than double the 2007 figure, and new developments continue apace. But our story is about one particular historical period: the rollout years, when ART first became widely accessible and its significance was becoming evident to a broad swathe of the population. At first glance, the advent of ART was momentous for two reasons: it saved dying people, and it was provided through new forms of health care.

The notion of the "Lazarus effect" belongs to those rollout years from 2004 to 2007, when AIDS was still known as a fatal disease and the medicine brought resurrection. According to the Gospel of Saint John, Jesus was called to Bethany to heal his friend Lazarus, who had fallen ill. But Jesus delayed, and he found Lazarus four days dead when he finally arrived in Bethany. His miracle of bringing Lazarus back to life is the metaphor for the effects of ARVs on people who were as good as gone. The metaphor is even more appropriate than most people realize, in that the healing power of ART came late to Africa, just as Jesus delayed his journey to Bethany. Peter Mugyenyi's *Genocide by Denial* is a gripping account of the deferral seen from the perspective of a leading player in the story of ART in Uganda, the director of the Joint Clinical Research Centre. Tales of dramatic restoration through ART are used to raise money internationally.[4] In Uganda, they were recounted to amaze, to reassure, and to convince in the period in which ART was a novelty. It was a miracle because of the assumption that AIDS was a death sentence and because many patients were so grievously ill by the time they started the medicine.

The new treatment was offered to Ugandans through innovations in care.[5] Whereas health care in Uganda, as in most African countries, was and is a matter of seeking treatment here and there, ART required affiliation to one program and regular checkups and refills at the same treatment site. From customers in drugshops and patients at the hospital, sick people became clients of HIV clinics. They joined and belonged to treatment sites that kept their records, monitored their health, and tried to insure adherence to medicine to avoid the development of resistance. Some clients even became volunteers, taking on tasks in providing care to others. Health care had never been so consistent over time and so "packaged" for so many people.

These two immediate aspects of ART were indeed momentous, and we return to them in the pages to come. But they were only the most obvious experiences of the first generation with the novel biosocial technology. More subtle were the consequences ART was to have on relations with families and partners and on the everyday practices of body monitoring, eating, working, medicating, and living. Less obvious, as well, were the changes that were happening in Uganda before the rollout—changes that were already forming the first generation before they ever began to swallow the vital medicine.

Exemplary Uganda

There is good reason to take Uganda as the country in which to follow the first generation of AIDS survivors. It was in Uganda that the African epidemic first became visible, and by 1987, Uganda had the worst HIV epidemic in the world.[6] Because the response to AIDS was so prompt, strong, comprehensive, and diverse, Uganda is often seen as exemplary compared with other African countries.[7] It was a pioneer in its immediate public acknowledgment of AIDS as a priority national problem when other African countries were denying or ignoring it. The openness of the National Resistance Movement (NRM) regime and the leadership it took in confronting the AIDS epidemic are legendary. One of the first national AIDS control programs in the world was established in Uganda in 1986, the year the NRM came to power.[8] By the late 1980s and early 1990s, self-help groups, nongovernmental organizations (NGOs), faith-based organizations, and donors were already active in providing education, support, and some health care. The "multi-sector approach" required the inclusion of HIV prevention and care activities in all areas of public and private enterprise: agriculture, education, media, road construction, and manufacturing. Thus, the first generation to benefit from ART in Uganda had been more exposed than citizens of other eastern and southern African states to massive information campaigns and a multitude of AIDS projects well before effective treatment rolled out.

Uganda's "success story" seemed to be confirmed by numbers: "the country's falling HIV prevalence rate became almost iconic, with the most widely circulated figures stating that the national HIV prevalence had fallen from 30% early in the epidemic to 10%."[9] The World Health Organization (WHO) estimated that HIV prevalence among adults (age fifteen to forty-nine) fell from about 14 percent to just under 6 percent from 1990 to 2007.[10] There were disputes about the epidemiological data,[11] but no one denies that there was a decline in prevalence. The much needed success story was further reinforced by reports of a fall in incidence.[12]

Testing for HIV was established by 1990. Although branches of the AIDS Information Centre, run by a US-supported NGO, were usually located at hospitals, testing was optional. Voluntary Counseling and Testing (VCT) required that the tester take the initiative. The Prevention of Mother-to-Child Transmission of HIV program was initiated in the year 2000 and has been rapidly scaled up as part of antenatal care in public health facilities. By 2005, a policy of routine testing was being established so that health workers could test patients' blood as part of diagnostic investigations. (Patients could still refuse to be told the results.) These two programs of testing place the initiative in the hands of health workers and opened the way for many more people to become clients by referral within a health unit. For the first generation, however, the first step on the path to ART was most frequently voluntary testing, often encouraged by a friend or family member. Many testing sites established "Post-Test Clubs," in principle for anyone who had tested, but in practice providing support for those who had tested positive.

Uganda was not only a pioneer in AIDS prevention and efforts to provide information and support to patients. It was also a regional center for research and treatment, building on the strong institutionalization of biomedicine from colonial times. Mulago National Referral Hospital has a distinguished history as the home of the first medical school in East Africa,[13] and in the era of ART it continues to play a leading role in training medical and clinical officers from the whole region on the provision of ART in African settings. The commitment of the NRM government to biomedical research and treatment was demonstrated in the establishment of the Joint Clinical Research Centre (JCRC) as a partnership between Makerere University and the Ministries of Health and Defense. Antiretrovirals were offered at the JCRC in 1996, four years after the center conducted the first trial of antiretroviral medications in Africa. In the beginning, very few people received therapy. While some high-ranking military (and probably government) officers were treated for free, most JCRC clients paid for the medicine, and the price was so high that only the wealthy could afford treatment. An initiative by the Joint United Nations Program on HIV/AIDS (UNAIDS) in 1999, Medical Access Uganda, ensured AIDS drugs to the JCRC and other gazetted treatment centers (such as Nsambya and Mengo hospitals and Mildmay Centre). But at $700 a month for triple therapy, even the rich could not always remain adherent.

Things began to change in 2001 when generics came onto the market. The Indian pharmaceutical company Cipla offered a generic triple therapy for $350 a month,[14] and prices fell from then on. The advent of generics brought prices down for patented medicine, as well. More and more people started ART on a fee-paying basis, although the monthly outlays required heavy sacrifices, and adherence was not consistent because people could not always find the money.[15] A few programs, such as Uganda Cares in Masaka and Médecins sans Frontières in Arua were offering free ART by 2003, and some people were lucky to be enrolled in research projects that gave ARVs.

At this time, several of us made a preliminary overview of the very uneven access to treatment in Uganda, with emphasis on the inequities in having to pay for treatment.[16] From there grew the plans for this study, which we nicknamed "ARVs for Fee and Free," because we wished to compare those who were paying for medicine, the majority of those on treatment at that time, with the fortunate minority getting them for free. By the time we finished our field research in 2007, many had moved from the first to the second category. It was this first generation that experienced the shift from paying for ARVs to getting them free of charge. That is, those who had managed to buy ARVs began to get them for free. Those who had never even started because of the cost finally got the chance.

Donors and Diversity

Two features characterized the scaling up of ART in Uganda: the heavy dependence on donors and the diversity of treatment programs. Donors have played a major role in Ugandan public health care since the present government came to power in 1986. Immunization, Essential Medicines, Safe Motherhood, malaria control, and many other programs depended on outside funding. When President Yoweri Museveni took such a progressive stand on AIDS, donors responded with unprecedented generosity, and the country became a nexus of global health interventions. Lacking the resources to offer ART itself, the government took a coordinating role and allowed others to supply the medicine, tests, training, and, to some extent, salaries and allowances.[17] In the early years of the epidemic, Uganda received more international funding for HIV and AIDS than any other African country.[18] In 2008–2009, the Ugandan government contributed an estimated 7 percent to the AIDS response, while multilateral donors covered 4 percent and bilateral donors covered 89 percent.[19] The United States, with its PEPFAR program, was by far the biggest single donor, contributing more than 80 percent of the funds for HIV and AIDS prevention and treatment. In the first three years after its inception in 2003, PEPFAR made Uganda one of its top three recipients; in 2005, it gave Uganda $148 million, more than any other country in the world.[20]

Even though a single donor provided the lion's share of resources, treatment programs on the ground were extremely diverse. There was already variety before 2003, and when it came into effect, PEPFAR's policy was to support many different projects—some faith-based, some secular NGO, some parastatal. The result was an AIDS care landscape in which "projectification" was intensified.[21] A plethora of acronyms reflect the many different organizations providing ART and other forms of support both within and outside the government health care system. Unlike in Brazil, Botswana, and other countries where treatment is provided primarily through government facilities, in Uganda, people gain access to ART from many different sources.

To reflect this diversity, we chose our interlocutors from seven different treatment sites. All have benefited from the surge in funding that occurred around 2004; some collaborate with one another in certain respects, but their histories and characteristics differ. For oversight, we can think of them in three categories, providing different sets of services to the first generation of people living with ART.

In the first category are two large institutions: the Infectious Diseases Institute (IDI) at Mulago National Referral Hospital, and the JCRC, the old center of expertise, with its regional branches (including the one in Mbale, where we also made contacts). They are rather impersonal because of their size, attracting clients from near and far because of their reputations. Here one may not necessarily get to know the personnel or be treated by the same doctor. The clients were not offered extra activities during the period of our study, given food rations, or visited at home.

At the opposite pole, in the second category, were the two geographically delimited high-service programs: Home-Based AIDS Care (HBAC) in rural eastern Uganda and Reach Out Mbuya in suburban Kampala. They were purposefully personal, assigning clients a supporter/monitor who followed them into their homes. Reach Out Mbuya involved people in all kinds of activities, from parades to Alcoholics Anonymous meetings and yoga lessons. HBAC was a research site for the US Centers for Disease Control, with carefully planned interventions. Its clients were organized in a representative council (Community Advisory Board), and they were all members of TASO, which had a range of activities.

The third category consists of two rural government health units in eastern Uganda: Busolwe District Hospital and Mukuju Health Centre IV. They were personalized in another way: they served fewer people, so the health workers knew their clients. In fact, they knew some of them anyway as neighbors or as patients in the general wards. The HIV clinics were part of general health services and were staffed by facility personnel who had (usually) been given a short training course. Home visits were not institutionalized, although they occurred sporadically when a donor program happened to provide allowances.

The programs our interlocutors joined reflected the political economy of treatment access in Uganda. They were all dependent on foreign funding for sustainability, a characteristic they share with AIDS control programs in many other African countries. Their diversity reflected the specific political response of Uganda, but some aspects are also found elsewhere. For instance, the large research project, HBAC, exemplifies the increasing role of global health research in providing high-standard treatment in Africa, albeit of limited duration.[22]

The foreign-funded interventions, especially PEPFAR, did not exclusively or even primarily target the public health system. In some ways, the NGO and international donor AIDS projects undermined the government health care system by drawing health workers away to better-paid jobs.[23] But as the examples of Mukuju Health Centre IV and Busolwe District Hospital show, donor funds also brought initiatives into government facilities; they provided training and insured the supply of ARVs, renovated buildings, and instituted new recordkeeping procedures. Sometimes they gave allowances for seminars and outreach visits.

In the debate about "AIDS exceptionalism," critics assert that too great a proportion of funding goes to HIV; other diseases and health services in general are neglected.[24] By its nature, our material does not illuminate this issue, since all of our interlocutors were benefiting from the outpouring of resources for AIDS. But the balance between treatment for HIV and treatment for other health problems was a problem for our interlocutors and one that merits investigation in other developing countries, as well. People on ART need care for opportunistic infections and for all kinds of other conditions, including those to which their ART medication makes them more susceptible. The availability and quality of these other kinds of treatment is thus a great concern.

Public institutional health care in Uganda is a mosaic of (free) government and (fee) private not-for-profit facilities. The waiting time is often long in the government Outpatient Departments; facilities are understaffed; and the drug supply is not always reliable. But there *is* a functioning and heavily used government health care system. At the same time, there is a thriving private sector of for-profit small clinics and drugshops, often registered in the names of public-sector health workers, that provide treatment conveniently for a large proportion of health problems. The public and private sectors are interdependent and complement each other. If the public sector were able to provide better service and higher salaries, people on ART would not have to use so much money on supplementary treatment.[25]

A Generation?

As a concept, generation is notoriously broad. In everyday language it refers to a stage in the life course ("the older generation"), kinship ("the parental generation"), cultural history ("the '60s Generation"), the sweep of human time ("past and future generations"), and creativity ("the generation of new ideas"). Anthropologists have long used generation to describe genealogical connections and to analyze succession, continuity, and conflict within families. In more recent years, they have taken up the notion of historical generation. Some set it together with kinship generation to examine how changing historical conditions interact with family relations.[26] Others, especially those working in Africa, have focused on youth as a social and historical category.[27] Several of these scholars are inspired by Karl Mannheim and by the interest in historical generations that emerged after the First World War.

In 1923, Mannheim published an essay that was later translated into English as "The Problem of Generations" and is seen as part of his corpus of work on the sociology of knowledge.[28] He argued that experiencing common historical events and conditions was formative for the way people come to have "certain definite modes of behavior, feeling and thought."[29] Just as classes share a particular social position, generations share a historical location. The period of youth and the time of coming into adulthood are especially formative, according to Mannheim. The historical experiences undergone then dispose young adults to rework the cultural legacy they inherit from previous generations. Mannheim's concept of generation was not based on chronological age, but it did contain an assumption of shared progression through the life course and a focus on the events that young adults lived through together.

The historian Robert Wohl, who wrote an account of the European generation of 1914, used the term "magnetic field" to capture the way that consciousness orients toward a particular set of iconic experiences. Deriving typically from great historical events such as plagues, economic crises, and wars, such experiences seem to signal a break with the past. The events "supply the markers and signposts with which people impose order on their past and link their individual fates to those of the communities in which they live."[30] Such events are always mediated in that they are represented; as June Edmunds and Bryan S. Turner write, "It is the intervention of collective agents who make traumatic events culturally significant."[31] That is, the social processes of representing and reflecting are what magnetize the field and create a historical generation. Our first generation is a historical generation in this sense. The frame of reference that created a sense of rupture with the past was the social appropriation of the AIDS epidemic and the advent of ART. These constituted the sense of "common destiny" that Mannheim highlighted and "oriented" perceptions in the magnetic field. The collective agents—the government, the donors, the NGOs, the spokespeople—represented the epidemic in changing ways but always as a phenomenon to recognize and respond to.

We use the term "biogeneration" to underline the biological and biomedical character of the events that magnetized consciousness. The "bio-" may also serve to remind us of a biological characteristic of its members: they were in the sexually and reproductively active stage of their life courses. We are not alone in linking the notion of generation to the AIDS epidemic. In 2011, the United States declared its intention to work toward an "AIDS-free generation" through its PEPFAR program. Its vision was to ensure that "virtually no children are born with the virus. As these children become teenagers and adults, they are at far lower risk of becoming infected than they would be today thanks to a wide range of prevention tools, and if they do acquire HIV, they have access to treatment that helps prevent them from developing AIDS and passing the virus on to others."[32] In PEPFAR's use, the term refers to a cohort born and following its life course under a comprehensive biotechnological program. It is a biogeneration in that its frame is the epidemic; it is defined by a biological fact—serostatus in relation to biological maturation—and determined by its relation to medical policies, procedures, and pharmaceuticals.

Our first generation is a biogeneration by virtue of sharing a relation to ART at a time that the biotechnology became widely accessible. However, our interest is less epidemiological than cultural and historical. While cohorts are defined from the outside by analysts (or policy makers such as PEPFAR), generations define themselves through their reflections on the world. For us, generation also implies questions about the members' experiences and subjectivity, their consciousness of their situation and of themselves as a generation.[33]

In the narrowest sense, our biogeneration consists of those who benefited directly from the rollout of ART—like our interlocutors. They embodied the experiences literally. But thinking of the epidemic and the advent of ART as phenomena at the center of a "magnetic field," we must recognize that their contemporaries were also influenced by the pull of these experiences. So widespread was AIDS at one point that nearly every family in the country was affected somehow. The effects of widely available ART spread beyond those who were actually taking the medicine. In fact, some of the first-generation activists were not on treatment and presumably were HIV-negative.

Pre-existing social conditions shaped the field magnetized by the great historical events. In imagining that field, we should think of the time just before the outbreak of the epidemic, which was the formative period for the first generation. The people on ART who told us their life stories were mostly in their thirties and forties.[34] Many remember something of the bloody years of the "regimes" after General Idi Amin's fall in 1979, but most grew to adulthood in the era after Museveni led his guerrilla army out of the bush in 1986. During their formative years, Museveni established a government that promised peace and progress, a respectable place for Uganda in the international community, and the development assistance that would facilitate this.

President Museveni's resolute leadership in response to the AIDS epidemic from his first months in power, and his welcoming of donor assistance, helped to legitimate his government. As one analyst put it, "In part, one might say, the state-building strategy of Museveni's National Resistance Movement, after a devastating civil war, was to mobilize around the AIDS epidemic in order to bring more of society under its purview."[35] Far from being a sign of weakness, donor dependence (or donor mobilization) became a strategy to strengthen the state. The young adult years of the first generation were years in which the NRM, which brought peace to most of the country, took up the battle against the next enemy: "slim" as AIDS was known in Uganda.

Talk of AIDS was part of these new times. From the village council to national organs, all public meetings had to include discussion of AIDS. National radio saturated its broadcasting with AIDS awareness messages. Before every news bulletin, traditional drums beat out a warning to remind listeners that there was danger; there were information segments in vernacular languages. Drama groups toured the districts; women's groups and schoolchildren sang about AIDS for visitors. Philly Lutaaya, a well-known musician, not only went public about being HIV-positive but created moving popular songs about AIDS.[36] It was not that all recognized the danger and took the warnings to heart, but everyone knew about AIDS through health education, just as everyone was getting to know it through personal experience.

After Amin's fall, new Christian denominations, which had been forbidden during his rule, were permitted as organizations.[37] Pentecostal and other Protestant churches, which had long been active in neighboring Kenya, began to multiply in Uganda. Even the two old established churches, the Roman Catholic church and the Church of Uganda (Anglican), felt the winds of revival as many members were "born again." Active Christianity had suffused life (and politics) since before independence in 1962. In fact, there was a wave of Christian revival in the 1930s. But the churches had been restrained during the years of turmoil under Amin and after. That tide was turning as many in the first generation came of age; they were young adults in a period in which old faiths were being enthusiastically renewed and new forms of religious devotion were flourishing. From the international evangelists who preached on Christian channels for those urban people with television sets to the hundreds of local pastors who proclaimed salvation to small congregations in modest mud-and-thatch churches, or gathered under a tree, the message of Christian faith was in the air everywhere.[38] Whether or not they were born again ("savedees") themselves, members of the first generation were familiar with the discourse of salvation, faith, and hope.

Christian revival and the response to AIDS affected each other in multiple ways. Some of the messages about HIV prevention fit with church teachings about chastity, monogamy, and faithfulness. Some churches and faith-based organizations were directly involved in support and even provision of medicine to HIV-positive people. Some Pentecostal healing churches promised the faithful that they could be cured of HIV without the help of medicine (a problem for treatment programs when they were persuaded to drop their medicine and for HIV testing sites because they returned again and again to see whether their prayers had been answered). But the most important confluence was probably the disposition toward transformation and salvation. For many in the first generation, the coincidence of spiritual and physical salvation fell naturally. In evangelical Christianity they found strength to accept their status and the resolve to take their medicine and work hard. In their miraculous return to health, they found affirmation of faith and help. Being born again in Jesus and born again as an enlightened client of an ART program were mutually reinforcing.

Paradoxical Consciousness

The notion of generation invites us to inquire into the distinctive consciousness that characterizes those who experience fateful historical events. In the spirit of Mannheim, we may ask about the worldview of this generation "in itself" (as a category we as researchers identify) and about the extent to which it has self-consciousness as a generation "for itself" (whether people think of themselves as a unique generation). These questions are particularly pertinent and difficult for the first generation living with ART. Conversations with our interlocutors, and literature about responses to AIDS in other African settings, point to a paradox of generational consciousness. On the one hand, openness and solidarity are idealized; on the other, secrecy and fear of discrimination are everywhere.

The first generation had its spokespeople, its activists, and its stars. Many had stepped forward well before the advent of ART. Some openly declared that they were HIV-positive; others campaigned on behalf of HIV-positive people, without highlighting their own serostatus. In the first category were the singer Philly Lutaaya, the Army Major Rubaramira Ruranga, and others who criticized AIDS policy on behalf of HIV-positive people. In the second category were tireless campaigners such as Noreen Kaleeba, the founder of TASO, and Peter Mugyenyi, the director of the JCRC, who built institutions and mobilized resources.[39] As is always the case, the active vanguard or carriers of the movement were a small segment of the generation, but they played a key role in representing the events and mobilizing others to recognize their significance.[40]

The practice of "witnessing" as part of AIDS education was well established before ART; HIV-positive people spoke about their disease at meetings, in schools, and in churches. Their stories served as warnings to avoid infection and as attempts to counteract discrimination by appealing for sympathy and support for those already sick. When ART became widely available, the testimony turned into tales of miraculous resurrection through the power of medicine. They were stories meant to encourage others to test and come forward for treatment and to adhere to their regimes assiduously in the promise of recovery.

Surely one of the most striking features of the response to AIDS has been the use of narrative both before and after ART. As Peter Redfield noted, AIDS is a disease that is particularly conducive to personal testimony.[41] Vinh-Kim Nguyen and his colleagues argued that giving testimony was decisive in obtaining medicine before it was readily available in Ivory Coast.[42] Whether told to a group of fellow patients at a Post-Test Club meeting or to a radio audience, testimony represents a key element in the consciousness of the first generation. HIV-positive people who had not openly announced their status listened to the stories and knew they were not alone. Journalists retold the stories for a wider public, in Uganda and abroad. One of the major national newspapers in Denmark serialized the story of Esther, later published as a book, so we could follow the development of her disease, her worries, and finally her good fortune in getting into a treatment program in Kampala.[43] Stories are used by projects and donors to mobilize support and document effects, as did Reach Out Mbuya in a small collection of clients' stories it produced.[44] Researchers gather cases to include in their scholarly works. We, too, encouraged interlocutors to tell their stories so we could write them down and use them to understand "the intersection of biography and history," in the famous phrase of C. Wright Mills.[45] If the British generation of 1914 expressed its consciousness of itself in poetry and other literary forms, the first generation in Uganda gave voice through public narratives of life with AIDS and ART.

Generational consciousness is more than personal accounts, however. It is a set of shared ideas and dispositions that we might call knowledge. Education about AIDS has played an enormous role from the beginning of the epidemic. It may not have changed behavior as thoroughly as the policy makers hoped it would, but it has provided information that has been absorbed, sometimes reinterpreted, and widely diffused. To the original messages about prevention were added dicta about living positively through healthy eating and abstinence from alcohol, tobacco, sex, and "overthinking" (worrying). Knowledge was disseminated widely, to HIV-negative as well as to HIV-positive people. In the same way, information about ART spread beyond those who were actually on the treatment.

For volunteers and health workers there were training courses, workshops, and seminars about AIDS, ART, and counseling. They were highly prized, not just for the allowances they offered, but also for the knowledge and the certificates of attendance they provided. AIDS had indeed become an industry and occupation, and the people it employed shared a discourse and a set of dispositions. Whether they were HIV-positive or not themselves, they were part of the magnetic field, and they expressed and disseminated important aspects of the consciousness of the first generation "in itself."

This knowledge is valued as a form of enlightenment, an indication of being modern and progressive. The rupture with the past is a break with darkness and ignorance about the disease. It is this self-awareness of being enlightened that characterizes the first generation and contributes to a consciousness "for itself," a sense of common destiny. As Hassan, one of our interlocutors, said, "At least for the current generation, we are fortunate that the disease is known. We have organizations like TASO that help us, give us support, and you get the chance to know the problem you have." Individuals look back on their own lives to the time before they knew. Elizabeth wondered whether she might have been infected through her work as a midwife, remarking that in those days it was not known that midwives needed to protect themselves. Many remembered how they enjoyed sexual affairs in the days of their youth, before they knew the dangers. And, of course, the advent of ART meant new knowledge about the possibility of surviving, as people found out about the medicine.

A new consciousness was emerging, but it was not evenly shared. On the one hand, as Mannheim emphasized, generations are not uniform within themselves. He wrote about generation units that had different social locations; they were contemporaneous but experienced and responded differently to historical events.[46] Thus, they might not share a generational consciousness. On the other hand, generations (or generation units) distinguish themselves in contrast to the "behavior, feeling, and thought" of previous generations and in this way form a sense of their own identity and uniqueness. For members of the first generation, a key distinction was the degree of enlightenment that a person or category possessed. They thought of themselves not so much in opposition to the parental generation as in contrast to the untested, the unenlightened, and the prejudiced. For the vanguard, the task was to include such people by making them understand and adopt a more progressive attitude.

But here is where the first generation presents its own special twist on the idea of generational consciousness. Enlightened people have to live thoroughly entangled in families and communities. They share values with, and are profoundly dependent on, relatives, colleagues, and neighbors. Although they knew that it was good to be open and discuss problems with others, they often did not do so, as we shall see in the pages to come. Even health workers who counseled AIDS patients to be open about their serostatus often did not reveal their own HIV infection.[47] One of the great ironies of testing and treatment programs, especially in the early years, was the exaggerated emphasis on confidentiality, combined with the injunction to patients to be open and reveal that they were HIV-positive.[48] With its early start on AIDS education and the massive resources it has received, Uganda is probably more tolerant and supportive of HIV-positive people than many other countries. But being HIV-positive is still discrediting in the eyes of many. So individuals and families want to control this information.

Generational consciousness is thus a complicated matter. The contrast between progressive openness and unenlightened secrecy is found not only between categories of people but also within the same person. While the activists and the AIDS stars speak out loudly and freely, most HIV-positive people identify with the enlightened discourse but prefer to keep quiet in a kind of enlightened secrecy. We met people who confided in us, or in their fellow patients, but never spoke about their serostatus to family and friends. This inhibits the possibility for massive expressions of common biogenerational interests, what could be called consciousness "for itself" in the sense of mobilizing resources to bring about change actively. It is hard to tell whether discretion will diminish as ART becomes even more widespread or whether it will simply become acceptable that people can use biotechnology without having to make such an explicit point of it.

Sociality

Considering social change in terms of generations requires care to avoid what Wohl called "generationalism" in the conclusion of his study of the 1914 generation. In exaggerating differences between generations, there is a danger of neglecting differences within them, such as those of social class and gender. Focusing on great historical events may overlook the givens of the immediate past. Generationalism, Wohl writes, "prevented those who fell under its spell from seeing that all lasting historical action takes the form of the transformation of that which already exists and results from the collaboration (as well as the conflict) of different age-groups."[49] In *Second Chances*, we use the notion of generation but try to avoid narrow generationalism. Much as people implied ruptures with the past, they were constantly trying to mend breaches in past conditions of life and to secure existing relationships. The dramatic transformations they all shared were not experienced directly; nor did individuals relate directly to representations by the vanguard. Rather, events and representations were mediated by the social relations in which actors were already embedded, including those with parents and children.

If there is one theme that is fundamental for understanding life with ART, it is the social nature of that life. The people we met and followed over the time of this study were always *social persons*, whether we were talking to them alone or meeting them in their homes among family and neighbors. In Uganda, people rarely live alone, and their life journeys, like their therapeutic journeys, are intertwined with those of other people. The demographic bottom line is that the total fertility rate is one of the highest in the world at 6.6,[50] which is to say that *on average*, Ugandan women bear nearly seven children during their reproductive lives. That means a lot of relatives—not only children but siblings, cousins, aunts, and uncles. Polygyny, divorce, and remarriage add further links in family configurations. So does the increase in children born outside marriage or cohabitation arrangements. Seldom do households consist simply of a husband and wife and their biological children. Relatives come to stay for short or long periods—for example, sisters or daughters who have left their husbands and children who have lost their parents.

In choosing to underline the social aspects of life for the first generation, and the relational nature of life journeys, we follow the emphases of our friends, families, and interlocutors in Uganda. Time and again, we have been struck by how people explain their experiences, decisions, actions, and plans in terms of other people. Certainly, individuals can make choices, exercise discipline, and care for themselves. Yet they talk about their lives often in terms of the help and hindrances offered by others: not "the community," as development rhetoric has it, but specific relatives, friends, and acquaintances. Dependence and interdependence are particularly underscored by poor and less well-educated people, the great majority of Uganda's population. In part, this is a conventional form of discourse, but it also reflects a reality of scarce resources and weak state welfare institutions.

The notion of citizenship, associated with the therapeutic rights of individuals vis-à-vis some polity, has gained ground in both development and academic circles. As a balance to that, we underline the intensely social character of accessing treatment and staying alive. Not only do people need family and friends to help them live with ART, but the treatment programs themselves have distinctive kinds of sociality. Nearly all require that people starting ART identify a treatment companion who will help them remember their medicine every day. These programs usually refer to their patients as clients, and we will suggest that "clientship" is a helpful term, which captures the use of services and the dependence, the sense of belonging, and the personal relations that were often important.

Other writers have pointed to the importance of everyday patterns of Ugandan sociality in regard to HIV and AIDS. Helen Epstein, a longtime observer, offers it as an explanation for Uganda's success in dealing with the epidemic even before ART, compared with countries of southern Africa. Citing the epidemiologists Rand L. Stoneburner and Daniel Low-Beer, she writes about the "powerful role [that] was played by the ordinary, but frank, conversations people had with family, friends, and neighbors—not about sex, but about the frightening, calamitous effects of AIDS itself."[51] In southern Africa, people were far less willing to talk about HIV with one another or to accept that it was everybody's problem, not just that of high-risk groups. Epstein gives credit to the AIDS information campaigns but also draws attention to structural differences between Uganda and southern Africa. With no history of settlers, land alienation, or massive labor migration; relatively sufficient and fertile land; and a low level of urbanization, Uganda is a country in which most people know their neighbors and live near their extended families. Epstein was making country comparisons, painting with a broad brush. But we think she was on the right track in emphasizing the "personalized, informal, intimate, contingent, reciprocal nature" of the response to AIDS.[52] And we suggest that these kinds of sociality continue to be key in the time of ART: for testing and getting treatment and for getting on with the life that ART made possible.

Second Chances

The rollout of ART meant that a biogeneration doomed to die was able to live. It is common to say that they got a second chance. In fact, speaking of second chances in relation to AIDS is so banal that an Internet search conducted for "second chances AIDS" in early 2013 gave about five million hits. But what does it mean to say that ART gave second chances to the first generation? How can we use it to understand the subjectivity—that is, the dispositions, concerns, and practices—of the first generation? There are elements, I suggest, of reprieve, of conversion, of contingency, and of reflection in the idea of second chances.[53]

A second chance is a reprieve. Those who take the medicine consistently get a stay of execution. Their symptoms diminish, and their deaths are postponed. A reprieve does not necessarily imply a different life; it could mean the opportunity simply to continue the life you had before the death sentence, a second chance at the same efforts, relations, pleasures, and worries that you had been resigned to giving up. A reprieve is an extension, a chance to resume and carry on. It is also a kind of recognition of human fallibility. People make mistakes or are victims of the mistakes of others. They are cast into despair and discredited. We must give opportunities for new beginnings to continue living with others, just as Hannah Arendt argues for the necessity of forgiveness in social life.[54]

The stronger meaning of second chances suggests a spoiling of life followed by the opportunity to try again and to live better. Loss is the occasion for conversion to a new life. In the Christian version of conversion, a person is born again, transformed by new beliefs, new practices, new fellowship, and a new relation to deity. One of the treatment centers our interlocutors attended, Reach Out Mbuya based at a Roman Catholic church in Kampala, clearly associated the second chance with a new life of hope. As Father Joseph, the project director, declared, "Every day is an experience of the presence of God who, through us, re-creates what was spoiled in each of us. Yes, AIDS, through concern and love, is a new beginning." At Reach Out, as at other faith-based AIDS organizations, medication, morality, and spirituality were interwoven. The new life on ART was to be a purer life of devotion and upright behavior. On the organization's 2005 calendar, every page was headed with the phrase, "We have a second chance, and that chance is now."[55] Through counseling, people who had believed they were doomed were encouraged to live new and better lives with medicine, awareness, acceptance, and support. As Line Jørgensen explains, "The central metaphors at Reach Out have Christian connotations and point to the dramatic transformation taking place when the individual meets the project."[56] Not all clients at Reach Out underwent a religious conversion (nor were all Roman Catholic), but the possibility was strongly present. Indeed, some of those receiving treatment from secular sources had also been born again and made the link between second chances through ART and religious salvation.

However, conversion can also be understood in the secular sense of transformation to "positive living," and this was even more common than religious conversion. Health care providers and counselors encouraged this kind of conversion, emphasizing that salvation was possible only to those who changed their way of life, embraced consistent medication, ate well, avoided alcohol and tobacco, and were responsible regarding sexual relations. Second chances meant taking responsibility for one's health, joining the congregation of the HIV-positive, and trusting in the medicine. Ideally, one should acknowledge membership in the fellowship of the HIV-positive by being open. Conversion implied a break with the past, commitment to new beliefs and disciplines, and membership in new institutions. It was this sort of conversion that informed the consciousness of the first generation, often infused with the Christian or Muslim convictions that were already present for most Ugandans. Some people were converted to positive life more thoroughly than others, but to have a second chance at all, you had to adopt at least part of the message. You had to take the medicine, and that meant becoming a client.

What happens to the sense of transformation and survival as time passes? Writing about people who survived the terrible events of Partition in India, Veena Das says: "life was recovered not through some grand gestures in the realm of the transcendent but through a descent into the ordinary."[57] In everyday life, the past was still present, not narrated, yet apparent in conversations and gestures.[58] For the AIDS survivors in Uganda, too, the second chance was a grateful "descent into the ordinary." Yet living an ordinary life with ART was an achievement more than a routine. The past was still present in another way in that they had to sustain their survival every day by taking medicine; they had to go for medicine refills and stand in line together with other infected people. Like the survivors of the Chernobyl nuclear reactor explosion in Ukraine, they had to go on struggling with physical symptoms in the context of all of the other difficulties of life.[59] As Ukrainians sought to make the "tie" that linked their health problems to the disaster and thus gave the possibility of entitlements, so Ugandans who survived AIDS attempted to achieve various kinds of support on the basis of their diagnosis through conversion to clientship. In both cases, the efforts of survivors had no guarantee of success.

Perhaps the most important element of second chances, one often overlooked, is their chanciness. Insecurity and uncertainty characterize life for most people in Uganda. The lack of sufficient health services, the absence of state welfare facilities, and widespread poverty mean that life is insecure and the outcomes of enterprises and problems are uncertain. "Gambling" is the common term in Ugandan English for trying to get by without a secure economic foundation, hoping that things will work out somehow, that something will come through. "Surviving" is the more positive idiom for creatively making do in difficult situations.[60] So the first generation of AIDS survivors rejoin the ranks of very many other people whose lives are not secure. The difference is that those on ART often have been unable to work at full capacity for years, may have lost a partner to the disease, and may still have bouts of illness.

Contingency is a form of chanciness that implies dependence on an uncertain event or occurrence or relationship. The first generation was reliant on historical contingencies such as the government ART policy and the goodwill of donors. Those on ART were dependent on their treatment sites, a matter of insecurity when rumors circulated that one, the HBAC project supported by the Centers for Disease Control, was going to close. These rather impersonal dependences were difficult to influence and seemed like forces beyond control. Much more immediate were the interpersonal dependences that are so fundamental to Ugandan sociality. Second chances were very much about the contingencies of involvement with other people. Unforeseen turns of fortune in the lives of others had consequences for better and for worse. Likewise, your own ups and downs are fateful for those who depend on you.

The experience of a second chance adds dimensions of intensity and reflection to many aspects of life—at least, for some people some of the time. The quality of "secondness" leads to second thoughts about things that might have been taken for granted. People weigh their relations to family members; they consider their sexual partnerships; and they think about children in another light, as we show in the middle chapters of the book. Even the most taken-for-granted aspect of existence, your own body, requires reflection, as do everyday habits of work and food. Such a common action as swallowing medicine, which every Ugandan has done since childhood, requires counseling sessions and monitoring.

Second chances are often some combination of reprieve, conversion, contingency, and reflection. They are reprieves in that they postpone death and offer an opportunity to pursue the life routines and projects begun or hoped for—the ordinary matters and the aspirations for children. They are a conversion in that they demand change; you must accept becoming a client, even if you do not adhere to all the disciplines of living positively. They are contingent on programs and people and on your own ability to deal with these other forces and agencies. And they provide food for second thoughts—reflections on everyday matters and relationships cast in new light.

Cases and Contexts

One of anthropology's most important contributions to global health is to examine interventions in the context of diverse lives, specific settings, and longer-term societal change. Using cases or situations to unfold contexts has been a classic methodology since Max Gluckman treated the opening of a bridge in Zululand as a condensation of the organization of power in the South Africa of the 1930s. Extending it out and making connections, piece by piece and link by link, Gluckman and his colleagues at the Rhodes-Livingston

Institute launched the methodology called "situational analysis" or "extended case."[61] To contextualize is to choose those threads, which by their relevance can be woven together to explain a phenomenon. As analysts, we make contextualizing moves in one direction or another, and we recognize that our interlocutors do so, as well.[62] Starting with one issue, we progressively draw in other elements, arriving at an understanding of the one, and painting a much broader picture of significance, just as Gluckman did beginning with the modest initiation of a rural bridge and ending with a critical synthesis of South African segregationist politics and society.

Anthropologists have already shown the contributions that cases and contextualization have to offer to the more universalistic approach of global health studies of the AIDS epidemic. In one of the first monographs about AIDS, Paul Farmer put the epidemic in Haiti in the context of national and global history and took cases of specific individuals as points of departure for arguments about inequity. João Biehl wove stories about HIV-positive people together with accounts by policy makers, pharmaceutical company executives, and activists. He contextualized the situation of a marginalized group within the national case of Brazil, which, like Uganda, is an exemplar in the field of global health. Didier Fassin showed how the understanding and response to AIDS in South Africa could be contextualized in relation to the country's political history.[63]

In *Second Chances*, we continue this work of contextualizing cases, asking somewhat different questions. How can we use the notion of generation to analyze the response to the epidemic within national history? How can we attend to differences in social locations within a generation and the diverse ways in which historical events affected people? What weight should we give to changing patterns of sociality in families and organizations? How should we approach the subjectivity of a life regained but still chancy?

Notes

1. The Joint United Nations Program on HIV/AIDS (UNAIDS) and World Health Organization (WHO) estimated that the number of people on ART rose from 44,000 in 2004 to 75,000 in 2005, 96,000 in 2006, and 115,000 in 2007. Coverage—that is, those receiving ART as a percentage of those who needed it, according to WHO guidelines— increased from 12 percent in 2004 to 33 percent in 2007: UNAIDS/WHO, *Epidemiological Fact Sheet on HIV and AIDS*.

2. Joint United Nations Program on HIV/AIDS (UNAIDS) and World Health Organization (WHO), *Epidemiological Fact Sheet on HIV and AIDS*.

3. This represents 58 percent of those in need of treatment at the current eligibility threshold according to Uganda AIDS Commission, *Global Aids Response Progress Report*.

4. Rasmussen and Richey, "The Lazarus Effect of Aids Treatment."

5. S. Whyte et al., "Therapeutic Clientship."

6. Barnett and Whiteside, *AIDS in the Twenty-First Century*, 149; Iliffe, *The African AIDS Epidemic*, 71.

7. Green, *Rethinking Aids Prevention*; Parkhurst, "The Ugandan Success Story?"; Parkhurst and Lush, "The Political Environment of HIV"; Allen and Heald, "The Political Environment of HIV"; Epstein, *The Invisible Cure*; Thornton, *Unimagined Community*.

8. The evolution of AIDS policy in Uganda is documented in Kinsman, *AIDS Policy in Uganda*.

9. Kinsman, *Pragmatic Choices*, 102.

10. UNAIDS/WHO, *Epidemiological Fact Sheet on HIV and AIDS*.

11. Parkhurst, "The Ugandan Success Story?"

12. Kinsman, *Pragmatic Choices*, 101–2. The success story was losing its shine by 2011, when the Ministry of Health showed an increase in prevalence to 7.3 percent of people age fifteen to forty-nine and, more alarming, a steady rise in incidence: Uganda Ministry of Health, *Uganda AIDS Indicator Survey 2011*.

13. Iliffe, *East African Doctors*, 60–91.

14. Iliffe, *The African AIDS Epidemic*, 148–49.

15. Byakika-Tusiime et al., "Adherence to HIV Antiretroviral Therapy in HIV+ Ugandan Patients Purchasing Therapy."

16. S. Whyte et al., "Treating AIDS."

17. Putzel, "The Politics of Action on AIDS."

18. Parkhurst, "The Response to HIV/AIDS and the Construction of National Legitimacy," 585.

19. Uganda Government, *UNGASS Country Progress Report Uganda*, 55–56.

20. See the website at http://www.avert.org/pepfar.htm, accessed 7 January.

21. Meinert and Whyte, "Epidemic Projectification."

22. Geissler, "Studying Trial Communities."

23. See Pfeiffer, "The Struggle for a Public Sector" for an analysis of how PEPFAR undermined the government health care system in Mozambique.

24. Whiteside and Smith, "Exceptional Epidemics"; Smith and Whiteside, "The History of AIDS Exceptionalism."

25. S. Whyte, "Creative Commoditization."

26. Cole and Durham, *Generations and Globalization*; Alber et al., *Generations in Africa*.

27. Honwana and De Boeck, *Makers and Breakers*; Christiansen et al., *Navigating Youth, Generating Adulthood*.

28. Pilcher, "Mannheim's Sociology of Generations," 482.

29. Mannheim, "Essay on the Problem of Generations," 291.

30. Wohl, *The Generation of 1914*, 210.

31. Edmunds and Turner, "Global Generations," 561.

32. US Department of State, PEPFAR Blueprint.

33. Burnett, Generations.

34. Of the forty-eight on ART who told us their life stories, six were in their twenties; thirteen, in their thirties; nineteen, in their forties; and seven, in their fifties. They may have been a little older than most people on treatment.

35. Swidler, "Responding to AIDS in Sub-Saharan Africa," 141.

36. Kinsman, Pragmatic Choices, 82–84.

37. About 12 percent of Uganda's population is Muslim, according to the census taken in 2002.

38. Christiansen, "Development by Churches, Development of Churches."

39. Mugyenyi, Genocide by Denial; Kaleeba, We Miss You All.

40. Edmunds and Turner, "Global Generations," 563.

41. Redfield, Life in Crisis, 191.

42. Nguyen et al., "Adherence as Therapeutic Citizenship."

43. Faber, Esthers Bog.

44. Dryden-Peterson and Kamunvi, Living with HIV/AIDS in Uganda and the Impact of Holistic Interventions: Clients Tell Their Stories.

45. Mills, The Sociological Imagination, 6.

46. The AIDS activists of the first generation might be said to form a unit. On generation units, see Mannheim, "The Problem of Generations," 304–12.

47. Kyakuwa, "Ethnographic Experiences of HIV-Positive Nurses in Managing Stigma at a Clinic in Rural Uganda."

48. Twebaze, "Medicines for Life"; S. Whyte et al., "Health Workers Entangled."

49. Wohl, The Generation of 1914, 236.

50. UNAIDS/WHO, Epidemiological Fact Sheet on HIV and AIDS.

51. Epstein, The Invisible Cure, 134.

52. Epstein, The Invisible Cure, 169.

53. Janet Seeley and Steve Russell pursue similar considerations about "getting back to normal," "social rebirth," and "transformation" after starting ART in rural eastern Uganda. They also conclude that there are different trajectories and no straightforward phases of separation, liminality, and reintegration: Seeley and Russell, "Social Rebirth and Social Transformation?"

54. Arendt, The Human Condition, 240–46.

55. Jørgensen, "We Have a Second Chance and That Chance Is Now."

56. Jørgensen, "Counselling, Coping and Conversion to a New Life," 68.

57. Das, Life and Words, 7.

58. Das, Life and Words, 97.

59. Petryna, Life Exposed.

60. S. Whyte, "Discrimination."

61. Mitchell, "Case and Situation Analysis"; Gluckman, Analysis of a Social Situation in Modern Zululand.

62. Dilley, "The Problem of Context."

63. Farmer, AIDS and Accusation; Biehl, Will to Live; Fassin, When Bodies Remember.

CASE I

Robinah & Joyce

THE CONNECTING
SISTERS

Lotte Meinert and
Godfrey Etyang Siu

CONNECTIONS

(overleaf)

Health workers like
these two clinical officers
are valued acquaintances.

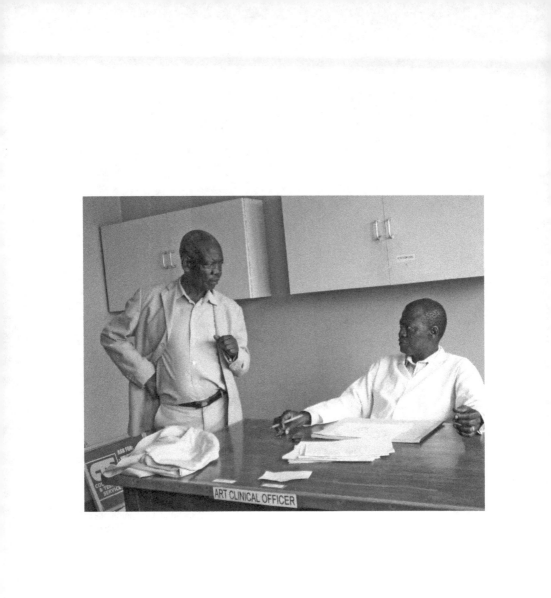

Robinah and Joyce were sisters, both in their early forties. They looked like night and day. Robinah was tall, skinny, weak, and quiet. Joyce was short, strong, active, and loud. It was a hot afternoon in December 2005, and we were seated in Joyce's small house, which belonged to the nearby primary school where she worked as a teacher. Rays of sunlight penetrated the rusty iron sheet roof through little holes, and you could tell from the smell that bats were hiding up there. A mobile phone hung on the door; books and papers were stored under a table; and the walls were decorated with posters on HIV and AIDS. It was not hard to tell that Joyce was a teacher and an AIDS activist.

Lotte had known Joyce since 1997 when she did fieldwork in the area. Then Joyce was alone with her one-year-old daughter, the last of her children still alive. The little girl was often sick, and one day Lotte helped bring the child to the hospital. She was admitted and put on drip but died two days later. Lotte began to suspect HIV but never talked about it with Joyce. A couple of years later, Lotte was back doing another study in the area, and during a focus group discussion Joyce suddenly remarked that she was HIV-positive. In the intervening years, it had become easier to speak openly, at least for some, and Joyce was beginning her career as an AIDS activist. In 2005, when Lotte and Godfrey asked her to participate in the study, she did not hesitate. Godfrey, who had grown up in the sub-county where Joyce was now a teacher, visited Joyce and Robinah regularly during the next eighteen months, at times accompanied by Lotte.

At that first visit, the sisters talked about their childhood in Kumi District, in eastern Uganda, where their parents were farmers. Robinah dropped out of school after a few years and married, as a second wife, into a family of cattle traders and businessmen. It was a big family, since her husband's father and his brothers were all polygynous. Together, Robinah and her husband had five children: one boy and four girls. When her father-in-law died, his sons inherited the young widows, as often happened in their part of Uganda. In time, they, too, fell ill and died, including Robinah's husband. "Today, if you went to that home, you would be shocked by the number of graves. I am the only one who survived," said Robinah sadly. After this experience and during the time of insecurity in northeastern Uganda that started in the late 1980s, Robinah moved to Kumi town, where she met another man, a soldier, and had a son with him.

Joyce married a soldier from northern Uganda. They had four children together, but three died, one after another. Joyce said, "My husband started hating me, and then he left to go and work as a security guard in Kampala. He used to send money, but at some point the money stopped coming." Joyce went to Kampala to find her husband seriously ill, and he soon passed away. Although she worked as a primary-school teacher in a village near Tororo, she could hardly make ends meet. Her baby sickened; every possible treatment was tried, but this last remaining child also died. "I remained alone with a lot of frustration," Joyce said. "Many fingers were pointing at me because I had lost all the people consecutively with the same signs and symptoms. It was through these experiences that I started wondering about AIDS."

One day, a colleague, who was HIV-positive, approached Joyce for a serious talk. He advised her to be strong-hearted, recall all of the suffering in her family, and take a test from the hospital. Joyce considered his advice, took the test, and found the courage to get the results. She was HIV-positive. "I joined TASO [The AIDS Support Organization] the next day and got a lot of support and hope from that." Joyce was put on a TASO program that provided safe drinking water and antibiotic prophylaxis, which helped her avoid infections for a long period. Remembering how her sister Robinah had lost her first husband, Joyce advised her to go for a test too. Robinah tested HIV-positive, as well, and her health started deteriorating quickly. She lost weight, vomited frequently, and had a skin rash and her hair started falling out. Robinah was living with their mother in Kumi district, and people in the community advised her mother to isolate her with her own plates, cups, and bedding.

At that time, Robinah's daughter was living with Joyce, where she was teaching. When the daughter started having dreams about her mother's death, she and Joyce decided to go to Kumi to check on Robinah. They found Robinah still alive but very ill and helpless. Joyce was disturbed by her sister's isolation and the discrimination against her; she started bathing her and cutting her nails, but she had to leave her and go back to work the next day. When Joyce returned home, she approached Simon, a neighbor and field officer in the Home-Based AIDS Care (HBAC) project run by the US Centers for Disease Control. Simon asked Joyce why she had not brought Robinah to stay with her and get help. Joyce immediately sent a message to Robinah in Kumi that there were people in Tororo who wanted to meet her.

Robinah gathered her strength and prepared to go to Tororo. Her family advised her not to leave because she was too weak and would not be able to make the journey. She was determined to go, but as she got ready, she could not control her diarrhea and dirtied her dress. She sought help from a brother, who wore gloves and washed the dress for her. When she was ready to go the next day, another brother agreed to carry her by bicycle to the nearest trading center, where she could take a *boda-boda* (bicycle taxi) to Kumi town to catch the bus. As she left, a group of men were watching her, and they blamed the boda-boda boy for taking such a sick woman away from home. She was likely to cause problems; if she died, it would be a burden for the family to bring her body back. But Robinah persisted and reached the bus station. The journey was to be the worst experience of her life. When she entered the bus, she felt everybody's eyes on her, noticing her emaciation, sores, skin rash, and lack of hair. As soon as the bus left, she had to ask the driver to stop so that she could get out to help herself. The driver was kind and stopped twice more because of her diarrhea. However, her condition was getting worse and worse. In Tororo, she found a boda-boda that could take her to her sister's village, but the diarrhea made the trip a nightmare. She only made it because of steadfast determination. On arriving, she found a group of people looking alarmed. They were quiet for a while, but later they said, "This one has brought problems for the teacher" (her sister). "Soon the word spread and people were coming to see me," Robinah said. "They were shocked, others were crying. They knew I was dying."

The next day, Joyce took Robinah to the HBAC clinic. "They examined me to find out that my body defense soldiers [CD4 count] were only 2. [The CD4 count is a measure of the immune system that ranges between 500 and 1,000 in healthy persons.] My tuberculosis test was negative, and I was given medicine for diarrhea and malaria and told to go home." After a week Robinah was started on ART. She had to fill in a lot of forms and sign consent papers. She was put on treatment from HBAC because she fit the inclusion criteria of its research project: a CD4 count below 250, membership in TASO, and full-time residence in the project's catchment area. (Robinah was considered a resident in her sister's household.) Joyce did not qualify for inclusion in the project because her CD4 count was not low enough when the project was recruiting patients.

It was rough in the beginning when Robinah was still so weak. The drugs' side effects were hard to tolerate; her feet and her fingers were numb, and she felt dizzy and weak. "I was staying in the home just like a child," Robinah recalled. "All support had to come from my sister, who earned only 165,000 shillings [at the time, about $94] per month." Some food rations were provided by TASO but not enough for the household, which counted seven people (the two sisters, two daughters and a son of Robinah, and two children of their brother and sister who were living in Kumi). Robinah regretted that she could not contribute anything during the first period in her sister's house.

The HBAC field officer brought Robinah's medicine to the house every week on a motorbike. A counselor from the project came to visit Robinah several times to interview her and advised her on feeding, side effects, traveling, involvement in social life, challenges, medications, and sexual relationships. To Robinah, the most important information concerned avoiding involvement in a new relationship. Both sisters were very determined not to let men into their lives. "Never again, there is no way we can do that with the suffering we have gone through," said Joyce in a way that left no doubt. And with these two—possibly exceptional—sisters, this decision did not change in the time we visited them.

Along with the medicine, the HBAC project provided mosquito nets and a jerrican to store drinking water. The sisters tried to lobby for food support from HBAC, because a shortage of food was one of their most difficult problems. At the time, neither had enough energy to farm the small piece of land around the house. Robinah recalled the negative answer from the project with some resentment: "they asked us whether it was the treatment or food that had taken us to HBAC."

After about three months, Robinah started to gain weight. The diarrhea also stopped, and her hair grew back. Then she began to worry about the restrictions of life on treatment. The HBAC program required her to remain in place, where her consumption of medicine could be supervised. Yet she wanted to visit the children she had left in Kumi. But she thought about her sickness. "After all, I would have died and left these children had it not been for these drugs," she said. "Then my worries stopped." The first visit ended with Robinah telling Godfrey that it was a privilege to have him come talk to her—it made her feel like a person again.

The next time Godfrey visited the sisters, in April 2006, Robinah had become even healthier, but Joyce was not well. Night was beginning to turn into day, and vice versa. They both welcomed him warmly, but it was mostly Joyce who talked. Despite her own trouble, she smiled at her sister and remarked, "Robinah is our miracle, as you see her over there. These people [Robinah and other AIDS patients in the area] were gone cases, but you cannot believe that they are the same ones now." Joyce and Robinah reflected on others in the neighborhood who were not doing so well and agreed that the problem was family support. "You know, with this disease you need to be loved and cared for, and that is what I did for Robinah—you can see how she is," said Joyce. Robinah smiled and added, "If you want somebody to be OK, you should love them." Robinah was busy on this day, and Joyce explained that after she had regained her strength, Robinah had become very active in cultivating. The sisters showed the crops of young maize, beans, and vegetables on their small piece of land. They had been receiving seeds from the organization Africa 2000, a connection Joyce had made as chair of the Post-Test Club.

After a while, Joyce also started taking ARVs. "My CD4 had fallen to 163, down from 360, and I was very upset. I had a high CD4 [count] and did not expect it to fall so rapidly. Maybe it was because of too much work. I have been too busy and was psychologically unsettled. I had a problem because my daughter [Robinah's daughter] conceived, and yet she is still in school. I think this is why my CD4 fell so fast." Joyce got into a TASO program, where she received doses of medicine for two months at a time; no regular CD4 tests were offered. For her, too, the drugs' side effects were tough in the beginning. Joyce had nausea, but she knew she had to endure, as her sister had done. She felt weak and had a paralyzed hand. Sometimes the numbness prevented her from teaching because she could not write, which worried her: how would she be able to provide for the family if she could not work? Sometimes when a colleague saw that Joyce was exhausted and unable to teach, she took over one of her classes.

Robinah got permission from HBAC to take a week's dose of the ARVs, then visit her children in Kumi on Monday and return to Tororo on Friday or Saturday to receive the next dose. When she passed through the villages on a boda-boda, the word quickly spread that *Isik*—"the sick one" in Ateso, the local language—had come back. Many people turned up to see her, hug her, and shake her hand. "People were greeting me, saying, 'Oh, God is good. What a miracle! What is the magic?'" They were convinced that Robinah had been employed somewhere and was now earning money, because her appearance and health were so good. "They asked me, 'Where did you get the job? Where are you working? You are now so healthy, and your standard reflects money.'" Her denial that she was earning money fell on deaf ears, but she continued to explain that the medicine was the secret.

When Godfrey visited the sisters next, Robinah was even better and seemed to have taken over the heavy work in the household. She thanked Godfrey for the sugar, soap, and cooking oil he had brought and invited him to sit inside the house. Smiling, she told him that she now had a CD4 count of 365—a miraculous number, considering that her count was only 2 when she started ARVs. Joyce believed Robinah was doing better than she was in responding to the medicine and in raising her CD4 count, although Joyce did not know her own count. Joyce lacked appetite while Robinah ate heartily. Joyce had been sickly and troubled by pain, skin problems, itching, and heartburn. She was bitter about what she was going through and said that at times she would rather be dead than have such pain. But she appreciated the support she was receiving from her family and colleagues.

Robinah helped Joyce arrange her pills in a small container with daily-dose compartments like the one Robinah was using from HBAC. She said,

> Robinah is like my medicine companion. Before I leave home for school, Robinah makes sure I have swallowed my drugs. But even if I forget to take them, Robinah can come herself or send the children to school to bring my drugs. One time I had forgotten, and I went to school. During break time, I went to the trading center. But I was surprised when schoolchildren ran after me, calling, "Teacher, teacher, we have something for you—your drugs." My sister had sent the drugs to the headmaster, who had sent children out to find me. Most of the time, they are supportive like this, but people can change. Most of my neighbors like me, and I am known as the AIDS doctor. This is because of what I do for them, especially the Post-Test Club. But one time I had problems with the neighbors, when our daughter conceived. When I learned that a boy from the neighborhood was responsible, I got furious and quarreled. Then some people started abusing me. They would say, "Her AIDS has now started."

Joyce had been mobilizing patients on AIDS treatment for an art project with a *muzungu* (white person). "The muzungu has been teaching a group of us to draw pictures to represent our experiences with our illness, and there will be an exhibition in Tororo in August," she explained. During the exhibition in Tororo, Robinah's picture was chosen to be shown at the Grand Imperial Hotel in Kampala, and she went along. She was proud and amazed that her illness experience could take her all the way to Kampala for the first time in her life.

Over the next months, a conflict developed between the sisters. Joyce was angry with Robinah because she let her pregnant daughter marry. Joyce said she was fed up with Robinah and her children and that she would not regret it if they went back to Kumi. She reminded Robinah that she would have been dead if it had not been for her effort. Robinah was hurt and wondered whether Joyce's anger had been accumulating over time and had to do with the fact that Robinah was in the "excellent" HBAC program. Robinah was doing well while Joyce was failing. Robinah's CD4 counts continued to rise and she gained weight, while Joyce had no CD4 tests because she was in a different program. She did not gain weight and went through a period of bad side effects. Robinah had the "right" CD4 count at the right time and was brought to the right place, while Joyce's CD4 count was not "right" (i.e., low enough) when the "excellent" project was recruiting patients. Robinah decided to ask the HBAC's doctors to transfer her to the treatment center near Kumi so she could leave her sister's home and return to her own. She told the doctors that she wanted to shift because of the children. They would not understand the real issue regarding the conflict with Joyce. But the doctors advised her to stay in Tororo because the ART program in Kumi was not well established yet, and she was not allowed to take the medicine from HBAC and live in Kumi. So Robinah decided to stay, but the sisters went through a difficult time; they did not talk or cook food together. Joyce said she was finding it increasingly difficult to look after so many people. But she was determined to live up to the responsibility she had taken on, even though it was a challenge.

The last time Godfrey visited the sisters, in May 2007, Joyce felt better, and the relationship between the sisters had been reestablished. They were again talking, cooking, digging, and doing their activist work together as the local "AIDS stars" in projects connecting neighbors, relatives, friends, and colleagues with HIV to testing, treatment sources, food rations, and other AIDS programs.

After our study ended, Lotte stayed in touch with the two sisters and learned of further developments in their relationship. Another of Robinah's daughters had had an affair with one of the teachers at Joyce's school and got pregnant. This disappointed and annoyed Joyce and caused a new conflict between the sisters, which affected their relationship and health. Robinah finally decided to move back to Kumi, although it meant making a long journey to Tororo every time she had to get her ARVs refilled. Joyce once said that the most important ingredient in AIDS treatment is the love and unity that family members, friends, colleagues, and others can show you as a patient. However, her own relationship with her sister revealed that the recipe was not without problems. Patients dependent on family unity could be vulnerable.

CHAPTER ONE

Connections

Lotte Meinert,
Phoebe Kajubi, and
Susan Reynolds Whyte

For Robinah, the way into the treatment program that saved her life was through personal relationships: her kinship tie to her sister Joyce and her sister's link to a neighbor who was a field officer in the HBAC program. In their accounts, Joyce and Robinah talked about how they took the steps to get tested and join a program by way of connections and with the support of other people. In principle—from a policy perspective—AIDS programs offer services to the population at large on an equal basis. But in practice, people learn about and gain access to these services through other persons. They *achieve* services with the help of others and are not simply caught up as individuals in a net thrown out by providers. Many people hear about testing and treatment options through various official channels and media. Yet the actual link between a program and a person is almost always mediated through a trusted social connection. Joyce had experienced her husband and children dying; she knew about HIV and AIDS. In her mind, she may have suspected an association between those losses and the symptoms she experienced. But in her telling of the story, she decided to go for an HIV test when a good colleague talked to her in private, made her reflect on her situation, and advised her to be tested. This emphasis on the sociality of decision making and action featured in most of the stories we heard about how the first generation came to take an HIV test and, in time, find a way into a treatment program. The weight given to the role of other people in helping to deal with problems was striking.

Personal relations involving proximity and reciprocity, expectation and obligation, are fundamental to getting things done in everyday life, as Patrick Chabal argues in his discussion of the politics of being and belonging in Africa.[1] While this is true everywhere, it is especially pronounced in situations where bureaucratic institutions do not function optimally and where kinship provides a moral and practical framework for life. In this light, it is not surprising that our interlocutors talked about their movement into treatment programs in terms of connections. Yet to say that social links are important is not enough. In this first chapter, we want to examine the issue of connections more specifically and more critically. We describe the nature of the social relationships that mediated access and consider those cases in which people spoke about access as if it could be accomplished without personal mediation. Then we discuss the downside of a world in which there is so much emphasis on connections—that is, the inevitable inequities that arise because some people are better connected than others.

The analytical insight that people reach treatment through the efforts and connections of their family and friends is an old one in studies of African health care. Based on research in Zaire, John Janzen launched the notion of the therapy managing group (TMG), an alliance of kin, friends, and associates who guided a patient to one source of treatment after another in the quest for therapy among alternative possibilities.[2] His point was that individuals did not reason completely autonomously in making decisions about treatment; rather, they were influenced and supported by people in their close networks. Janzen argued that the concept's value lay in focusing on the social process of treatment seeking.[3] The alliance might include non-kin as well as family members, but the assumption was that all members of the network had a relatively enduring relationship to the patient.

Technical Know Who

To the concept of the TMG we add another, taken from Ugandan popular culture: the notion of "technical know who" (TKW), which refers to the widespread conviction that it is through personal contacts, and not only through knowledge (technical know-how), that things get accomplished. People and structures are activated and institutions are made to work effectively when you have a connection. When a sick person is going to a health center, concerned others will ask whether he or she knows anyone there, because everybody understands that having a link to someone who is employed at the health center—a doctor, a nurse, or even a guard or a cleaner—will make a difference in gaining access to treatment and avoiding long waiting hours. On the basis of her fieldwork in eastern Uganda, Hanne O. Mogensen writes: "I came across people who had never had the courage to turn up at a health facility. It can be difficult to find out where to start, where the line is, where to go next, who to ask, how to respond, how much to pay for what, where to get the medicine and so on. Knowing somebody—anybody—whether it is the gatekeeper or the anthropologist, may help one move in the right direction."[4]

The usefulness of personal contacts is not limited to health care. Technical know who works in all sectors of society: to get a child admitted at one of the better schools in Uganda, it is very helpful to have connections to the school's management. People looking for work ask their friends and relatives for possibilities to connect and "fix" them in a job. The reliance on personal connections is part of the patterns of clientship and patronage that we discuss in chapter 2. But for the moment, we simply want to explore the ways people talked about getting tested and joining programs.

In strict terms, TKW deployed in relation to ART would entail being helped by a contact among the employees of a program, as Robinah was helped by Joyce's neighbor, the HBAC field officer. But knowing any health worker, even one who did not work for an ART program, was a very important kind of connection. People talked about how relatives or friends working in the health sector provided advice, suggested sources of treatment, and generally offered a kind of support that they felt was based on expert knowledge. In many cases, there was an overlap of TMG and TKW, when a health worker in the near network provided guidance or a family member or friend knew someone working in a program. The importance of the TMG and the use of TKW confirm the notion that access is mediated, whether we speak of the support and encouragement of close relatives, as Robinah received from her sister Joyce, or the contacts to health workers, as Joyce had to her neighbor, the HBAC field officer.

The dispersion and variety of AIDS programs and treatment sources in the Ugandan landscape is very uneven. In large urban centers, a dense jungle of programs offer various services of testing, counseling, and treatment. In some other places, the ART landscape looks more like a desert, with a few oases offering relief. But in both the desert and the jungle, finding one's way into the health system or to a specific program is much more likely to be direct and smooth if a connected person, who knows the road, can walk the way with you—or if you know someone at the destination.

In other words, there is a difference between availability and accessibility. Although ART may be available in principle at a treatment site in your area, it may become accessible only when you are able to get in touch and talk to the staff. That step must seem feasible to you personally, which often means being helped and reassured by someone you trust.

The First Link to the Test

A crucial step on the way to an ART program is an HIV test. Testing was a necessary prerequisite in the search for treatment, and nearly all of our interlocutors spontaneously described how they came to know for sure that they were HIV-positive. For the members of the first generation, "voluntary counseling and testing" was the common pattern—that is, they had to take the initiative and present themselves at a testing site where they received counseling before and after getting their test results. Only a few of our interlocutors underwent "routine counseling and testing," the policy adopted later that involved testing at the initiative of health workers as part of the process of diagnosis and treatment (e.g., during a hospital admission). So the first generation had to *decide* to test.

Like Joyce, people recounted experiences of sicknesses that failed to respond to treatment; partners and children who had passed away from a mysterious disease; and suspicions about the partners of partners. For a few people, worries and speculations about these things moved them, apparently autonomously, to take a test. But most people, like Joyce, mentioned a conversation with someone else as the push toward testing. They named family members, neighbors, colleagues, and friends, who encouraged testing and sometimes suggested a specific venue where a test could be had.

Robinah tested on the advice of her sister Joyce (after Joyce had tested positive herself). Other interlocutors also related that some close relative made the suggestion to test. After her husband died, Harriet was admitted to the hospital twice and her co-wife fell ill. "This is when my brothers decided to take me for testing," she recounted. "They said, 'Let's take you for the test, because you are sickly all the time from malaria, and yet you have been such a hardworking woman.'" Norah had just lost a small child when she started coughing terribly. "I had so much pain that I was feeling like the chest was split and I was spitting terrible sputum and had also started thinning," she said. "At this time, I was living in Kaberamaido with my husband, but my mother became so concerned and bothered about my situation. She called me and said, 'My daughter, you come and I check you, you could be having a problem.' So my mother organized and sent me to Soroti hospital for an HIV test, where I was found to be positive." The way Harriet and Nora spoke about the decision to test showed that they did not claim responsibility for making the decision alone; they attributed it to others. They only consented to what was suggested or decided by their relatives.

The place of health workers in these kinship networks was prominent. As Steven Feierman and John Janzen write: "The person who combines the two roles of healer and therapy manager is especially influential. Most of the people who know the patient's personal circumstances do not have technical medical competence. Most of the people with technical competence do not know the patient. The healer-relative holds technical as well as personal knowledge and therefore plays an especially important role."[5] Sometimes a close relative knew a health worker. For Helen, it was her brothers who had a contact. They did not accept the suggestion of another family member that she be tested at their district hospital in western Uganda. Instead, she said, "They took me to our friend in Mulago Hospital [in Kampala], to a doctor who is a friend to my young brother, and he advised us to go to Kadic Hospital to be tested."

In several cases, a close relative was a health worker. Ivan's wife was admitted to a hospital where her stepmother was a nurse. He said that she had advised his wife to take an HIV test. On the surface, this looks like an example of a health worker initiating testing, but in Ivan's telling, his wife was following the advice of a woman she calls *mama*.

The advice of health workers as friends also figured in the accounts of deciding to test. Hope was depressed and worried after her partner died:

I had a friend who is a nurse. She saw me losing weight because I was not eating, and I was thinking too much — of course, worried. I became very weak, and if I did not have that nurse working in Mulago, I think I would have died. She called me to her home and asked what the problem was until I told her the truth. She explained to me that I could not die. I told her that I may die today or tomorrow and asked her to look after my children. She comforted me and advised me to go for HIV testing."

The soldier Saddam (case II) said he tested on the advice of a good friend who was a medical assistant in the Army. In these examples, health workers promoted testing not as professionals in a health facility but as knowledgeable members of networks, what Janzen called therapy managing groups.

Allies in Seeking Treatment

Once they had tested HIV-positive, our interlocutors had to find their way into a treatment program. Sometimes years passed between getting a positive test result and actually joining a program. Most people did not take their first test with the program they eventually joined. And, of course, most members of the first generation tested before free treatment was widely available. Jackie (case VI) tested at the AIDS Information Centre in Kampala but did not take any further steps for some time. "I kept quiet after the first test because by then the medicines were very expensive and only affordable by the rich," she said. "I just got firm and didn't tell anyone because I knew I could not afford to buy drugs." But when Jackie did in time find her way to an ART program, she did so, like most, through the mediation of another person.

The details of connecting to a treatment program resembled the stories about being encouraged to take a test. Supportive friends and family members knew about, or knew someone working in, a place where ART was provided. A connection with a health worker was also common in this step. William, a construction worker from Luweero, contacted his brother, who owned a school in Kampala and who advised him to test at the Joint Clinical Research Centre (JCRC). When he was found to be HIV-positive with a low CD4 count, he was asked whether he was prepared to start treatment there on a fee basis. "We knew we could not afford to buy the drugs," he said. "I told them, 'Let me consult my brother.' Then we went to Dr. Jack at Mulago [National Referral Hospital], who took us to IDI [the Infectious Diseases Institute]. He is a very good friend of my brother. He has children in my brother's school." It was through this connection that William accessed free treatment at the Infectious Diseases Institute.

Ivan, whose wife had tested at the advice of her stepmother the nurse, talked about the day his wife was discharged and the couple returned home. "I have a friend who works with HBAC. He is a neighbor here," Ivan said. "When he saw us coming from the hospital, he asked me privately whether we had heard about HIV/AIDS. It seems he had suspected. I told him everything, being my friend, and this helped us because HBAC was recruiting people to include in their program. He took my wife's name and recruited her. She started on ARVs."

The youngest interlocutor in our study, James, who was twenty-five, was receiving industrial training in connection with his studies when his leg became swollen and painful. The human resource manager at his workplace referred him to the private clinic with which his employer had a health care contract. There the doctor tested him for HIV. But James's workplace did not cover ART costs, and he was there only temporarily in any case. He finally got connected to a treatment program through a former classmate, Henry, who was a lab tech student at Makerere University. "I visited him," James said. "Henry's friend saw me and realized that my health was not good. They discussed about connecting me to the IDI, and that is how I joined [that program]."

There are many more examples, but these underline the point that most people talked about getting into a program as a matter of connections. We think that in at least some of these cases, health workers were simply doing their jobs. Ivan's neighbor was supposed to recruit participants for research on home-based health care. But Ivan spoke of it as a personal favor. Maybe Ivan did not actually know about the HBAC program; maybe he had heard about it but did not know how to get enrolled. Or perhaps he thought that the link through a neighbor would ensure better attention to his wife. In any case, like many others, he spoke of her joining the program as mediated by someone he knew.

Confidence in Bureaucracy

The great majority of our interlocutors mentioned connections when they talked about how they tested and joined a treatment program. But a few were personally familiar with health institutions or were insiders in organizational bureaucracies that seemed to work, and they spoke as if they had made direct contact with HIV/AIDS facilities and had confidence that the programs would serve them. Matayo was a lab technician in an HIV testing unit. When he fell ill, he went to a private hospital covered by his employer, where a doctor recommended that he test. When he was found to be HIV-positive and in need of treatment, he started buying medicine at JCRC. In time, the organization for which Matayo worked contracted with the JCRC to cover the cost of treating its staff, so Matayo no longer had to pay for his medicine there. Then there was Julia, a nurse who developed tuberculosis after her husband died. In 1998, when HIV testing became available in the hospital where she worked in Pallisa, she tested. No treatment was available, and she tried to concentrate on working and supporting her seven children. Three years later, a friend, who had also tested positive, told her about the JCRC in Mengo/Kampala. "Let's try Mengo—it's about buying drugs," the friend said. Julia claimed they were well received there, although they apparently had no connections.

Tom, a soldier, gave a picture of Army health care as functioning well, at least in the early phase of his illness:

I used to get constant malaria, terrible malaria, starting from the time I was in an ambush operation for fifteen days waiting for Kony rebels. Sometimes I would go and drink and feel better and think that it was just a hangover. *Kumbe!* [But no!] It was the real thing. I was advised to visit our medical personnel in Mbale, who sent me to Bombo [a military hospital] for an examination and HIV test. I went and checked in on 5 May 2005 in Bombo. I was told that I was HIV-positive, and I felt all my life gone low. I was so disappointed, and that is when I remembered all my lifestyle. I said OK, *kama mbayambaya* [the struggle continues]! I was counseled that I should not get worried, and I was told to go for a second test. . . . I again went to Bombo, and they took my blood on 16 September 2005, and I waited for results, which I got on 26 September. My CD4 [count] was 145, but I did not know what that meant. Then I went back to Mbale with a letter to our medical personnel. The letter said they should transfer me to Tororo barracks, which is near Mukuju Health [Centre], because our barracks administration has an arrangement with [that center]. I started at Mukuju on 22 December 2005.

In contrast to his friend and fellow soldier Saddam, Tom did not mention any personal connections in the process of testing and joining a treatment program at Mukuju Health Centre. To him, the impersonal rational bureaucratic system appeared to work.

People who worked for organizations were more likely to view testing and treatment as directly accessible; through such employment, they became knowledgeable about the workings of bureaucracy. Some might even be acquainted with people providing the services, so they did not have to worry about TKW.

The Paradox and Inequity of Connections

There is an inherent contradiction in global health policy between the desire for equity and the promotion of patients' initiative. The mediated access to AIDS programs through social connections exemplifies the latter. It underlines the significance of human agency and sociality in making a health system work. All of our cases about using connections substantiate that HIV-positive people are active, socially embedded seekers of health, not passive recipients of donors' beneficence. Yet mobilizing connections reinforces inequalities that are already present in the population, because some people are better connected than others; some have large, influential networks, while others have limited social networks and may not know the "right" people.

Because we recruited most of our interlocutors through treatment sites, we got in touch with people who had been able to make connections. When we initiated this work in late 2005, estimates were that fewer than a third of those eligible for ART were receiving it. Even though the percentages are moving in the right direction, there are still not enough medicines and human resources to get all those people who need ART into treatment. The people who did gain entry to programs were those who had the necessary means and contacts. A little more than half of our original forty-eight interviewees started out paying for their medicine. That means they had more economic resources than most Ugandans (even though none were in comfortable financial circumstances). They were better educated than average; thirty-seven of the original forty-eight had studied beyond primary school. This was not a quantitative study; we note these characteristics, however, to put the issue of equity and connections on the table. We cannot say much about those who did not have the connections and did not achieve treatment. But considering how connections function illuminates the workings of advantage and inequity.

Other research in Africa underlines the link between social networks and health outcome. Steven Feierman and Elizabeth Karlin, working in north-eastern Tanzania, found that the most vulnerable children were those whose mothers lived alone.[6] Health workers blame parents for taking children to traditional healers and delaying biomedical care. But the children at risk were not those who were given alternative treatment first, but those who did not receive any kind of treatment because their mothers had a weak social network: "those who continue to search for therapy together with a managing group, and continually change therapies, do better than those who fare alone. It is the seeking of medical care until the desired effects are attained that results in the healthy patient."[7] The broader the TMG, the more chance that a variety of treatments will be tried. If the therapy alliance includes a health worker, a patient has better chances. Epidemiologists working in Guinea-Bissau showed that among children admitted to the pediatric ward in Bissau's main hospital, the risk of dying within thirty days was 48 percent lower for those whose mothers knew a doctor than for those whose mothers did not.[8]

The struggles that some people undertook to get treatment reveal obstacles that may have blocked others. John (case VII), the railway worker Godfrey followed, provides a telling example. He is a member of the "working class," as we shall see, with the advantage of a regular income, and he had completed secondary school. But he did not appear to have a health worker in his close network, and his path to sustained treatment was far from straight. In his telling, he first looked for a treatment source where he could feel comfortable. In 2001, he developed a cough and weakness; fearing that he had tuberculosis, he went to a clinic in Kampala. "They said they did not have the machines, so they did not check, but the doctor looked at me and directed me to go to the research center at Mengo [the JCRC] for the test," he said. "But being a man from Jinja, I decided not to go to this place because I did not know it and I was alone. I thought about where else to go, and I decided to have the test done back in Jinja." It was there that he was found to be HIV-positive.

John did not know anyone well enough in Kampala to tell him about sources of HIV treatment there. He went to a private clinic and got tested but did not start treatment. While some of our interlocutors preferred to seek treatment in Kampala, where the biggest and best facilities are found, others, like John, traveled to their home area when grave illness found them. However, John was soon transferred to work in Kampala, which is where he almost died the following year. He lost his appetite and weight; he coughed; and his stomach swelled up "like a person who has been poisoned," he said. At last, his brothers and wife took him to Mulago, the national hospital. He recounted the terrible experience:

My brother, the way I was handled there. You cannot believe. Those people rejected me there. I was sent away. They saw my health condition and maybe thought, "After all, this one is dying." They said, "This one should be taken home because he has no hope." So we left the hospital and came toward town in a "special hire." [a taxi hired for a specific trip rather than the more common vans, also called taxis, that ply a fixed route]. I was badly off, and my brothers were considering returning me to the village just to wait for my death. But they disagreed with my wife—she said no. Even me, I said no, as I still had some sense. We appeared stranded [undecided] on where to go as the vehicle headed to the city center. It was a hired car, and the driver challenged us to decide quickly. But this driver was too good. . . . He was too sympathetic to my situation and expected that I should be taken to another hospital. But my brothers did not seem to want that. So this driver took personal responsibility and decided to drive to Nsambya Hospital, saying, "At least I should take you to Nsambya and dump you there, rather than leave you go to the village."

Contingency is at play here. If John had not ended up in the taxi of a concerned driver, he might have been taken home to his village in eastern Uganda to die. Instead, he was well received at Nsambya, a Catholic hospital, where he stayed for nearly three months. One of the physicians who treated him there, Dr. Xavier, started him on "a certain drug" for AIDS and told him to take it always, even if other doctors gave him other medicine. John was paying for this drug, whose name he did not know. It helped at first, but he then relapsed into even more severe illness. He went back to Nsambya, and Dr. Xavier suggested that he try a private clinic in a suburb of Kampala. John said,

> You know, at that time I wanted health, and I was ready for any advice, so when I was told to go to this clinic, I did not hesitate. When I went there, I found Dr. Xavier. I was happy to find him because he had been very concerned about my health. Dr. Xavier introduced me to another doctor, who happened to be his brother. He told me, this man is going to treat you. So his brother took over, and I can tell you, this is where I saw what they call a professional doctor. That man is so good—the care, the way he handles you and talks to you. You know with this sickness, even just talking to the patient in a good way without harassing him can help him get better. It can break the too many worries.

Fortunately for John, he was still collecting his salary and could continue to buy medicine. But the treatment was expensive, and when he again began to feel ill, he decided to try Mulago Hospital once more:

> I thought I should try to get some free treatment from there, since for all this time I had been paying for treatment. I wanted admission—but my brother! The same experience as the first one happened. [Mulago] again turned me away, this time claiming that I looked a bit fair and did not deserve to be admitted, as there were more acute cases. I was surprised because to me I was also doing badly. I was sick.

John returned to the private clinic and continued to buy ARVs. Sometimes his doctor brought them to the clinic; sometimes John bought them on prescription from pharmacies in the Katwe neighborhood.

It was not until 2004 that John went to the JCRC because the sickness was still troubling him. He explained that he had gotten more information about the center and was living in Kampala, unlike the first time he had been referred. He was taken on as a paying patient. To his surprise, he met Dr. Xavier, who had taken a job there. But even though he knew the doctor by then, the connection was not very personal. Under circumstances discussed in chapter 7, John was forced to drop his treatment. He was desperate. When Godfrey asked whether he had discussed the problem with his doctor, he said that he had been told that Dr. Xavier was not there. He tried to get Dr. Xavier's telephone number, but privacy policies prevented the JCRC from providing it. Thus, even John, a person with relatively strong resources, experienced the insecurity of not having good connections in the first years of his therapeutic journey. He found an ally in Dr. Xavier, but the relationship clearly was more professional than personal. If John's journey to clientship was so beset with impediments, it is not surprising that many others failed to achieve membership in a program at all.

Connections are important not only for joining a treatment program but also for getting linked to other kinds of support. Robinah benefited from opportunities that came through the Post-Test Club chaired by her sister Joyce. In a landscape of projects, people were looking for information and contacts. As we conducted our study, people saw us as possible contacts, too. Some asked whether we could help them get food aid. One man hoped we could get him into a research project for discordant couples. Another, who was paying for medication, asked Godfrey to find a way for him to get a subsidy. When Godfrey could not help, the man shrugged and said, "You never know—keep trying." This sense of the possibilities in connections infused sociality with hopefulness, sometimes muted and sometimes explicit.

Connecting the First Generation

Mediation between patients and health services was particularly important for the first generation on ART in Uganda. They discovered their serostatus at a time that HIV testing was almost exclusively voluntary, so individuals had to take the initiative; in their telling, they were usually encouraged by someone they knew. Most people in the first generation were aware of testing, but needed others' mediation actually to go for the test.

Once they tested HIV-positive, people went on the lookout for personal connections to health workers and others "from within" who could hook them up with a treatment program. Connections and TKW have always been an important part of Ugandan sociality; for the first generation on ART, however, that importance was greater because the treatment programs were still relatively few and scattered. For many patients in the first generation, the specific connection—the very person who got them into a treatment program— came to play a special role as savior, because being connected to ART made the difference between life and death.

Connections made second chances possible. But at the same time, the focus on connections also draws our attention to the vulnerability of basing treatment programs on contingent socialities. The global concern with the accessibility of health care takes on deeper dimensions when we realize that, from the user's point of view, access to a program is not just a matter of cost and location. It is also a matter of social connections.

Notes

1. Chabal, *Africa*.
2. Janzen, *The Quest for Therapy in Lower Zaire*.
3. Janzen, "Therapy Management."
4. Mogensen, "Finding a Path through the Health Unit," 224.
5. S. Feierman and Janzen, "Introduction," 19.
6. S. Feierman, "Struggles for Control," 83.
7. E. Feierman, "Alternative Medical Services in Rural Tanzania," 402–3.
8. Sodemann et al., "Knowing a Medical Doctor Is Associated with Reduced Mortality among Sick Children Consulting a Paediatric Ward in Guinea-Bissau."

CASE II

Saddam

TREATMENT
PROGRAMS

Phoebe Kajubi and
Susan Reynolds Whyte

CLIENTSHIP

(overleaf)

Donor-financed filing
system for the ART clinic
at Busolwe Hospital.

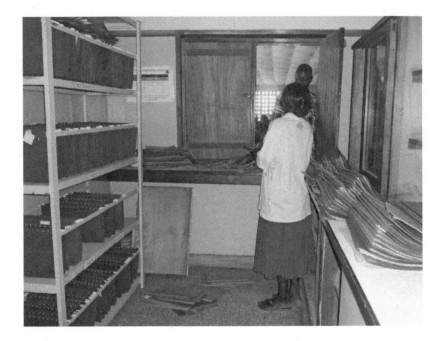

Phoebe first met Saddam in December 2005 at Mukuju Health Centre, where he sat with his friend and fellow soldier Tom waiting his turn at the antiretroviral therapy (ART) clinic. Saddam's ease with the situation was evident when Phoebe asked whether he would be willing to participate in our study. "You can interview me right now," he said. "We really want to help medical people like you." Later, when one of his senior officers called to find out where he was, he explained, "I'm with these doctors from Mukuju who are working on HIV/AIDS; they are interviewing us about the disease to see how treatment can be improved." Even after Saddam found out that Phoebe was not a medical doctor, he continued to be obliging.

Saddam was forty-five years old and born in Masindi, where his mother still lived. He was a career soldier who had dropped out of secondary school to join Idi Amin's army, fled to Juba in Sudan when Amin was overthrown, and returned to enlist in the National Resistance Army in 1986 when Yoweri Museveni came to power. During Army operations in eastern Uganda in 1988, he met and married his wife; they had three children together but separated in 2004. When Phoebe met Saddam, the oldest child was staying with his former wife, while the other two were with Saddam's mother and sister in Masindi. Over the time Phoebe knew Saddam, those three children moved in with him one by one.

Saddam first realized that he was sick after losing 40 of his normal 128 pounds. He thought he had been bewitched by his colleagues. A civilian friend took him to Busolwe, a place well known for witchcraft, which had people called Bakunja, who were famous for killing by mystical means. "They can send you their 'things'—for example, such a witchdoctor can plant a bean for killing you. The bean is monitored how it grows because it represents you; when it dies, you also die," he said. "I, too, tried that kind of witchcraft." He spent almost a million shillings [about $578] on healers (often called "witch doctors" in Ugandan English), who asked for goats and chickens to cure him.

It was at this time that another friend, a clinical officer in the Army, suggested that Saddam go for an HIV test. He first went to The AIDS Support Organization (TASO), where he was referred to Tororo Hospital. He waited for his results for three months. When they were finally ready, a nurse called him for a confidential talk. She asked him, "If we give you the results, what will you do if you are affected?" Saddam said, "nothing," reasoning that "he was a man." The nurse told him that he was HIV-positive and gave him some forms to take to TASO. There he was given a card and medicine, probably the antibiotic Septrin (co-trimoxazole). The medicine did not help him at all, he said; they had similar medicine at the health facility at the Rubongi Barracks in Tororo District, where he lived.

He went back to his friend, the clinical officer, and told him his results. The friend asked him whether he had money so he could take him where there was real treatment, and Saddam affirmed that he did: "We went to the JCRC in Mbale . . . and talked to the doctor. They took my blood, I paid 73,000 shillings [$42] and was told to go back the following Wednesday for my results. They also took my [weight]." On his return visit, he was given the results of his CD4 test and started on antiretroviral medicine (ARVs) that very day. The doctor assured him that within two months he would be going for Army operations again in Congo. Saddam remembered the doctor's words of reassurance: "There are people who are carried in here, but for you, you are walking." He was paying 28,000 shillings ($16) for a two weeks' supply of ARVs. He also bought syrups to boost his appetite and ate well; within two months, his weight had increased from 88 pounds to 120 pounds, and he was switched to another combination of medications along with his regular Septrin. "I bought milk, good food, and I made sure I took fluids," he said. "I drank passion-fruit juice and ate fresh fish; when I have money, I eat well. I haven't fallen sick. The reason I lost weight was because I didn't know I was infected; all along, I thought I was bewitched."

Saddam continued to buy medicine for only two months. His health improved, but he became angry and bitter that he was infected with HIV. He was annoyed that the healers had taken his money for nothing—and, perhaps, about the expense of ARVs. He went back to his home in Masindi, where he stayed for seven months. When he told his mother that he was HIV-positive, she encouraged him to return to Tororo, "You go back and work so that you will get money to buy drugs," she said. "Your children are still young. Who is going to help them?"

When he eventually returned to the barracks, he was imprisoned as a deserter. But after two weeks, the committee sat and decided to release him for fear he would die in jail. He started work, but his name had been struck from the payroll, and he was not receiving a salary. His friend, the clinical officer, advised him to get back on ARVs, but he had no means to resume buying medicine. He said,

> So that's how I went to Mukuju Health Centre. They were always announcing on the radio the names of hospitals that were giving free AIDS drugs.

So I went and talked to the doctor, and he recommended me to start getting drugs free from Mukuju. That was last year [2004], although I don't
remember the month. I showed the doctor my CD4 form. They give me
drugs for two months whenever I am going for safari [a journey] because
they don't want me to miss. Whenever I move out of the camp, I move
with the drugs in case the time for taking them comes when I am out of
the camp.

Saddam affirmed that his bosses and colleagues in the Army knew that he was
HIV-positive. When Phoebe asked him whether he had had any problems
with the ARVs, he responded, "I have no problem with the drugs, if only the
project can help me with food, since I am having problems with money. I wish
they could give us milk."

Five months after the first interview, Phoebe, unable to reach Saddam by
phone, went to the barracks to confirm that he would continue in the study.
At first he did not recognize her, but when he remembered who she was, he
said he was grateful that she had kept her promise to check on him. Saddam's
household was growing. His eldest boy had run away from his mother in
Masindi to stay with him, claiming there was too much poverty at his mother's place. At the next visit, two months later, Saddam's daughter from Masindi
had also joined him in the barracks. Although he had not started receiving his
salary yet, he had been put back on the payroll. Phoebe inquired about how he
managed to support a family without a salary. He replied, "We soldiers know
how to survive in our own way, but it is not easy." He asked Phoebe whether
she could do something to help get food supplies, and she advised him to contact the clinical officer at the health center where he was getting his medicine.
Just then, another soldier came into the house. Saddam insisted that Phoebe
talk to him. "He is like me," Saddam said, meaning that the other soldier was
also HIV-positive.

The next time Phoebe visited Saddam, in September 2006, Jenipher accompanied her. Saddam had many complaints, even about Phoebe. He wondered why she never called him and why she was never available when he
tried to call her. He grumbled about the low monthly salary he was being paid
(80,000 shillings [$44]) and attributed it to corrupt Army officers who took
money that was meant for soldiers in low ranks. He complained about the
government, which he said was responsible for the poverty among soldiers,
who were forced to cultivate crops to supplement their meager incomes and
feed their families. He was bitter because of a planned move to retrench soldiers who were non-effective, including sick soldiers, who were to be given

three months' salary and told to go home. "What are we expected to do?" he asked. "How are we going to survive?"

Because of his poor health, Saddam could not go on any missions in Congo. He had been involved in only two Army operations: to pick up casualties and dead soldiers in Karamoja and southern Sudan. He was pleased that his health worker supported him with all kinds of medicine. "The conditions are very bad where we go out to get the bodies, but I always go with my medicine," he said. "For example, the last time I was away for months, my clinical officer gave me medicine for the entire time I was there. He also gives me quinine tablets and other medicine." Whenever he was troubled by any kind of illness, he got the medicine he needed from Mukuju Health Centre. He commented that quinine had really sustained him and helped him to be in good health. According to him, the military hospital at the barracks might not have medicine, though he was not sure.

On another visit, Susan joined Phoebe. Saddam had called Phoebe the week before and asked her when she would be checking on him. He looked thinner and worn out:

I have lost weight. One time, I weighed 67 kilograms [150 pounds], and then reduced to 55 kilograms [120 pounds], and the last time the weight had reduced further to 54 kilograms [118 pounds]. I am in a lot of pain. My legs hurt so much that I cannot sleep at night. I lie in this chair, and [my daughter] massages my legs. I can walk to Tororo town, but I cannot sleep at night because I am in a lot of pain. I was given Valium, but when I take it, I don't sleep until around 4 AM. Like last time, I walked to Tororo and from there I got transportation to Mukuju Health Centre. The problem is that Henry [Saddam's clinical officer at Mukuju] was not there, and I am not used to the other health workers who were attending to us and therefore could not confide in them. Henry had talked about taking my CD4; he told me it would cost 21,000 shillings [$11.50], but I didn't have the money, so my CD4 has never been taken again since the first time.

Saddam went to his bedroom and brought out his medical documents in a large envelope. The receipts showed that he had started taking ARVs in 2003 and was paying about 25,000 shillings per week. One paper showed that his CD4 was 213 in 2003.

We mentioned to Saddam that we knew his clinical officer had returned from leave and offered to take him to the health center. When we arrived there, Henry was seeing outpatients, so we waited for him for a few minutes. There were still a large number of patients, but he came to talk to us in his office. Saddam updated him about his health, and Henry explained that the drug Saddam was taking was responsible for the pains in his legs. He told Saddam to get 10,000 shillings [$5] and come for the CD4 test on a Wednesday. He asked him to bring his children for the HIV test, although Saddam said that they were in good health.

The health center actually had three different ART programs: the JCRC-TREAT [The Regional Antiretroviral Therapy program] collaboration; Plan International's Prevention of Mother-to-Child Transmission program; and the Ministry of Health (MOH) rollout program. We had assumed that Saddam was on the JCRC program, since that is where he originally started buying ARVs. Saddam was not sure himself, although he had noticed "MOH" written on his file. When we asked Henry, the clinical officer, he confirmed that Saddam was on the government MOH program.

The four of us walked to the building for HIV/AIDS activities. There, a senior clinical officer working for the PLAN program was attending to the waiting men, women, and children. He introduced himself, and Henry took out Saddam's file. The two health workers discussed switching Saddam to another drug, since the Triomune was giving him such pain in his legs. Earlier, Henry had told us that the MOH program did not have the medications Saddam needed and he was going to borrow them from the Plan International program. Saddam was given Viramune, Duovir, magnesium compounds (for his ulcers) and Septrin and instructed to buy the vitamin B complex because it was out of stock. He surrendered the seven tablets of Triomune he had with him and promised to return the rest to the health center later.

Prior to the next visit, in November 2006, Saddam again called to find out when Phoebe would be checking on him because he wanted a ride to the health center to pick up his medicine. Saddam and other soldiers sometimes walked from the barracks to Mukuju, 15 kilometers away, to get their refills. He said that a number of soldiers were on ARVs, but it was hard to know how many because everybody went for treatment on different days. He knew about six, and some soldiers on ARVs got food supplies. When Phoebe asked whether the Rubongi Military Barracks Hospital was providing ARVs, Saddam said he was not sure but strongly believed there were none.

During the November visit, Phoebe asked Saddam to take her to see the barracks hospital. They walked between the residences of high-ranking officers. Most of them were away on Army operations; mainly women and children were around. Many houses had iron sheets instead of glass in the windows, and there were bullet holes in the walls. The barracks hospital was very neat, and the compound was mowed. Sick soldiers basked in the sun;

inside the hospital, there were more women with children than men waiting to be attended to. Soldiers saluted Saddam and called him *afande* (officer).

The nursing officer, herself a soldier, talked about the ART program at the barracks hospital. Rubongi started providing ARVs in June 2006, she said:

> We provide only Triomune 30, Septrin, and fluconazole [for meningitis] to those who need it. We started with ten and now have forty people here on ARVs. Some are getting the drugs from far places, and they have asked to be transferred to the military hospital here. We supply our clients with ARVs and Septrin on a monthly basis. There are about sixty people getting Septrin from here, including some soldiers who access ARVs from TASO. Even when soldiers run short of ARVs, we can give them for two weeks with a covering letter so that their treatment centers don't accuse them of skipping their drugs.
>
> For tests, we depend on the Mbale AIDS Information Centre, where they charge 5,000 shillings [$3] for a CD4 test. The cost of a CD4 test at the Mbale JCRC is 10,000 [$5]. Taking a CD4 test from TASO involves going through a very slow process. But people still go to TASO because of the treatment for opportunistic infections and skin infections they get from there, which we don't provide here.
>
> Another thing is that our clients ask for additional support, such as food items given in Mukuju, because they think that the Ministry of Defense has a lot of money, which is not true. Nutritionally, they feel, we are not supporting them.

At the end of the conversation, she pointed at Saddam. "He is one of those who are accessing ARVs from another place," she said. "We have encouraged them to transfer here, but they still go elsewhere." As Saddam and Phoebe walked away, he said he did not want to get medicine from the barracks hospital because it would be dispensed weekly, and no treatment was provided for opportunistic infections (although he did sometimes get Septrin there). He commented sadly that he had hoped Phoebe would come with a car and take him to Mukuju Health Centre to pick up his medicine because his refill was due in three days. He asked for money for transportation to take him to Mukuju, but Phoebe told him that she had just enough for her own transportation. He thanked her for the sugar she had brought for the family. He also mentioned that his children were missing a mother figure in their lives, and left Phoebe wondering whether he had implied that she should take that role.

Two months later, when Phoebe visited Saddam, he seemed thinner but also happier. He was not telling bitter stories or complaining about his job, his poverty, or his treatment. She asked him about his health, and he said that his CD4 count, which had been taken in November, had increased from 213 to more than 300. He realized that he did not look well but insisted that he was very fine and challenged Phoebe to go to Mukuju Health Centre and check for the CD4 results from his file—file number MOH/72. Saddam reported further that he now got medicine every other month. He had picked up the current dose in December and would be returning in February for a refill.

The last news of Saddam came from Jenipher, who replaced Phoebe when Phoebe left the country for a few months. He had been transferred to Masindi but by chance had gone to Tororo that day to pick up documents from the barracks. He had moved with all his children and was pleased to be near his family home. Despite his earlier attachment to his clinical officer at the Mukuju Health Centre, he reported no problems changing to another ART clinic. He was getting the same medicine and treatment from a hospital near Masindi and was in good health. He soon excused himself and said that he needed to leave to get what had brought him to Tororo.

CHAPTER TWO

Clientship

Susan Reynolds Whyte,
Lotte Meinert, and
Jenipher Twebaze

Saddam's remark that we could just go to the Mukuju Health Centre and check the CD4 test results in his file (number MOH/72) suggests a radical change in Ugandan health care: it indexes membership in a treatment program that keeps records and follows people over time. This transformation is marked in discourse by a shift we noticed around the turn of the millennium in the way health workers spoke about their patients. Specifically, they began to refer to them as "clients." To be a client of an ART program is to belong to a treatment site and an organization that registers your information, provides you with regular services, and has certain expectations of you. It is a kind of contractual relationship that differs significantly from the usual encounter between patients and health workers, or between customers and the attendants in the drugshops and small private clinics that provide most of the health care in Uganda. As Robinah (case I) said about the Home-Based AIDS Care (HBAC) program, "I am their person."

The first generation was a generation of clients; they got a second chance to live because they joined programs—with all that this entailed in terms of expectations and entitlements. In this chapter, we continue our exploration of sociality in HIV treatment. We suggest that new social forms emerged as ART became more widely available—new but familiar if we consider the double meaning of clientship. We investigate the nature of the exchanges between programs and their clients and the extent to which people reflect on their places in the landscape of different programs.

The Two Meanings of Clientship

When health workers and policy makers began to refer to patients at AIDS clinics as clients, they presumably had in mind the reciprocity between providers and users of services. Architects, lawyers, and social workers have clients; the term suggests a contractual relationship based on professional standards, not only money. A client is not merely a customer, as are many Ugandan seekers of health care who patronize drugshops for medicine to treat themselves.[1] Nor is a client only a patient. While patients should be passive and quiet, clients are interlocutors who have expectations about services. There is a neoliberal tinge to "client" in this sense, which suggests user-friendliness and respect on the part of service providers, a far cry from the indifference or rudeness to patients for which government health care was notorious. A client receives professional services; in health care, this would mean proper examination, diagnosis, and monitoring over time, not one-off presumptive treatment based on reported symptoms. The word "client" flagged the exceptionalism of ART programs in relation to normal public health care; they offered another standard of service that included regular medication and a long-term relationship with the patient.

Clientship has another, and older, meaning, as well. A client is the dependent of a patron—in Roman history, a plebeian under the protection of a patrician. The relationship is hierarchical in that the patron provides access to scarce material resources needed by the client in exchange for less tangible prestations, such as loyalty. It is personal and has an emotional component. Eric Wolf cites Julian Pitt-Rivers's description of patron-client relations as "lop-sided friendship."[2] Social science approaches to patronage or patrimonialism follow Max Weber in distinguishing systems based on impersonal rational bureaucracy bound by law and family-like personal systems of redistribution to dependents. Scholars of governance in Africa use the term "neo-patrimonialism" to describe the intertwining of the rational-legal bureaucratic systems established during the colonial period with patron-client patterns.[3] Donor-funded projects, including AIDS projects, fit into the pattern of neo-patrimonialism.[4] Project resources such as cash, contracts, equipment, jobs, the location of new infrastructure, even the perquisites of workshops and transportation allowances, flow through relations of patronage and clientship. At the same time, the projects are logically frameworked, benchmarked, quality assured, and evaluated through standardized mechanisms that belong to the realm of rational-legal bureaucratic authority. Our material shows how elements of patron-client relations are evident in the way people actually use the organizations providing ART and other benefits for those infected and affected by HIV.

We use the term "therapeutic clientship" to explore the relationships of the first generation to programs and health workers. Awareness of the double meaning of clientship alerts us to the ways in which the new social forms of long-term treatment programs tend to evoke older patterns of obligation and lopsided friendship between big men and dependents. In both kinds of clientship, vital resources are accessed through enduring social relationships to a powerful authority, with expectations by both parties about the morality of exchange.

Therapeutic clientship complements the notion of therapeutic citizenship, which Vinh-Kim Nguyen used to call attention to the relation between HIV-positive individuals and wider national and international polities.[5] With its emphasis on rights in a polity, therapeutic citizenship is useful for understanding the positions of the donors, activists, advocates, policy makers, and, to some extent, providers. They make claims on behalf of others for inclusion in a world community of therapy, as Peter Mugyenyi, director of Uganda's JCRC, did so effectively in relation to PEPFAR.[6] Citizenship is a more abstract relationship between categories of individuals and forms of governance. Clientship corresponds more closely to what Nguyen refers to as "local moral economies," in which "individuals call on networks of obligation and reciprocity to negotiate access to therapeutic resources."[7] In Uganda, while the vanguard spoke out for the first generation as therapeutic citizens, most people on ART were not talking about their rights and claims in the abstract sense. They were worried about much more immediate entitlements, favors, and assistance from people they knew or wanted to know.

We want to use "therapeutic clientship" as a heuristic term that will help us ask questions about a new but familiar form of sociality. We are interested in the links through which people connect to programs, the nature of clientship as expectation and obligation, and the "transactables" that are exchanged in such a relationship. How do they assess and compare programs, and how do they try to affect the exchanges they make?

Paperwork

Clientship in the sense of using professional health services is indexed by paperwork, an essential part of rational bureaucratic procedures. The association between paperwork and health care is not new. In government health units, the health worker writes down the diagnosis and prescription on a "Medical Form 5" or in a cheap school exercise notebook kept by the patient. The act of writing distinguishes treatment at government health units from that purchased at Uganda's many small drugshops, where school exercise books are used as the source of paper to make the little cones into which loose pills are packed. Writing is an appreciated form of acknowledgment,[8] which is part of what constitutes the higher quality of care in a professional bureaucratic facility. Its function is to show the dispenser which medicine has been prescribed. Patients are supposed to keep these records and bring them next time; sometimes they do, but the papers usually are not treated with great care and tend to get lost, after which the patient simply buys another exercise book. For people on ART programs, paperwork is more comprehensive and precious. Not only do they keep the papers documenting their registration, treatment history, and appointment dates but, exceptionally, the treatment facility keeps a file on them, as Saddam so clearly knew. One of the donor-funded innovations at Busolwe Hospital's AIDS clinic was a modern filing system for organizing the records of all registered clients.

Having your file at the AIDS clinic shows that you belong there, you are "their person." It indexes a kind of contractual obligation—or, at least, an intention—on the part of the clinic to provide treatment. Jenipher was present at a clinic when a "bad client" was being scolded for drunkenness and general indiscipline. The clinical officer showed him the precariousness of his belonging by handing him his file and telling him to go home. The "bad client" had to plead with the health worker to take the file back again and keep him as a member of the treatment program.[9] Belonging to a program was so exclusive that getting treatment from another, even for a short time, required paperwork. Letters of referral were necessary as part of the careful accounting to the donors and the attempts to monitor the adherence and clinical history of every patient.

Patients were clients of other organizations in addition to their medical program, which also had bureaucratic elements that included paperwork. Those who tested positive for HIV received a card on which was written "for continuing care," code for "HIV-positive and eligible to join AIDS programs."

Such a card was a ticket for joining a range of support programs that helped with food rations, blankets, income-generating projects, and various kinds of medical care. The oldest and best known of these is TASO. Many of our interlocutors, like Saddam, were enrolled in TASO after they tested positive; sometimes they were given membership forms to fill out immediately after getting their results. The program was particularly active in eastern Uganda; during the time of our study, TASO was reregistering its members, a bureaucratic process that seemed impressive to Hassan (case VIII). He explained that he used to have only a number at TASO but recently had been issued a card. He had been called to have his photo taken and told that the Ministry of Health would retain one copy of his picture. Perhaps the Ministry of Health was recognizing and obligating itself to the people whose photographs it kept, just as the treatment facility kept the files of its clients. Hassan showed his new health card, with his number, and his TASO membership card, with another number, valued tokens of registration and belonging.

Cards, forms, and files were mentioned by all of the people we followed. It was not uncommon for people to show us their papers to underline something they were telling us about their treatment, just as Saddam did when he went to his bedroom and brought out the envelope with all his records. Others pulled out cards or papers to check on their next appointment, or, as we will see in chapter 10, the details about medicine consumption. The fact that so many people remembered the exact dates of their treatment initiation and tests can partly be attributed to these home "archives."

Personalization

While paperwork was part of the new "service" meaning of clientship, getting those papers was often described as a process mediated by personal connections. And realizing the benefits that the paperwork was supposed to ensure was often thought to depend on the goodwill of the individuals administering them. Dorothy, a prison officer, was disappointed with her counselor at TASO. "He is not helping me at all," she complained. "I knew that in TASO they were giving blankets, food, and many other things, but when I asked him why I was not getting them, he said that it depended on the patient. He is a difficult man. I don't know why they cannot change [counselors] for me." The idea that clientship allows access to scarce resources through personal relations to a powerful person was thus intertwined with the provision of services to members of a bureaucratic organization.

Belonging to a treatment program can involve relations that are more or less personal. In small rural programs and in those in which peer counseling and home visits featured, it was difficult to control information about being HIV positive. People knew one another and saw who was being visited and who was waiting at the ART clinic. In contrast, the big clinics in Kampala, such as the JCRC and the Infectious Diseases Institute (IDI), at Mulago National Referral Hospital, were quite anonymous. People did not see the same doctor each time they came. If counseling was needed, they saw whichever counselor was available. Some people appreciated this anonymity because it allowed discretion. Yet it was striking that even in the large, anonymous settings, people tried to personalize relations. They used pre-existing connections to staff or tried to develop new ones when they could. James, a university student, was adept at getting around the maze of departments at the national hospital when he needed tests and treatment not provided by the ART clinic. He cultivated friendships there, something that was probably easier for him to do as an educated person. As he put it, "Maintaining life is not the responsibility of one person, and those other people who help you maintain it should not be your enemies."

At the small rural and home-based programs, possibilities for a personal relationship with the health worker providing medicine were much greater. Often the health worker lived in the same area, so one might even have known him or her in another capacity. There were cases in which health workers personally got someone they knew to test and enroll in a program. Some people praised their health workers warmly as good people, as caring and concerned. They mentioned things health workers had done that they took as indications of personal favor rather than simply following procedure, as other eyes might have seen it. One woman spoke this way about the officer in charge of the AIDS clinic. "Mr. Mwangale is happy with the improvement in my health," she said. "He cares so much for me, comes and checks on me, and he gave me days when to visit the clinic—that is, every Thursday. If I don't go, he comes and checks on me or he sends someone to do it." (Thursday was the regular clinic day, so it was hardly a personal favor to ask her to come on that day, but that was how she perceived it.) Several expressed such exclusive trust in their health workers that they did not want to be attended by anyone else. When his clinical officer was on leave, Saddam did not go to the clinic, even though he was suffering painful side effects from his medicine. Hassan asked God to bless the staff at the district hospital's AIDS clinic and ensure that they would always be there. He remarked that, because they came from the same village, he had known some of them for a long time. Herbert thanked God for three things: a friend who helped him pay school fees; a wife who looked after his many children (from other wives); and his clinical officer, who gave him medicine to survive and even lent him money.

The personal relationships people had with health workers sometimes seemed rather hierarchical, with clients dependent on the beneficence of a professional, and sometimes egalitarian, with friendly interaction beyond the medical relationship. When he was not at the health unit, the clinical officer for whom Herbert offered thanks to God used to spend time at Herbert's shop, and they often ate lunch together. The one that Hassan blessed talked to us as if Hassan were a patient who needed special attention to stay on his meds, while Hassan saw the health worker's visits to bring him his ARVs as a gesture of friendship. Like many relationships, personal links to health workers seemed to have a quality of indeterminateness or of possibility. That meant there could be uncertainty, difficulty, and disappointment, as well as confidence. Ivan was given a counselor who lived in the same area and who became very impatient with him when he was slow to adjust to the regime of taking ARVs regularly. "*Hullo*, this lady could quarrel! I even reached an extent of saying, 'Why can't I leave these drugs and die?'" But Ivan did not want to report his counselor to the program officials because he was afraid he would be blamed if she was fired. "You know, when someone loses a job because of you and you are from the same village, it can be terrible. So I decided to keep quiet," he said.

This points to a more general issue concerning clientship. It is not just a matter of whether or not you belong, whether you have papers, a number, and a right to treatment. It is a question of what belonging means for expectations, rights, and obligations. The usefulness of the term "clientship" is that it points to a concrete field of relationships, which can be differentiated and specified. There are various kinds of programs with different services for their clients. There are particularities of personal relationships to which the parties bring different resources. The relations between clients and their patrons or service providers can be analyzed in terms of exchange, just as Patrick Chabal argues that political relations are characterized by structures of reciprocity. "Such relationships of exchange are unequal, based as they are on a clear reality of power," he writes.[10] ART clientship is also based on unequal exchange, yet there is a very clear sense of expectation and obligation that reflects a moral logic at work in these relationships. The reciprocity in clientship leads us to inquire about what is given and what is received.

The Stuff of Exchange

Of the forty-eight people we originally interviewed, twenty-seven had started on ARVs on a fee basis. Characteristic of the first generation, ten had already moved on to free programs by the time we talked with them. In doing so, they also moved from relationships of direct and immediate exchange to ones of more generalized reciprocity. Ivan reflected that when he was buying his medications, they were given to him according to the amount of money he had rather than the amount of medicine he was supposed to take. Purchasing medicine, with its immediate exchange, casts the patient as more like an anonymous customer. In this scenario, Ivan was hardly a client in either sense of the word: the drug provider did not extend professional services by showing concern beyond the monetary; nor was the provider a patron with whom Ivan entertained a continuing lopsided friendship.

The free programs involve more generalized reciprocity; what is given and received does not have to balance out in the short term but should involve mutuality over time. While the personal relationship between a client and a health worker is often important, exchange also may extend to other staff, fellow clients, potential clients, and other programs providing other kinds of support.

Of all of the material and immaterial things that flow in relations of clientship, the antiretroviral medicine is the most important. The provision of medicine comes with obligations on the part of recipients that constitute an exchange. There is a contract, which is often written. Since most people begin a daily regime of the antibiotic co-trimoxazole (Septrin) before being put on ARVs, health workers can assess their ability to live up to their side of the bargain. By keeping appointments at the clinic and showing adherence to Septrin, clients demonstrate their competence for starting on ARVs once their health is impaired enough. In all of the free programs, clients must undergo preliminary educational and counseling sessions—"studying ARVs"—before they begin ART. At this point, they may be asked to bring a treatment companion and to sign an agreement. Thereafter—and ideally, for the rest of their lives—clients exchange time for medication in that they must keep appointments and wait, sometimes for hours. They must submit to monitoring by showing the remaining medicine before getting refills so health workers can check for adherence. "If you don't do it right, they will stop you," one man said. In fact, they may not even start you if you do not seem willing or able to be punctual and compliant.

The discipline that clients exchange for medicine is documented through paperwork and converted into numbers that health workers use in their own exchange relations with authorities and donors. To receive more medicine, equipment, salaries, and further opportunities, treatment programs must provide evidence that the health workers are doing their jobs well. Thus, the unequal relations between health workers and patients are embedded in more comprehensive structures of hierarchy and clientship.

Beyond discipline in exchange for medicine, clients give a disposition of openness in return for advice and reassurance—ideally, at least. They offer their narratives or fragments of stories in return for moral support and sometimes to negotiate terms, as Saddam did to get supplies of medicine to take on military assignments. To be a good client and to realize the benefits of clientship one must tell about one's bodily and social situation. The communication in ART clientship does not always live up to ideals of patient-centered counseling, but it is radically different from the perfunctory verbal exchange of most health care in Uganda.

Openness as an element of exchange extended to discussing HIV and the benefits of treatment with others. Joseph, a client of Reach Out Mbuya, put it explicitly: "For us, we don't pay anything. Instead, the only reward we give back is to encourage others, also telling them about the problem and asking them to join." Program patrons appreciated these efforts. The clinical officer who took such a personal interest in Hassan told Susan that Hassan brought people to be tested. He spread the word about ARVs, comparing them to *ebigwasi*, the blessed sacramental millet balls consumed at offerings to the ancestors in their part of eastern Uganda. Hassan was not an activist, but his efforts to publicize his ART program were a part of his exchange with the patron he liked so much.

The clients who could be considered activists were a minority, but an important and high-profile one who formed part of the vanguard of the first generation. Their openness and storytelling led to exchanges far beyond the medications themselves. These "AIDS stars," who became proficient at telling the tale of their escape from death and their second chance on ART, found new opportunities and new horizons opening. Joyce (case I) loved talking about the work she was doing as the chair of the Post-Test Club. "Through the Post-Test Club we have managed to get many people to come and test, and even access help. Many people are appreciating this disease now because we have come up to show that even when you are infected you can still be helpful, and there is hope." Joyce explained that members like her sister Robinah were witnesses for the Post-Test Club; when people heard about her return from the very edge of the grave and saw how well she looked, they were encouraged to test and join treatment programs. Robinah's world expanded through her spoken and illustrated testimony as she joined an AIDS drama group that toured the area, met foreigners, and traveled to Kampala with her drawings about life with HIV. The same was true for Brenda, who rose from her deathbed and used her second chance to pursue studies at Uganda College of Commerce in Tororo. When the American ambassador came to visit the HBAC program in Tororo, he was taken to Brenda's home to meet a living example of the significance of US Agency for International Development support.[11] She thus gave to her patrons in the treatment program the stuff that they could pass on to their respective patrons.

Being an AIDS leader and spokesperson put Joyce in position to play the part of patron herself, just as Amy Kaler and Susan Cotts Watkins have shown for community-based distributors of family planning in nearby western Kenya.[12] Joyce said she had become popular and well known for her campaigning about HIV. As chair of the Post-Test Club, she had been able to facilitate access to projects that distributed seeds and provided resources such as pigs and goats or cash to invest. She was the one who chose who would benefit from the new opportunities, and she realized that she had to distribute such resources with care to avoid obvious favoritism.

For a few of our interlocutors, being a client opened the possibility of becoming an employee, a topic explored further in chapter 7. The need for "task shifting" to lighten the burden on health workers correlated well with the GIPA (Greater Involvement of People Living with HIV and AIDS) Principle adopted at the AIDS Summit in Paris in 1994. Many treatment programs recruited "expert clients" among their patients who assisted with testing, paperwork, weighing patients, counseling, and packing medicine. Like AIDS activists, the expert clients worked as volunteers and hoped that this might put them in a position to take up opportunities as they appeared. For the expert clients, those opportunities typically took the form of workshops, training, and allowances. Their hope was that some kind of paid job might materialize, even if only for a few months. Antiretroviral therapy gave people a second chance with families, partners, and children and all of the matters of everyday life. But the treatment programs and auxiliary support projects themselves offered chances for those who were able to position themselves in relation to donor interventions and expand their spheres of exchange.[13]

Clientship involved the exchange of medicine, compliance, dramatic stories, and job opportunities between unequal parties. Something else was being reciprocated, as well—something in the nature of acknowledgment, respect, or regard. The power of the patrons and service providers made this aspect of the exchange hopeful for clients. To have a file at the program office, to have your photo with the Ministry of Health, was to be made visible to a powerful organization. To belong to a program was to be noticed, to be recognized as a person with needs, and to have an expectation of entitlement. It is not that people always felt they were treated with enough respect or that they always received everything they were entitled to, but they did attain grounds for tentative optimism.

Programs Compared

Unlike countries such as Botswana, Uganda did not have a standard ART package provided mainly through the national health system. The projectification of AIDS care, with its many versions supported by and implemented through different agencies, meant that clientship could be more or less comprehensive. It involved different kinds of exchanges in that resources and obligations varied. Clients on the comprehensive programs had more obligations; they had to live in the catchment area and be home when field officers came to check on them: the higher the level of service, the more surveillance. (Those who were paying for their medicine did not have their adherence checked at all; they were customers more than clients, and their exchanges were simple and direct, involving fewer requirements on their part.)

People might not know which donor sponsored which program, but they were aware of different levels of service. Saddam lived near the Rubongi Military Barracks Hospital, which had an ART clinic he might have joined, obviating the need to find transportation to the Mukuju Health Centre for refills. But he was convinced that the barracks hospital was not as good and expected its staff would give him supplies for one week at a time instead of for a month or two, a common tactic when clinics were running low on medicine and rationing them. He was aware that there were several donors at Mukuju, which alone suggested more human and material resources.

The ARVs themselves differed from one program to another. The barracks hospital provided only Triomune, while Mukuju Health Centre was able to switch Saddam from Triomune to Viromune and Duovir. Only large and better-financed programs had second-line treatment. Some included treatment for opportunistic infections and were better supplied with the necessary medicine for other related health problems. Programs like HBAC and Reach Out Mbuya provided regular free testing of CD4 counts as part of their service to clients. But Saddam had to pay for the tests because his program did not include CD4 monitoring. Neither were CD4 tests part of the treatment program at the barracks hospital; the nursing officer was knowledgeable about prices because she had to refer her clients elsewhere. Those who could not afford the extra expense simply did not have their CD4 counts monitored. At Busolwe Hospital and other Ministry of Health facilities supported only by the Global Fund, most clients had never had their CD4 counts taken. During the time of our study, many were initiated into treatment on the basis of the clinical stage of the HIV disease rather than a CD4 count.

In addition to differences in medical treatment, programs varied in terms of other kinds of support. As the health worker at the barracks hospital noted, food supplements were offered in some programs (though not by the Ministry of Health, which sponsored Saddam's treatment). Many people got their medication from one program and other benefits from another. Their membership in a clinical program was enduring and vital, while belonging to other programs was often short-lived. The activities and benefits changed as projects and donors shifted. At one time, blankets were provided to deserving HIV-positive members; at another, members might receive seeds and other agricultural inputs.

Sometimes members of a single family were clients of different programs, as we saw with Robinah and Joyce. Robinah was a client of the "deluxe" HBAC program, while Joyce received her medicine from TASO. Robinah was visited weekly at home by HBAC staff, who brought her medicine, while Joyce collected her ARVs and saw a health worker or counselor every two months. MamaGirl and MamaBoy (case IV) were both clients of HBAC, but MamaGirl was also a member of TASO, which provided food rations for a period, while MamaBoy was not. Philip's wife, who lived in a camp for displaced people in northern Uganda, was receiving treatment from TASO in Kitgum while Philip was a client at Reach Out Mbuya in Kampala. "There is an Italian doctor there, and they now also give free drugs," Philip said. "But there are not so many machines there as here. They cannot do as many tests, and she is not doing all that well."

People who switched programs could compare them based on firsthand experience. Among our interlocutors, these were almost all people who had started on a fee program and moved to one that was nominally free, as Saddam had done. As clients in free programs, they had to exchange their time for medicine. They mentioned the hours spent waiting to see the health worker and to collect their medicine from the dispensing counter. Dorothy had started paying for her medicine, then moved to free treatment at TASO, but opted to return to fee-based treatment because "there are long queues at TASO, and sometimes you do not get all the drugs." Moses remarked, "I would like to be on free drugs, but the problem is time. I hear those who go there spend the whole day in long queues, but at JCRC, you don't spend more than ten minutes."

Clients cannot expect the same privacy that customers enjoy. Martha, a paying patient at the JCRC, was critical of free programs. "Here I just come, pay, get my drugs and go to work," she said. "Here nobody would ever see you coming to pick drugs, but at TASO, everybody would know because they make you sit there, read files, then call you to pick up drugs after so many hours. It is tiresome and unnecessary revealing someone's health status as far as HIV is concerned." She did not agree with TASO's policy of involving other members of the family in a client's treatment. As the breadwinner she wanted to keep her secret and not have her health problems "paraded" before her dependents. The necessity of accepting the conditions of service delivery reveals the power relations between ART providers and their clients. Despite the efforts to establish more respectful patient-centered care, the resources controlled by ART programs are so vital that clients with insufficient money must live with the inconveniences imposed on them or drop out.

The dependence of patients on their ART providers is replicated on a much larger scale in the reliance of the country as a whole on donors. Without external funding, there would be no first generation of clients. Our interlocutors did not bring up the problem of sustainability—certainly not at this more general level. This may have to do with the timing of our study in the early years of the rollout, before funding problems seemed to threaten. Worries about the future instead centered on the particular treatment program of which one was a client and the prospect of having to shift. Ivan, a client of the HBAC program, had heard rumors that it was going to close and that its clients would be moved to TASO. When an HBAC employee denied those stories, Ivan seemed relieved. "At least there is hope for us that we shall live longer," he said. "Otherwise, we were worried about going to join TASO." (After our study ended, HBAC did close, and TASO had to take over the treatment of more than a thousand HBAC clients.) Hanifa had read newspaper reports that the IDI would run out of ARVs in three months but said that she still had her file with JCRC and TASO and would try to continue at one of those programs if things got bad at the IDI. In other words, people thought in terms of clientship and possibilities in the projectified landscape of care.

A New Form of Sociality?

The first generation became experienced in a form of sociality that had hardly existed before in Ugandan health care. Patron-client relations were familiar; patterns of access to resources through relations to "big people" had long been common. What was novel was the conflation of those relations with rational bureaucratic forms in the arena of health services. By joining and engaging in the lopsided exchanges that gave them access to lifesaving medicine, patients became clients of chronic treatment programs. Involving commitment both by patients and providers, the clinics had a durable contract character indexed in files and other paperwork. The sociality of clientship came in different versions, with different requirements and exchanges. The proliferation of treatment programs appeared to offer choice, but actually choosing and changing from one to another did not seem so easy. Alongside the treatment programs—and, in some cases, pre-existing them—various support organizations for those infected or affected by HIV offered other opportunities that were accessible through patronage-like relations.

Notes

1. S. Whyte and Birungi, "The Business of Medicines and the Politics of Knowledge in Uganda."

2. E. Wolf, "Kinship, Friendship and Patron-Client Relations," 16–17.

3. Erdmann and Engel, "Neopatrimonialism Reconsidered."

4. Cammack, "The Logic of African Neopatrimonialism"; Swidler, "Dialectics of Patronage."

5. Lisa Richey has suggested that therapeutic citizenship and clientship supplement each other, especially in poor communities where counselors and other front-line health workers act as brokers: Richey, "Counselling Citizens and Producing Patronage."

6. Mugyenyi, *A Cure Too Far*; Mugyenyi, "Flat-Line Funding for Pepfar"; Mugyenyi, *Genocide by Denial*.

7. Nguyen, "Antiretroviral Globalism, Biopolitics, and Therapeutic Citizenship," 126.

8. S. Whyte, "Writing Knowledge and Acknowledgement."

9. Twebaze, "Medicines for Life."

10. Chabal, *Africa*, 50.

11. Meinert et al., "Faces of Globalization."

12. Kaler and Watkins, "Disobedient Distributors."

13. Swidler and Watkins, "Teach a Man to Fish."

CASE III

Suzan

THE NECESSITY
OF TRAVEL

David Kyaddondo and
Susan Reynolds Whyte

MOBILITY

(overleaf)

"Nja Hutine," which means "Come,
Let's Go," is the motto on a taxi
that transports people and things,
including chickens.

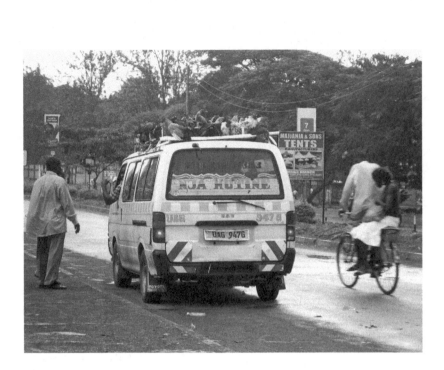

"I started the journey at 6 PM. I came with the Coca-Cola truck, because all the buses had stopped by then. They had refused to bring me, and I pleaded with them. They wanted 20,000 shillings [about $11], but I had only 15,000. I explained to them that I was coming to the hospital, and they accepted." Suzan was talking about how she had borrowed 15,000 shillings to come to the Infectious Diseases Institute (IDI) in Kampala, anticipating that her sister, who lived in the city, would give her the transportation money to return to her home in Lira, 250 kilometers to the north. Because she stayed so far away, we had decided not to include Suzan among those we would follow beyond the initial interview. But in the ensuing year, she made a habit of stopping by David's office, which was within the hospital, every time she came to collect her medicine. Her struggles to make the journey regularly, even though anti-retroviral therapy (ART) was available at her local hospital, involved negotiations with the drivers of trucks and buses to move between the sites where her family, livelihood, and treatment were located.

Suzan was from Lira. That was where she had met her husband, a man from the neighboring district of Apac, an orphan, who was staying with a chief in Lira. After he finished his training as a carpenter, they went to live in Kampala. First he was taken on at a workshop in the industrial area; then he got his own furniture workshop not far from the university and the Mulago National Referral Hospital. So Suzan knew the city and the hospital very well. The couple stayed in Kampala for almost twenty years, with occasional trips to Lira, where Suzan's parents lived, and to Apac, where her husband had built a house on land that had been his father's. In those years they had five children. The first born died of sickle cell anemia; the last born died of malaria. Suzan remarked, "I think she was not alright," implying that the baby might have been HIV-positive.

In December 2000, Suzan's husband fell sick and was admitted to the hospital. He recovered, but pain in his back remained. In April, the couple decided to "go to the village"—that is, to visit his family home in Apac—because they had not been there for a long time. But there was not enough money for the entire family to make the journey, so he went with their son. When he reached Apac, the back pain became much worse; he was taken to Abel Hospital and then to Lacor, the best hospital in northern Uganda. Suzan received a call in Kampala, then went to her husband's workshop and sold some furniture quickly to get money. At Lacor she learned that he had meningitis "that had reached the brains." She was there when he died. She journeyed back to Kampala to collect the children and take them north for their father's funeral, but afterward she returned to Kampala so they could finish the school term.

Life in Kampala was expensive. Before her husband died, Suzan had been trying to earn money by selling fried buns (*mandazi*). "It was OK in Kampala when we were two," she said. But after her husband's death, Suzan saw that it would be better to go back to the north, where she could cultivate. She sold the remaining furniture and even her husband's tools and rented a hut in Lira town, close to where her family lived. There she stayed with her daughter, Flora, so the girl could be close to a school. Flora was sickly and could not walk long distances. Suzan also had a house in Apac, on her dead husband's land, where she farmed. There her teenage son built a house, maintaining his right to the land of his father. "I leave the girl in Lira with my people and go back to Apac to dig," Suzan explained. "If I don't go back, they can take my land. *Mzee* [elder man], the brother of my husband's father, tried to get it. I went to the sub-county—they even brought him the law book; they asked him why he was disturbing the widow. I have a son. Where will he live? I have to keep the home." Suzan grew cassava, which she took to sell in the market at Lira. Her son worked during his holidays, growing yellow beans to sell for school fees. At that time, many people in Lira and Apac were displaced because of the Lord's Resistance Army war (an armed conflict in northern Uganda that lasted from 1986 to 2006). Suzan rented out some of her land to refugees in a nearby internally displaced people's camp. The flood of refugees into Lira town drove up the price of rent. Her small one-room hut used to cost 2,000 shillings a month, but the rent shot up to 5,000.

When David first met Suzan in early January 2006, she talked about the terrible losses she had suffered the previous year. First, her brother had died; he was a soldier, and it seemed that he "stepped on some local medicine" (he had been bewitched). Then her grown daughter, her second born, died, leaving an eight-year-old daughter. A month later, she lost her father. "I am saved. That is why I am running an easy life," she said. "Otherwise, when those three people died, I almost ran mad. But when I kneel down and pray, it cools my heart."

During that dreadful year of 2005, Suzan had also suffered with her own sickness. It had begun to show itself in late 2004. She tired quickly working in her garden in Apac and was exhausted after fetching water. "I said, 'I am now a widow. I need to check my blood, because I don't know what this man did.'" First she went to the hospital in Lira for an HIV test, but the "machine" was not working. She was advised to go to the Joint Clinical Research Centre (JCRC) in Kampala. After testing positive there, she was found to have abdominal tuberculosis and was admitted at Mulago for two weeks. Upon discharge, she stayed for three months with her sister, who was living in Kampala. It was the sister's husband who paid the 86,000 shillings for Suzan's first antiretroviral medicine (ARVs) from the JCRC. When the time came for the next round of treatment, she was told to pay 50,000 shillings, but her sister and brother-in-law could not manage. So she was transferred to a free treatment program under the IDI at Mulago Hospital starting in July 2005.

As Suzan was telling this story, she searched through her handbag and pulled out a bundle of receipts and medical forms to show the receipt for the expenses at the JCRC. Among them, she found the bill from a private clinic in Lira for her daughter, who had recently died. Her voice choked up as she showed it: "the doctor was giving some drugs for TB, but I had a problem of money. She had missed her TB drugs for a week. . . . When she passed away, the doctor refused to give me the body [until I paid what I owed]. That is why I had to sell the bicycle and the goat." The paper showed that she had to pay a deposit of 80,000 shillings, then 40,000 shillings more.

For the whole of 2006, Suzan regularly made the journey from Lira to Kampala. Picking up her medicine at the IDI was the primary goal, but David came to see how she combined this with three other purposes, which she pursued with the help of relatives in Kampala. There was the matter of her son and his future, the health of her sickly daughter, and her own attempts to secure a livelihood. The first time she turned up at David's office on her own initiative, he thought that she had come to ask for his assistance. She told him that her son had not done well on his secondary school exams, but one of his paternal uncles had helped him gain admission to a catering and hotel management institute in Kampala. Her sister promised to pay his fees, and he was able to stay with a sister of his dead father. Coming to Kampala enabled Suzan to see him and to bring food from Apac to the household that was keeping him.

Suzan's daughter Flora, now twelve, was HIV-positive and had been taking Septrin (co-trimoxazole), according to the standard practice. In May, Suzan brought her to the Pediatric Infectious Disease Clinic at Mulago, where her CD4 and viral load were counted, and she was started on ARVs. Because she had to be checked regularly, Flora stayed for extended periods with Suzan's sister in Kampala, an arrangement that Flora enjoyed. But she had a clinical appointment shortly before her primary leaving exam in Lira and had no money for transportation back to Lira, so she had missed her exams at the end of 2006 and had to repeat the final year. Sometimes Flora made the journey from Lira to Kampala alone. Her mother put her on the bus in Lira, and her brother met her at the bus park in Kampala.

When her son went to Kampala to study, Suzan found it difficult to cultivate enough to make money from their gardens in Apac. Instead, she tried selling cooked food at a market near Lira. Truck drivers came early to eat, so at dawn she walked the four kilometers from her home to the market to prepare and sell hot meals. But this was tiring and not very profitable. She realized that she could make more money buying used clothes at the Owino market in Kampala and selling them in Lira. She had little capital but gave the example that in July, when she came for her appointment at the IDI, she bought clothes for 2,500 shillings, which she sold in Lira for 4,000 shillings.

The constant trips were difficult in themselves, but Suzan always made sure to pass by David's office when she was in town. Once she was hurrying to catch the bus back to Lira and hired two motorcycle taxis to carry herself and her luggage to the bus park. But the driver with her luggage was a thief; he sped away and disappeared. She called David from the bus park, at a loss because the luggage contained the two-month supply of ARVs she had just received from the IDI. He suggested that she come to his office the next morning so he could accompany her to the IDI to explain what had happened. However, she did not turn up until 2 PM. She explained to David that she had decided to try on her own before coming to disturb him. She went to the IDI in the morning to ask for replacement medicine; the doctor accepted the explanation and gave her a new prescription. "But at the pharmacy, it was war," she said. "They wanted me to prove that the drugs had been stolen, and they wanted to give for only one month [which would have compelled her to make an extra trip]. I explained that this was happening for the first time, and they finally gave me [the ARVs]." On a later occasion, in January 2007, Suzan came for her appointment but decided to wait until the next day. She had peeped into the pharmacy at the IDI first and saw that an unfriendly dispenser was on duty, who usually did not want to give her medication for more than one month. She hoped that someone else would be at the counter the next day.

As Suzan told David at that first meeting when she had gotten a lift on the Coca-Cola truck, she always tried to negotiate the fare, appealing for sympathy because she had to go to the hospital. She had gotten to know the drivers at one bus company, and they allowed her to ride for 12,000 shillings instead of the standard 15,000 shilling fare. They even let Flora ride for free "because they know my problem," whereas other bus companies charged the child half-price. Suzan kept her bus receipts in her small blue diary. The company had several buses and different drivers, so she showed the operators the receipts to prove that she paid a special price. Once she completely failed to get money for her transportation and called her husband's uncle in Kampala. He told her to take the bus on credit and he would give her money for the fare at the Kampala end. But when she reached the city, he was not there. After a few days, she got the money and paid the bus driver. Another time, she missed her usual bus from Lira and got a lift with the Nile Breweries truck. The driver wanted 15,000 shillings, but she told him she had only 10,000. He agreed to take her on the condition that the woman to whom she was carrying food in Kampala meet the truck with the balance of 5,000 shillings. Suzan borrowed the driver's phone (paying him 500 shillings for the air-time unit) and made the arrangement. In the end, the driver was kind and settled for 2,000 shillings from the woman, who waited for them on Kitante Road in Kampala.

The constant need for transportation money plagued Suzan, and she struggled to earn enough so she would not have to depend on her relatives to cover the cost. When she came to the office in July 2006, she could hardly speak because two teeth had been extracted. She motioned David to come outside, where her daughter, Flora, presented a chicken to David. It was still small, and Flora advised David to feed it for a month before eating it. Suzan also handed him a letter (Letter 1).

Apart from what it revealed about Suzan's appreciation of David, this letter was another demonstration of her enterprising spirit and her constant efforts to scratch together the fare for her treatment travel. (David gave her the money as a gift rather than a loan. Suzan reminded him of one of his close relatives who had also lost her husband to AIDS and was left to fend for her children without a stable income.)

Through the year, David wondered why Suzan did not try to obtain ARVs from Lira Hospital, which was near her home. It was clear that Suzan had considered the possibility, but it was difficult. "They can give to only fifteen people, and then they say it's over, go and buy," she said. "I have a cousin sister who is a nurse, but she has to come here for the drugs. The tests are not there. You can see the doctors, but they tell you to go and buy." Later, Suzan mentioned a friend who had started ART at Lira and died within a month. She seemed to think it was because the treatment there was not good enough. She said she had heard that the Ministry of Health had investigated and found that the hospital's doctors were selling ARVs in their private clinics. (We never confirmed this.)

By the beginning of 2007, Suzan's opinion of Lira Hospital had improved. She had fallen very ill at their village home in Apac and went to stay with her brother in Lira, counting on better support from her own family than she

24 July 2006

Hullo,

How is the morning? Our side we are yet fine. I have been around and I was in need of talking to you, but I was on a sharp pain that day.

Now sir, I am with a request to you to assist me to borrow [lend] me something like 20,000 [shillings] which I want to buy some clothes from Owino. I take it to the village for sale. I have to make sure I pay that money back. Mostly in instalments, if I have to be coming for my drugs. I really feel ashamed for me to ask that from you, but I have [thought] left and right— no other way. I am around because the one who gives the money for going back had gone to Apac [in northern Uganda] for a workshop. But they came back on Saturday. I am in need of doing something to help me for my transport. How to start has been a problem, that is why I am to disturb you Sir. And Dr. apart from [that] which [I] have asked now, don't make it a must that if I came to you, you have to give something. No Dr. you have been helping me a lot. I just like how you handle me, how you talk to me. I feel very well. I feel that is a part of my treatment. I pass just [to] say hullo to you and [get] your comfort only Dr. No more Dr. Thanks may the Almighty God bless you and your family in whatever you are doing AMEN.

Yours faithfully,

Suzan

received from her late husband's relatives. First she went to a private clinic, where she paid 7,800 shillings for a medicinal syrup and twelve capsules of ampicillin (an antibiotic). When she failed to improve, she went to Lira Hospital. She was tested for malaria and given twenty-four antimalarial tablets, for which she did not pay anything (except the cost of transportation). She recovered and during her last conversation with David she said that ARVs were now available in Lira. By that time, Uganda was receiving even more donor support, so the rollout was gaining momentum. Moreover, as security had improved in northern Uganda, the sister with whom Suzan had stayed had established a home in Gulu to farm her husband's land, so one of her primary anchor points in Kampala was no longer there. Suzan was considering asking the IDI for a referral letter so she could start getting ARVs from Lira Hospital, thus eliminating the problems of transportation and having to leave her home unattended while she was in Kampala. But when she mentioned her plan to her son, he begged her not to do it. He thought the hospital in Lira could not be trusted—it might run out of medicine at times. The boy promised that when he finished his course and found a job, he would pay for transportation so his mother could continue getting her medicine in Kampala.

After our study ended, Suzan kept in touch with David. She did switch to Lira Hospital for her treatment and even became a community HIV and AIDS counselor for a project in her village. Her daughter was staying with her son in Kampala, continuing her education at a Kampala school.

CHAPTER THREE

Mobility

Susan Reynolds Whyte,
Michael Whyte, and
Jenipher Twebaze

Suzan's constant worries about money for transportation, like the account of Robinah's grueling journey to treatment and salvation (case I), underline the importance of mobility for the first generation living with ART. For twenty years, it had been understood that HIV spreads through countries and regions by means of human mobility.[1] Long-distance truck drivers, soldiers deployed here and there, traders searching markets, fishermen between landing sites, tourists on holiday from the strictures of everyday life—all of these voyagers form connections between sexual partners at various points on their itineraries. As the epidemic entered the new era of ART, and concern shifted toward ways to get people into treatment, mobility became another kind of problem. Treatment is about fixing people in a program, disciplining them to come for their medicine every month, monitoring their health systematically, and stabilizing their lives. To achieve treatment, some people, like Robinah, must accept being relatively immobilized. Others, like Suzan, must move between the places where they get medicine and those where they get on with their lives.

In the first chapter, we examined the roles of relatives and friends in the therapeutic itinerary, suggesting where to go and making connections to programs. But there are further dimensions entailed in therapeutic clientship, the new form of sociality that the first generation experienced. Not only must people find a treatment for HIV; they must stay on it for the rest of their lives.

The journey does not end with a cure. It requires continuing movement of people, medicine, and resources to maintain the treatment. Clientship, the exceptional arrangement of belonging to a long-term treatment program, is at odds with the dispersed and fluid pattern of Ugandan sociality. In this chapter, we examine the interplay between the stability of ART clientship and the mobility of Ugandan life. We outline the ways in which treatment programs require both fixity and mobility, and we trace the movement of clients among the coordinates of treatment, homes, houses, family support, and sources of livelihood. Not only are people themselves moving, but the situations in which they navigate are also shifting. People on ART are engaged in "motion squared," moving within a landscape that is in motion.[2] We argue that the challenge of clientship is to maintain stability of treatment in circumstances in which family members, livelihoods, and even the ART programs on which people depend may change. Thinking about mobility in this way ensures that we consider time as well as space. To receive treatment, one must be in the right place at the right time. This depends partly on how often one has to report for medicine refills. To stay in treatment, people adjust to changes—and, indeed, create changes—in their social environments over time.

What people strove for was a tactical congruence among livelihood opportunities or requirements, family support, and treatment connection. Suzan's loyalty to the IDI rested on the support of her sister and, later, her son in Kampala and the opportunity to buy used clothes in the city, which she could trade at a profit in the north, where she lived. When Saddam (case II) was transferred to Masindi, his life came together in that he moved close to his family home and joined a treatment program there.

The Two Topographies of ART

In principle, it is possible to map out the locations where ART and other sources of support are available in Uganda. The Uganda AIDS Commission took on this task and, aided by GIS technology, produced an extensive atlas in 2005.[3] It showed that there were 147 sources of ART in 2004, up from 62 the year before, with at least one in every district and with a dense concentration in Kampala. This bird's-eye view reveals the geographical inequity of ART's availability, with Kampala standing out as a "potent place" loaded with possibilities and organizations. By contrast, outlying districts such as Kitgum and Yumbe have only a single source serving a large area.

Most citizens of Uganda do not navigate this kind of topography of availability. No one has the kind of oversight implied in the Uganda AIDS Commission's atlas. Even if people do know that ART is available from a given source, that knowledge alone is not enough. As we have seen, testing and becoming a client are socially mediated. People join given programs and manage to remain clients because they navigate within another kind of topography. They seem to have in mind a kind of social geography of Uganda (and sometimes the world beyond) that features the positions of relatives and friends and possibilities of accommodation, care, support, and livelihood. They think about where they can stay while getting medicine and where they can find care and support while taking the medicine. Instead of a strategic policy maker's overview—what Henrik Vigh calls the GPS landscape[4]—they have in mind a social environment that consists of a set of pathways that fit their own mutable situations.

These two topographies may seem incommensurable: one is a grid of institutions that, in principle, are available to the public; the other is a maze of potential personal networks and subsistence tactics. They must be made to interdigitate for people moving into treatment and moving on with the new lives that treatment makes possible. Becoming a client, being locked into a treatment program at one location, has to fit with ties to other locations that provide homes, accommodation, nurturance, and livelihoods. And contingencies are such that when one thing changes, others become problematic.

The Fixity of Programs

Certain aspects of mobility had to do with the treatment programs themselves and people's perceptions of their virtues. With their various rules and requirements about residence, amounts of medicine supplied at one time, categories of people treated, and services offered, the programs both fixed people and required them to move. Because people became clients tied to a particular clinic, they had to obtain their medications and be regularly checked at one place—an exceptional, even revolutionary, requirement in Ugandan health care. In principle, some programs with branches in many places, such as the JCRC, could write letters permitting clients to pick up medicine at, or even be transferred to, another branch; in practice, this was considered difficult and happened rarely among our interlocutors—although several considered the possibility. Perhaps flexibility will increase as ART becomes less exceptional. But for the first generation, clients had to go regularly to the programs in which they were members.

Residence requirements characterized two of the treatment programs we studied, whose services were limited to inhabitants of a clearly defined geographical catchment area. Reach Out Mbuya in Kampala and the Home-Based AIDS Care (HBAC) research program in Tororo had monitoring systems that required people to be in place. In Mbuya, "Community AIDS and TB Treatment Supporters" visited clients weekly for six months to ensure that they were taking their medicine. In the HBAC project, field officers on motorcycles called on each client weekly to bring medicine and assist with medical and counseling needs. This also allowed continuing surveillance for the research projects in which these clients were subjects.

Both of these programs were immensely appreciated. They were free; they offered many services; they were reliable. Robinah and others mentioned that relatives living in the catchment areas had called them to move there from other parts of the country to qualify for affiliation. Philip left three wives and twenty children in an internally displaced people's camp in northern Uganda to stay with his eldest daughter in Mbuya and begin treatment. Mary came to live with her sister in the area because her uncle was already in the program, so the family knew about it. Rachel and her husband (case X) moved to Mbuya Parish because the husband's brother was in treatment there.

In the first months, as people were stabilizing in treatment, the residence requirement was not onerous. But later, when they had regained strength, some felt restricted. Lotte Meinert wrote about a well-educated woman on the HBAC program who would have liked to move to a larger city, where she could find work commensurate with her qualifications.[5] Robinah had left children behind on her deceased husband's land in Kumi and could not visit them for more than a few days because she had to be in Tororo District to receive her medicine. For clients of these residence-based programs, travel for work or family reasons required negotiation with the treatment provider.

Most programs treat clients from their area but draw no sharp boundary within which they have to reside. Health workers are aware that some of their clients come from long distances. At the rural Mukuju Health Centre and Busolwe Hospital, staff reported that patients traveled from neighboring districts. One of our interlocutors resided in Kenya and crossed the border to receive treatment at Mukuju. Michael Mwangale, the clinical officer at Busolwe, talked about a teacher in Kampala whose village home was in the Busolwe area and who wanted to join the program. He refused partly because he thought the teacher would fail to get money for transportation to come to the clinic regularly; it is a four-hour journey from Kampala. Mwangale saw the mobility of his clients as a major issue and explained that he had been told to write referral letters to other treatment centers if people wanted to move or stay with relatives far away for long periods of time. Antiretroviral medicine is given for one month at a time, although sometimes ARVs are given for two if a client has a convincing reason for not being able to come to the clinic and if the clinical officer trusts him or her. Mwangale recounted one case after another of people who wanted to travel and asked for a longer supply of medicine. He knew their reasons—to visit relatives in Kenya, to trade fish on the lakeshore, to stay with a family member who could provide better food, to live with a son in Kampala—and because he knew so many people in the area, he could check up on their stories. Those who were unable to fetch their monthly medications because of illness or lack of means sent someone else to pick them up, and he generally accepted this. He was understanding about the difficulties of travel and spoke sympathetically about the efforts of poor families to get medicine: "like yesterday, I saw an old man come riding from far away on an old bike to get drugs for his daughter."

The problem of distance was greatest at the big Kampala treatment centers, where clients came in the thousands. The renown of facilities such as the IDI and the JCRC attracts people from afar, such as Suzan. Although health workers there seldom have the personal knowledge of their clients that Mwangale had in his rural hospital, they were also aware of the difficulties of distance. Sometimes they were willing to give a two-month supply of ARVs to clients who lived very far away so they did not have to come so frequently, as the friendlier dispensers did for Suzan. The doctor at the Mbale branch of JCRC remarked that it was difficult for most patients to come for their medicine every month; now the center gives enough ARVs for two or even three months at a time to ease the expense of travel.

Recognizing the problems of travel and increasing numbers of patients, the largest organizations opened new branches to provide ART at other facilities. In an attempt to "decongest" and bring services closer, the IDI began to support the dispensing of ARVs at two municipal clinics in Kampala in May 2006. The JCRC continued to open treatment centers in large towns and to expand The Regional Antiretroviral Therapy (TREAT) collaboration with government facilities. The health worker at the JCRC Mbale clinic reported that the number of its clients fell when the JCRC opened a clinic in Soroti, the next district to the north. At the military barracks hospital where Saddam was posted, fifteen of the forty people on ART had transferred from more distant treatment centers.

Yet as we have seen, proximity was not the only characteristic of treatment facilities that carried weight with clients. Like Suzan, people sometimes bypassed programs closer to where they lived to obtain or maintain membership in a more distant one they appreciated. Not only the services and degree of professionalism offered, but also simple familiarity, evoked confidence that outweighed the savings in time, convenience, and money of getting treated closer to home. Many people mistrusted their local government health facilities because of years of experience with medicine being out of stock and lack of staff. Confidence, trust, and technical know-how were thus important elements in where people accessed their treatment.

The element of discretion was important for some who traveled to distant more anonymous treatment centers.[6] While attractive to some, the familiarity of rural health facilities, where one might meet neighbors and know some of the health workers, was anathema to others. Confidentiality, so central to the ideology and exceptionalism of AIDS treatment, is very difficult to maintain in such circumstances.[7]

One more characteristic of ART programs affected mobility: their specificity in terms of categories of people and treatment offered. Most programs did not manage adults and children in the same clinic. The number of clinics offering pediatric ART is slowly increasing, but the first generation started on treatment when ARVs for children were available only in a few places. Even if Suzan had transferred to the ART program at Lira Hospital, her daughter would have had to continue at the pediatric AIDS clinic in Kampala. Rachel and her husband were both enrolled at Reach Out Mbuya, but their HIV-positive child was being seen at the Pediatric Infectious Diseases Institute at Mulago, in another part of town, because Mbuya did not treat children at that time. John (case VII) was getting his ARVs from the JCRC Kampala, but his HIV-positive wife and child were affiliated with the clinic at Nsambya, the Kampala hospital where John's wife had received antenatal and maternity care and been found HIV-positive. The families were shuttling to clinic appointments at different places, which was especially difficult in John's case because his wife and children were staying in his home village in eastern Uganda. Moreover, programs might give only certain kinds of treatment—for instance, ARVs but not treatment for malaria. Or they were not open on weekends. So people moved to other sources of care for their other health problems. The Ministry of Health rollout provided only generic first-line treatment, so someone who needed second-line treatment had to go elsewhere. Government health units did not have the facilities to conduct tests such as CD4 counts or viral loads. (In fact, Busolwe Hospital did not even have HIV test kits for at least six months.) Patients either had to travel to where these tests were available or go without. These were all ways in which the limitations of the programs required clients to make other stops on their therapeutic journeys.

Homes

The topography of treatment facilities is overlaid with a social topography of kinship. People are oriented in terms of where their parents, siblings, children, spouses, and in-laws are to be found. In the next chapter, we discuss the dynamics of support within families; here we consider those aspects of kinship that have to do with location. The principles of patriliny and virilocality are fundamental for understanding the coordinates on social maps. Men inherit land from their fathers, and women go to live at the homes of their husbands, where they cultivate their husbands' land. While these principles are not always honored, they are the background for understanding many of the mobility patterns into which ART must be made to fit.

The term "home" usually refers to the houses and family members established on rural land inherited by sons from their fathers. It evokes a sense of belonging to a place and family members, an enduring connection to a locality linked to living and dead kinsfolk. Even urban people have rural village homes in the sense of family links and rights to land. When city people say they are going home to the village for the holidays or that they are building a house in the village, they refer to this link to a father's or husband's father's land. Elizabeth, a midwife, had moved to many places because of her husband's job as an officer in the Army. When we met her, she was a widow and was living in Mbale but explained that they had made a home on her husband's family land in Lira and went there to stay when she had leave from her job. At death, the grave—the last home—is almost always made according to patrilineal principles at the father's place or, for properly married women, at the home of their in-laws.[8] Even city dwellers are taken to their village homes for burial. Very few are consigned to urban cemeteries or interred on land they might have bought in town. The opposition between home and house was made famous in the highly publicized case of S. M. Otieno, the Kenyan lawyer whose widow wanted to bury him near their house in Nairobi, in opposition to the wishes of his paternal relatives, who finally succeeded in burying him at his father's home in western Kenya.[9]

In one way or another, considerations about home—belonging to a place and a family—figure prominently in the stories our interlocutors told and in their accounts of mobility. Suzan might have stayed on in Kampala after her husband died but went back to northern Uganda, where she and her son could sustain their rights to her dead husband's land. Having a house and farming there asserted their maintenance of a home and the rights of her son to inherit his father's land. When John lost his job in Kampala, he moved back to his village to start a small business, commuting to Kampala for his medicine. When Dominic's child died (case XI), his former mother-in-law, with whom his estranged wife stayed several hundred kilometers away, brought the baby's corpse in a suitcase for burial on its father's land. When Robinah was mortally ill, people thought she should stay at home to die and not inconvenience her family by making them transport her body from Tororo. Nearly every story, including the original forty-eight life stories, contained references to a home as a point of orientation in therapeutic journeys, even for those who lived elsewhere.

In principle, daughters do not inherit land but move to the homes of their husbands at marriage, where their sons will inherit land. However, in most Ugandan societies, women retain close links to their natal families, where they seek refuge if their marriages break down or if they fall gravely ill. Their children may stay for shorter or longer periods in the homes of their maternal relatives, even though children belong to the clan and home of their fathers.[10] So although land is inherited patrilineally, and children are said to belong to their fathers, relations through women are important. Wives belong to their husbands' homes, but as daughters they still belong to their fathers' homes, as well. Suzan's movements reflected this double belonging: she was traveling between her source of treatment in Kampala, the home of her dead husband in Apac, and the place where her own family stayed in Lira.

This basic patrilineal virilocal pattern is conjugated, complicated, and even ignored in many ways. Men sometimes buy rural property and take up residence away from their fathers' homes. In some localities—Buganda, for example—daughters may inherit land. Men may be given land by their mother's family. People move away from their rural homes because of their work, or they go to stay with relatives in town to search for jobs. Divorce is common; women living virilocally must leave and usually go to stay in the homes of their fathers and brothers or sometimes with another relative or in urban areas. Likewise, when a husband dies, his widow often leaves (although this is not always so, as case IV shows).

Virilocality in itself means that daughters and sisters are dispersed. Divorce, work-connected mobility, and mortality intensify dispersion. Hanne Mogensen argues that women often must move to stay connected and, at the same time, maintain a degree of disconnection that allows them possibilities for their own lives and livelihoods.[11] Add to these factors the extremely high birthrate, which means that most people have many relatives, and it is understandable why people's social topographies are rich with coordinates in many different locations. Nor are these coordinates themselves necessarily stable.

Suzan once stayed with her sister when she went to Kampala to visit the clinic. But in early 2007, her sister left for northern Uganda. However, her son, who had been staying in Apac, had gotten a place at a training institute in Kampala by then. For her, mobility was squared—that is, the social landscape in which she was moving was itself shifting. The changing location of relatives figured in her considerations about whether to continue getting treatment at the IDI.

Accommodation

A house, in contrast to a home, is a shelter, a place of accommodation that can be rented or borrowed or provided to employees. It does not have the same necessary connection to kinship, descent, and land. Accommodation away from home was a concern for many of our informants; houses, like homes, were crucial points in mobility patterns. While Suzan maintained rights at her dead husband's home, she also rented a hut in Lira town close to her own family home, where her daughter could stay near school. The logistics were complicated. While her daughter was attending school in Lira, she was receiving ART from the Pediatric Infectious Diseases Institute at Mulago Hospital in Kampala. The girl commuted frequently, staying with her mother's sister when she was in the city. In fact, she missed her exams in Lira because she was in Kampala when they were given. The steep rise in rent in Lira town, attributed to the influx of people displaced by the war with Joseph Kony's Lord's Resistance Army, was a burden, but having a house in a convenient location was a high priority. Convenience for Suzan, as for many others, had to do with proximity to the support of her own family, her children's schools, and, probably, opportunities for small business offered by the town. Such considerations had to be balanced against the distance to sources of ART and the location of other possible family assistance.

In finding convenient accommodation, some people were helped by family members who owned houses in towns and trading centers or knew the housing situation in the target area. Rachel and her husband, Steven, moved to the Mbuya catchment area after they tested positive for HIV. Steven's brother, who was already a member of the Reach Out Mbuya program, found two rooms for them in his neighborhood. Hassan (case VIII) left his rural home to stay with his sister in two rooms of their father's building in Tororo. This meant that he was farther away from Busolwe Hospital, where he was a client, but his sister could cook for him, and he earned some money repairing shoes on the sidewalk in front of the building. Fortunately for him, the clinical officer came to Tororo regularly because his wife and children stayed there, so he often brought Hassan's medicine. (Health workers were mobile, too, and given the personal attachments people developed to their treatment providers, this figured in their movements.)

A few of our interlocutors had little to do with most of their relatives and rural homes. For them, accommodation was crucial. Noah, in treatment from Reach Out, said that his family in Bwaise was difficult. They were thirty-seven children (from different mothers), but all were on their own. The land was insufficient, so Noah took up brickmaking and, later, scrap metal trading. He rented a small room in a mud-and-wattle building in Mbuya with a loan from the Reach Out program. He said:

> My biggest worry is the house. Since I don't work, I have no earnings. I pay 15,000 shillings for this house. I have heard that my landlord may even break this house down for renovation—that is, if it has not been sold to a rich person. It is the single most important thing in my life now. I am very worried, given that the landlord is not so friendly. . . . There was a time when I was too sick and people thought I was dying. They even mobilized transportation to return my body [to the paternal home]. But when they came, I was not dead, and I told them that I will not go there. I refused to be returned home because I know that my [step]mother who is there will not take care of me. They can even kill me or leave me to die. In my life now, the only thing that will force me out of [Mbuya] is accommodation. Otherwise, since I have started on the drugs, I can't move away. You can't get this type of drugs anywhere else, and if I am sick, I can easily reach the clinic. I don't want to change my place of residence often, because here everyone now knows me and likes me. When they hear that [I am] not feeling well, you soon see someone coming [to give me money for] transportation.

For Noah, Mbuya was a "sweet place" that offered treatment and social support, while his rural home was "bitter."[12] His house in Mbuya was what kept him alive, in the sense that it allowed him to remain where he felt secure. Yet even though Noah had rejected his rural home, his brothers still feel an obligation to bury him there.

For about 1.5 million people in northern Uganda, accommodation was in bitter places during the years of the Lord's Resistance Army war. They were forced into camps for internally displaced people and only began to return to their rural homes in the years after the cessation of hostilities in 2006. For the HIV-positive people among them, mobility and immobilization had special consequences. Concentration in camps meant that access to ART was relatively easy in many locations once it became available for free. Moreover, patients benefited from other kinds of project support, such as visits by project volunteers and the "positive identity" that was fostered by patient groups. Once they dispersed back to their rural homes, they had to face the same problems of transportation to treatment sites as our interlocutors from southern Uganda. Because government health care facilities were in a shambles in the rural areas outside the camps, and because people on treatment were familiar with the clinics in the camps, many people on ART hesitated for some time to return to their rural homes. When they did, they reported that the transition was difficult. As bitter as the camps were, they had some trace of sweetness for the clients who lived so close to their clinic coordinates.[13]

Livelihood and Location

The location of work, the topic of chapter 7, was a primary coordinate in the new topography of life that had to include treatment sites. Members of the "working class"—that is, those who were paid a regular salary—were subject to transfer or temporary assignments far from house, home, family, and treatment. For all employees, regardless of their serostatus, transfers and travel are elements in workplace politics. But they took on special significance for those concerned about being away from their fixed coordinates at the treatment program.

For some people, the mere possibility of a transfer was worrying. Dorothy, a prison officer, was upset when she heard about plans to transfer her away from her source of treatment, as well as from her husband and children. She was relieved when the transfer did not materialize but then worried when she was informed that she would be sent to Luzira, the big prison in Kampala and far from her home in Tororo District and her ART clinic, for a three-month training program. Benjamin, who worked for the Uganda Revenue Authority, asked to extend his annual leave because he felt sick and weak. His boss had promised to put him on light duty, but he feared that if he kept making excuses and missing work, he would be transferred away—maybe even to a place where people did not understand such problems and where there were no facilities offering ART.

For others on salary, journeys were already a reality with which they were trying to live. It is striking that many of our interlocutors, like Benjamin, mentioned that their immediate bosses tried to accommodate their health problems. This included understanding about the problems mobility might pose to their treatment regimes. The two soldiers, Tom and Saddam, were posted to the barracks near Mukuju Health Centre so they could easily get their ART. John's boss took him off duty for a long train journey when the bag containing his medicine was stolen. Perhaps the most dramatic example is Steven, Rachel's husband, who managed to work in southern Sudan while getting his medicine from Kampala, sometimes with help from his boss. Clearly, not all workplaces were so accommodating, but employers' recognition of the requirements ART set for employees on treatment reveals a great deal about the consciousness of the first generation.

People trying to get by through trading and small-scale business activities also had to move around to earn livelihoods. For some, this was so strenuous that they finally had to give up. Hanifa started on ARVs in 2004, buying them from the JCRC in Kampala. At the time, she was a trader, going back and forth to Kigali in Rwanda with various supermarket merchandise. The first month, she took her medications with her on the journey to Kigali. "I went with my medicines, but they got finished before I returned," she said. "I missed about four days, and I got so sick. When I returned, I went straight to the hospital. I didn't even go home. I just phoned to tell my family that I had been admitted. It is that time I stopped going to Kigali, because I realized that *safaris* [journeys] were straining my life. Also, three of my friends had died because of safaris. I got scared of the safaris and said to myself, 'Nobody sent me for money'"—that is, no one had demanded that she take the trip to get money. The problem was that giving up the Rwanda trade meant she often did not have money to buy medicine. Fortunately, like so many others, she was able to switch to a free treatment program.

The Costs of Journeys

Having to travel regularly from a place of work or residence to the source of treatment was a problem for nearly everyone. Even those in the geographically delimited programs of Reach Out Mbuya and HBAC sometimes had accommodation in the catchment area and homes elsewhere to which they traveled. Suzan's case was extreme, with its logistics of Coca-Cola trucks and special deals with bus drivers. But many people talked about the expense, time, and discomfort that characterized their traveling. Most moved by bus (for long distances) or *kamunye* (passenger vans that carry about fifteen people and ply fixed routes). Others were carried on the backs of bicycles.

Transportation needs money; therefore, it was a constant worry for most people. Roscoe lived in Pallisa and struggled to buy his medicine, pay for tests, and manage school fees for his children. He had trouble finding the

6,000 shillings for transportation to Mbale, where he was receiving treatment, so his wife picked up his medicine when she went for her own (free) treatment. However, this meant that the health worker did not see Roscoe regularly, which concerned her, since he was suffering severe side effects from the medicine. Goretti lived in Busolwe but had to travel 50 kilometers to Mbale to collect her medicine. She had to put aside money from her meager salary to ensure transportation and looked forward to the time when her drug regimen would be available at a hospital nearby. For a time, John was staying in Tororo District but getting treatment in Kampala. He told Godfrey that transportation was "just a gamble." At one meeting, he recounted his most recent journey:

> I came by the goods train from Tororo because I had no money for the transportation fare. I just go to my friends [who work for the railway], and they will give me a lift, as they are going to Kampala. But moving by train is difficult, my brother. For example we arrived at night, having left so early in the morning. The cargo train I used was coming to Jinja, and it arrived at 3 PM, but since it was ending in Jinja, I had to look out for another one going to Kampala. Fortunately, there was one leaving at 6, and I had to wait for it. It finally left and arrived past 9 pm. So it was difficult, but since I have no money, I have to endure.

Our interlocutors emphasized the ways they managed the costs of transportation; other research suggests that transportation costs may undermine adherence to ART, even in nominally free treatment programs.[14]

Beyond the money, long journeys cost strength; they are arduous, especially for ill people, as Robinah's account so sharply shows. Benjamin described what it was like to make the journey from his home in Busia to the JCRC Mbale at Christmastime. By the time he reached Mbale, he said, he "was so tired and having body ache. You know the problem with public transportation and especially during Christmas season. It is bad. We were so packed in the taxi, yet I was sick. I was being squeezed with other passengers, but I just had to endure."

Given the difficulties of travel, people spoke with warm appreciation about the efforts made to help them move. Harriet, who lived about 20 kilometers from Busolwe Hospital, said that her son carried her on his bicycle and that other children living in Busolwe insisted she stay with them to be near her treatment.

Dispersed Coordinates and Fixed Treatment

Mobility is not only required to pick up the next month's supply of medicine at the treatment site, although that can be problematic enough, but also because people's social coordinates—their points of orientation and possibility—are dispersed and shifting. This is nothing new. Women have always moved at marriage; people visit relatives and sometimes stay for months; children are sent away for education; work opportunities are available elsewhere. These aspects of sociality have always been about place. What is new for the first generation is the temporal and spatial fixedness of being a client in a treatment program. Fitting the demands of therapeutic discipline to the necessities of family support and livelihood, and to the desires to visit and expand social horizons is where problems and conflicts arise. Reacting to changes in the social coordinates and, potentially, to shifts in treatment programs and to the waxing and waning of bodily health may all motivate mobility. The chapters that follow take up the coordinates that orient movement and must be adapted to one another.

The first generation experienced these matters intensely because early treatment sites were few in number and unevenly spread; it took time for them to expand. As more sources of free treatment appeared, and as people like Suzan gained confidence in the clinics near their homes, complications brought about by mobility were reduced. But they will not disappear as long as clientship, the new form of therapeutic sociality, remains fixed to places and times.

Notes

1. Iliffe, *The African AIDS Epidemic*, 61; Barnett and Whiteside, *AIDS in the Twenty-First Century*, 147–48.
2. Vigh, "Motion Squared."
3. Uganda AIDS Commission, *National HIV/AIDS Atlas*.
4. Vigh, "Motion Squared," 427.
5. Meinert, "Regimes of Homework."
6. Meinert et al., "Faces of Globalization"; Kisuule, "The Social and Cultural Context of the HIV/AIDS Epidemic in Rural Areas of Jinja District."
7. S. Whyte et al., "Health Workers Entangled."
8. S. Whyte, "Going Home?"
9. Cohen and Odhiambo, *Burying SM*.
10. S. Whyte and Whyte, "Children's Children."

11. Mogensen, "Ugandan Women on the Move to Stay Connected."

12. Meinert, "Sweet and Bitter Places."

13. Wilhelm-Solomon, "Challenges for Antiretroviral Provision in Northern Uganda"; Wilhelm-Solomon, "The Priest's Soldiers."

14. Hardon et al., "Hunger, Waiting Time and Transport Costs."

CASE IV

MamaGirl
& MamaBoy

FAMILY MATTERS

Hanne O. Mogensen and
Godfrey Etyang Siu

FAMILIES

(overleaf)

Households often include
a grandmother and
her daughter's children.

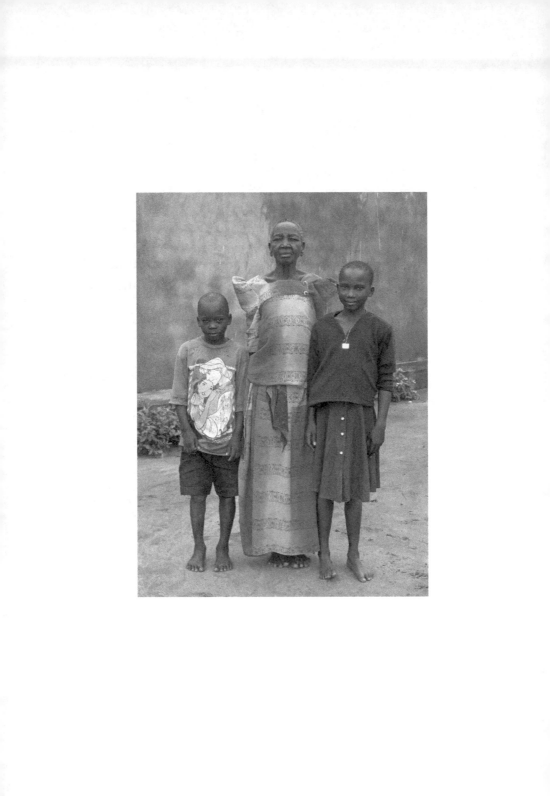

It was a big homestead in the eastern part of Uganda, with several permanent brick houses and just as many small thatched huts. The biggest and nicest was painted light blue and yellow. In this house, built by her late husband, lived MamaGirl. Her father-in-law had just passed away when Hanne and Godfrey visited the home in late 2005, and many relatives were still sitting by fires near the grave, mourning the deceased and cooking maize porridge. The two researchers were welcomed into MamaGirl's living room, which had newly painted walls and numerous couches and chairs—and a motorbike. Mama-Girl herself turned up a few moments later, sweaty and with dirty legs, as if she had just come from the garden. She looked happy, healthy, and confident, and the size of her biceps left no doubt that she was able to dig and do hard work. As we soon learned, her occupation had always been farming, supplemented since 2001 by a part-time career in politics as a member of the sub-county's Local Council (LC) 3.

When her husband died in 1997, MamaGirl realized that he might have suffered from "this new disease" and decided to go to The AIDS Support Organization (TASO) for counseling and testing. She did test HIV-positive and kept going to TASO every two weeks to get as much treatment as possible and remain strong. She was still OK back then, she said, except during a period in which people were saying, "Doesn't that woman smell from having all those rashes?" In 2002, Home-Based AIDS Care (HBAC) began working in the district, and MamaGirl's TASO counselor managed to get her taken on as a client. When her CD4 count fell below 250, she started on antiretroviral medicine (ARVs). That was in 2003, about two years before our first visit.

MamaGirl was born in 1967 in a neighboring sub county and finished primary school in 1986. She was supposed to go on to secondary school but could not because her father was killed during the insecurity that accompanied Yoweri Museveni's takeover, and there was no money for school fees. She went to stay with an uncle in Kampala for a short time, then returned home and got married. Her husband had already separated from his first wife, with whom he had two daughters, but later this wife wanted to return. The husband harshly told her that he did not want her as a wife anymore and that she should leave the children with him. When MamaGirl tried to intervene, he said that his first wife had done so many bad things to him and abused him for years. He admonished MamaGirl, "Why are you entering into things you do not know anything about? You just stay quiet." He beat the woman until she left. MamaGirl took over the responsibility for the two small girls and cared for them so well that people thought they were her own. Now and then their mother would visit them. When she came for the funeral of their husband in 1997, she decided to stay. MamaGirl emphasized that she had welcomed her co-widow back: "I told her, you stay here, and we will take care of the children together." MamaGirl had one living daughter. She had been pregnant five times but miscarried once, and three of her children died at a young age.

The family of MamaGirl's husband was large. He had four full brothers and a sister (who had also died of AIDS). There were many half-siblings, as well, since her father-in-law had five wives and many children with each. Her mother-in-law was his first wife, and the father-in-law was buried in the compound where the old lady lived with two of her sons and their families and her two widowed daughters-in-law. A number of orphans also lived in the homestead, mostly from the families of her father-in-law's brothers. "Their sons [paternal cousins, or "cousin-brothers," of her husband] produced so many children whose parents have now died," she said, "and I am a God-fearing person, so I cannot reject them." Three of these orphans, classificatory children of her dead husband, were under her care.

MamaGirl's husband, like several of his brothers, had a good job. He worked in Kampala for an important government department. When he died, she received a payment from his pension fund of 3.8 million shillings (about $3,115), a relative fortune, which representatives of the fund emphasized was for her alone. But the windfall was a bone of contention, envied by his brothers and her co-wife. It evaporated quickly. MamaGirl spent it going to TASO in Tororo every two weeks and buying medicine for the many sicknesses she had in the years after his death. In 1999–2000, she bought medicine from the South African company Swissgarde that, she said, "kept the virus in my body low." She seemed slightly uncertain about the medicine—it was for HIV/AIDS, but she did not know exactly what it was. She had been connected to the people selling it through her sister, whose neighbor was also buying the medicine. MamaGirl remarked, "They worked in a somehow secret way, asking who had told me about them." (Swissgarde is a multilevel marketing firm that sells through personal networks rather than retailers. It deals in nutritional supplements and does not sell ARVs.) The price of the medicine kept increasing: at first, it cost 46,000 shillings a month, then, over time, rose to 500,000 shillings. MamaGirl bought the medicine for about six months until she ran out of money. "These drugs gave me a few problems with my brothers-in-law," she said. They kept asking her what she was doing with the money. When she explained about the expensive medicine she had been buying, they complained she was wasting their brother's money on a disease that has no cure and asked why she did not leave them the money and wait to die. "But were it not for that money, I would have been dead already," MamaGirl said repeatedly. Instead, she managed to stay alive until the HBAC project started providing free ARVs.

Hanne had known the family for years, and before this first interview she had passed by to ask MamaGirl whether she would be willing to participate in the study. She had found only the co-wife, MamaBoy, who explained that when she returned after their husband's death, she had also joined HBAC. She was accepted by HBAC as a member of MamaGirl's household and did not even have to go through TASO. (Index HBAC clients were taken from TASO membership lists, while other members of their households were automatically tested and included if found HIV-positive.) MamaBoy's test showed that she was not yet ready to start on antiretroviral therapy (ART); she was given Septrin and had her blood tested every month. Now she and MamaGirl were staying together and jointly looking after the children. "So things are OK," she said, "except that we do not cooperate well. MamaGirl has chewed our husband's money. We were given a pension of almost 4 million to help the children, but MamaGirl just spent all that money on herself." She added that MamaGirl was the sister of one of their brother-in-law's wives. "Those two sisters, they know medicine that can chase co-wives—and they don't fear using it," she said. When Hanne left the home that day, her interpreter, a woman from a neighboring village who was distantly related to the brothers-in-law, accompanied her. She commented, "The two women are somehow cooperating, but not too much. Co-wives are like that. Some people agree that it was OK for MamaGirl to keep the money, since the other woman had been gone for many years, but others disagree." The interpreter also explained that sometime after the co-wife returned, she gave birth to a child. "The boy is now so big that he has started walking," she said. "Nobody really knows who the father is, but people say that it's the brother-in-law of MamaBoy [the brother of her late husband]." Neither of the co-wives had mentioned that boy in the course of the conversations.

Four months after the first interview with MamaGirl, Godfrey returned to her place and found the co-wives at home. They were delighted to see him, thanked him for the sugar and bread he had brought, and started preparing food for him. He immediately noticed that MamaGirl looked sickly and had lost weight. She confirmed that she was not doing well. "There is something happening in me which is worrying me," she said. "It comes like menstruation and has been going on for six weeks now." A few days before, she had told a

visiting HBAC field officer about the problem. The next day, he brought medicines for her, but it was too early to tell whether they were working. When
MamaBoy entered the room and joined the conversation, MamaGirl did not
appear bothered—on the contrary, the women seemed used to sharing problems and concerns.

Later, Godfrey suggested that he talk a bit more with MamaGirl in private,
and they sat under a tree near the house. She told him that she had been
reelected to a third term as an LC3 councilor, but the campaigning had been
very hard on her. She suffered many insults because Museveni's National Resistance Movement (NRM) was not popular in the eastern part of the country,
and her status as an HIV-positive woman had been used against her. The
campaigns were exhausting; she had lost weight and used a lot of money.
Because she did not receive any salary as a councilor, she had decided not to
run in the next elections.

When asked about her relationship with her co-wife, she said it was OK.
They were sharing their problems, working in unity with no major conflicts.
"We do everything together for the family," she said. " We know that no one
else will help us and that we have to help each other." They had had big problems raising school fees for the oldest girl, and they only managed with help
from MamaGirl's sister.

The relationship with the brothers-in-law was still bad. Recently, Mama-
Girl had hired some men to plough. She was supposed to pay them 5,000
shillings but only had a 10,000 shilling note; the ploughman promised to
change the note and return with her balance. He never did, however. He just
told her to ask her brother-in-law, who owed a debt to the ploughman, for
the money. When the brother-in-law heard of the incident, he was furious.
"Why do you always try to antagonize me?" he snarled. "You already lost your
husband so leave me alone. If that so-called Slim of yours has failed to kill you,
it will be me to kill you instead!" Other people tried to support her and put
an end to his abuses, but he seemed to have something against her. "He feels
jealous that we are able to take care of many children, some of whom are not
ours," MamaGirl said. "He always expects us to serve him food, even when
there is sufficient food in his house. It is as if there is something he wants from
me." She seemed to be implying that the brother-in-law was assuming the
superiority of a husband; by custom, brothers of the deceased could inherit
their wives. Perhaps he felt threatened by the women's relative independence.

In the end, Godfrey had a short conversation with MamaBoy, who confirmed that the relationship between the co-wives was good: "we work hard,
do our tasks together, and look after the children whom the man left for us.

We have nothing else to do and nowhere else to run to. Also, MamaGirl regards me more highly these days. You know, that time, when we had a lot of money from our husband's pension, I tried to advise her, but she did not listen, and she ended up using the money in a bad way. But these days, she listens and does not do anything without consulting me first." When asked whether she knew how MamaGirl had spent the money, MamaBoy seemed careful not to point a finger at her co-wife; instead, she said that MamaGirl had been misguided by one of the brothers-in-law on how to use the money and that she had used some of it for treatment. "But we are not really doing badly," she added. "Not in terms of food. We do not receive any help from our brothers-in-law, but we still have the strength to work for our children." She did indeed look strong, but thin.

When Godfrey turned up to visit the women again two months later, MamaGirl said she was impressed that he had kept his word to return, as if she had not expected he would. She was on her way to an LC3 meeting but had delayed because she was waiting for the field officer to deliver her medicine. Because the council's chairman understood the delay, MamaGirl had a little time to talk to Godfrey. She seemed both happier and healthier than she had been at the previous visit. The treatment she got from HBAC had worked, and her bleeding had stopped. She was also still doing well on ARVs, and the HBAC staff were delivering the medications promptly.

Since the previous visit, MamaGirl had started benefiting from a goat and piggery project initiated by the nongovernmental organization (NGO) Africa 2000. Priority was given to longtime TASO clients. She was very pleased and optimistic about the project. She also talked about a coming poultry project she hoped to join. As a member of the sub-county's council, she had further been involved in registering orphans in the district and was hoping that help would come her way for the orphans in their care. The relationship with the brothers-in-law had been improving; one recently had been surprisingly friendly, offering to buy her a soda and cake when they had met at the trading center. Her mother-in-law was around during the interview, working in their shared compound. The co-widows seemed to have a good relationship with the older woman.

The following month, MamaGirl had gone to an LC3 meeting at the sub-county headquarters when Godfrey arrived, and it was MamaBoy who happily welcomed him. She said they were all doing fine; that she had no problems and felt strong enough to work in the garden every day. MamaGirl was not quite so strong, and sometimes she did not dig. But this was also because she was consumed by her political duties: she was busy attending meetings, mobilizing people, moving up and down. This was good because it sometimes gave the women extra cash and a chance to benefit from projects, but Mama-Boy also felt that it was exerting too much pressure on MamaGirl's health.

During a later visit, MamaBoy gave the impression that she was no longer impressed with MamaGirl's political activities. "She has gone to the sub-county headquarters with her usual issues," she said in a tone that revealed she was fed up. Godfrey probed a bit, and MamaBoy explained:

Well, you know there are many challenges. Some are about survival, but others are not. Recently, we exchanged bitter words about how we live in this house. You know we share domestic chores, but she spends most of her time moving around, and I remain at home doing most of the work. I cook and prepare everything for the family and for her. She only comes to eat. But one day, I had not prepared dinner because I was too exhausted and it was late. When MamaGirl returned from wherever she had been and did not find food, she quarreled over it. I did not take it lightly, because I felt she did not appreciate my role in this home. I told her that I am not her servant and that she should be glad that I had forgiven her for misusing the money of our husband. MamaGirl said I should recognize that her work as a councilor also brought benefits to the home and that I had relied on her since I came back. But the few shillings her work brings to the home are not more than what I manage to contribute. And when TASO was still bringing assistance like maize meal, sugar, and oil, it was never enough. We still had to supplement from the gardens, where I was the one doing the work.

As Godfrey was leaving, he talked briefly with the mother-in-law, who thanked him for looking after her daughters-in-law.

After talking to MamaBoy, Godfrey went to the sub-county headquarters, where he found MamaGirl. She was happy to see him and to tell him about her work with the council. She was involved in mobilizing people for development projects that were due to come and spent most of her time away from home. Godfrey asked whether this did not put too great a strain on her health and family, but she played down the possible effects on her health and made no reference to the conflict with her co-wife.

Four and six months later Godfrey paid his last two visits to the family. MamaGirl seemed less busy with her council work. The kitchen of the co-wives had collapsed, and they were now cooking in their mother-in-law's kitchen, which meant that sharing everything they had was inevitable. It worked out well. Sometimes it was even the mother-in-law who helped them when they did not have enough food. However, the old lady became increasingly sick during this period. She had never really recovered from the death of her husband. It was mostly MamaGirl and MamaBoy who took care of her—other people in the home did not help them with the feeding and caring work. "One of the brothers-in-law has clearly been jealous for a long time about us sharing the kitchen and meals with our mother-in-law," MamaGirl explained. "He thinks we are parasites depending on grandmother for food. But in reality, we are the ones helping her. She seems to have been left entirely to our care. It was like a trap, because we have not had a kitchen of our own since it collapsed last year. If only we had our own kitchen, we would be in control. Now they are expecting us to look after the grandmother while always abusing us."

Godfrey explained to MamaGirl that the research project had come to an end and that he would not be returning. She seemed puzzled, as if she did not understand this and thought of him not as a researcher, but as a friend of the family. Seven weeks later, she called Godfrey to inform him that her mother-in-law had died and that the burial would take place on the following Saturday. He was sad that the kind old woman had passed away but had to tell MamaGirl that he would not be coming to the funeral and that he wished them the best.

CHAPTER FOUR

Families

Susan Reynolds Whyte,
Hanne O. Mogensen,
and Jenipher Twebaze

The story of MamaGirl and her co-wife, MamaBoy, illustrates a theme that is central to all of the cases we came to know: shifting alliances within families. The human immunodeficiency virus and the responses to it, including ART, have reconfigured families across Uganda. This re-forming is not something that happens once and for all; it is an ongoing process. Relations between the two co-wives were distant at first, although in MamaGirl's version, she took the moral high ground in offering to accommodate the co-wife whom her husband rejected. While he lived, the husband refused to allow his first wife to stay; it was his death from AIDS that opened the opportunity for her to take a place as his wife (widow) and be reunited with her children. In MamaGirl's telling, she showed generosity by accepting the estranged first wife back into the family home to live with her in the house their husband had built in his village so that they could care for the children together. And it was because of this that MamaBoy was able to benefit from the HBAC program as a co-resident of a client.

In the first three chapters of this book, we examined the sociality of treatment—both the new form of clientship and the persisting importance of everyday social relations. We showed how efforts to gain access to and live with ART depend heavily on kinship ties. Not only is treatment contingent on family support. It also affects those relationships, as we saw in the case of Robinah and Joyce (case I), whose sisterhood was practiced more intensely, in terms of both care and conflicts, because Joyce brought Robinah to stay with her and access treatment. Moving in with a relative is a concrete example of re-figuring families. It reminds us that kinship is practiced in households where people eat, sleep, and work out the details of a domestic economy. The people we considered in the previous chapter, on mobility, were shifting from one household to another, often maintaining footholds in several. In this chapter, we examine the ways in which those living with ART conceived, practiced, and reconfigured kinship relations both within and between households. We argue that families can be understood as a changing network of possible relationships rather than as units of undifferentiated solidarity. Second chances are heavily dependent on these contingencies of relationship, for better or for worse.

This view of the family fits with recent developments within studies of households, as well. Earlier, they were seen by social scientists as solidary units of cooperation, sharing resources for production and consumption. Partly under the influence of feminist scholarship, a view of the household has emerged that "sees it as a locus of competing interests, rights, obligations and resources, where household members are often involved in bargaining, negotiation and possibly even conflict."[1] This assumes that households are internally differentiated, and the positions of members can be analyzed in relation to one another. The complaints by MamaBoy that her co-wife did not appreciate her domestic work and expected a hot meal to be ready when she came home at night resemble the disgruntled comments we have often heard about husbands.

The mobility of Ugandan life means that household composition is fluid, and widespread poverty makes the management of domestic resources a matter of contention and concern. Nor are households autonomous in terms of domestic economy. Time and again we found examples of people who received financial and other help from family members in other households to pay school fees, buy medicine, and provide temporary accommodation. Economic interdependence characterizes relations within the household and, often, relations with members of other households.

In considering how relatives support, neglect, and antagonize one another, it is important to remember that Ugandan families are large. While the average woman bears 6.6 children, there were examples of women who had ten or twelve. Moreover, the fathers of many of our interlocutors had multiple wives so they had numerous brothers and sisters. Harriet's father had nine wives and sixty children; Dominic's (case XI) father had fifty-five children; Hanifa's father had thirty-six children; Major Charles's father had five wives and fifty-six children; Paul's father had forty children with different wives. In most Ugandan languages, kin terms are classificatory—that is, they include more kinds of relatives than, say English or Danish systems, which are more descriptive. Paternal cousins are all called brothers and sisters, just as father's brothers are called father and their wives are all called mother. There are many relatives with whom to develop more or less warm relationships, and a family will be localized in many different households.

The Amity and Practice of Kinship

Two approaches to the study of kinship are useful for understanding its significance for the first generation living with ART. One emphasizes the ideology of solidarity among kin; the other points at the way relatedness is actually practiced and thereby made into a social reality. Together they can help us grasp what is happening as people seek and offer help in some quarters while neglecting others or even treating them antagonistically.

One of the greatest of the early scholars of African kinship systems, Meyer Fortes, wrote about the ideal that informed kin relations of common blood (consanguinity). He called it the "axiom of amity": the moral expectation that kinsmen should share, help in times of trouble, and take responsibility for one another. They should show their unity by eating together and using resources jointly. Fortes recognized that the principle of amity was not always realized either within or across generations. Bitter conflicts could erupt and might last over many years. His point was that amity is a moral ideal rather than a consistent characteristic of family life. [2]

Subsequent research in eastern Uganda has emphasized the continuing importance of this ideal, even when it is honored mainly in the breach. In West Budama, where MamaGirl lived, a song celebrates family unity and solidarity: "We are one. / We are one family. / People in the clan are there for each other." In the neighboring area of Kwapa, Meinert found that "unity" within families was seen as a virtue so important that it was considered a resource for health. [3] In nearby Butaleja District, the leader of one clan had a rubber stamp made in Kampala that printed the words "*Bagombe hwendana*" (the Bagombe [clan name] love one another). In case love fails, a proverb reminds people that they are stuck with their kin: "kinship is like your buttocks: you can't cut it off." [4]

In our study of the first generation, we found confirmation of kinship amity as an ideal. The way people spoke about the support or lack of interest of their relatives revealed a strong sense of the morality of giving money, care, shelter, food, advice, comfort, and company. To give and receive in these ways showed others that one was a virtuous relative, and people were recognized and admired for that, just as people were criticized for stinginess and neglect. Harriet, a widow who had been sickly, was taken for testing by her brothers. When the results came, they supported her. "What really made me strong were my brothers," she said. One of them brought her to stay with him near the hospital and admonished his wife to feed her well: "if you don't take care of my relative—who knows, we might also fall sick. You might be here thinking that she is going to die, and then God helps her and she gets better, and then you also get infected and she looks after you."

No one among our interlocutors was repudiated or neglected by relatives just because he or she was HIV-positive and sickly, although we did find a few cases in which some members of a family thought others were "discriminating" or not taking adequate care. Generally, the extra challenges of HIV and ART exacerbated existing tensions and strengthened ties that were already sound. When bad words were said or imagined about "having AIDS," it was usually because relations were already strained or a quarrel about something else had flared up, as when MamaGirl's brother-in-law abused her in connection with the money for the ploughman.

Recognition of the supportive role of the family is a well-established theme in scholarly work on the response to AIDS. Researchers have pointed out that in most places, families have not rejected people with AIDS and have shown resilience in meeting needs even when resources are scarce. However, many of these researchers, especially earlier in the epidemic, wrote about families in general terms, as if they were homogeneous units: "the urban family," "the extended family," or even "the African clan."[5] In contrast, the line that we are following is to differentiate relationships among kin to show how infected and affected people form alliances and develop tensions with some and not other family members.[6] In practice, the amity of kinship does not extend to all kin, or even to all consanguines. In actualizing kinship, people are dealing with specific relatives, not with families as a whole. Given the size of Ugandan families, and their dispersion in households sometimes at considerable distance from one another, this is inevitable, although scholars have not given it much attention.

The notion that kinship, or a sense of relatedness, emerges from everyday practice has been put forward by Janet Carsten. One of her points is that the sharing or distribution of substances is a concrete way to enact relatedness. Breastfeeding a baby and eating together are some of the strongest examples, but sharing houses or money are also ways to enhance that feeling of commonality she calls relatedness.[7] Taking the point of view that relatedness is not just given by biology but actually performed allows us also to analyze instances in which people who might have been included as kin were not. People with whom a biological link could have been emphasized may be left aside, or those people may themselves drop out of the active chain of kin because of distance or lack of interest or for some other reason. Jeanette Edwards and Marilyn Strathern made this point about English kinship,[8] and it holds for the way Ugandans on ART activated kinship links differentially.

Relatedness is a tool for approaching how people actually use family relationships in living with ART. Instead of assuming what a family is, it requires us to notice process and diversity, the particular kinds of sharing, helping, and communicating that are at play in relationships people point to as "family." It helps us to see families as networks rather than as groups or units. Looking at practice entails examining everyday life in households, as well as the specific assistance that people in other households offer. It is with this kind of perspective that we can grasp the figurations and reconfigurations that emerge in living with ART.

Gender, Blood, and Marriage

Fortes contrasted the solidarity of those who shared blood (consanguines) with the kinds of relations entertained with relatives by marriage (affines), which he described as more contractual, based on agreements, exchanges, and the balancing of debts. (Here he seems to have been thinking especially of men's relations to their male in-laws.) Where consanguineal ties are enduring, affinal ones are subject to rupture. Unlike your buttocks, relations by marriage can be severed. This is certainly evident in today's Uganda, where formal marriages are on the decline and partnerships dissolve, often leaving children who never live with both biological parents. Yet to some extent, the distinction between affinal and consanguineal relations is overridden within households, where husbands, wives, and consanguines from both sides may be living together. Within households, people eat from one pot and share household resources—at least, to some extent. MamaGirl, her co-wife, and her mother-in-law were affines, but the practice of cooking and eating together, sharing a kitchen, and helping with everyday chores created a sense of relatedness between them.

Still, ideology and assigned status are important in the way people enact kinship and assess possibilities. A fundamental point is that they act as kin from positions as men or women. Especially in patrilineal societies, gender is key in negotiating the rights and obligations of different family members. As we mentioned in chapter 3, sons usually inherit rights in their fathers' land, while daughters are expected to move to the homes of their husbands, where they have use rights to his land. On the one hand, it seems that men have more enduring links to a home than do women. But on the other, women may have somewhat more room to maneuver in that they retain links to their parents' home (their consanguineal relatives) even after they make a new home with their husband (and other affinal relatives).

The epidemic put these issues in a new light. The old, common perception, once articulated by Aidan Southall, was that women were more fully incorporated into their husbands' families, and marriage was more enduring, among the Nilotic ethnic groups (e.g., Teso, Padhola, Acholi, Langi) than among the Interlacustrine Bantu ones (e.g., Ganda, Soga, Toro).[9] These patterns were already changing when sickness and death from AIDS began making inroads. Women and orphans had to seek support wherever they could find it. A woman's rights in her husband's home are put to the test when he dies; there are many reports that male agnates attempt to evict widows and take over land and other property. "Chasing away" the widow may even be rationalized if she is thought to be HIV-positive (maybe even suspected of having infected her husband). Public health messages warned against the widespread pattern of men "inheriting" the widows of their brothers, and this caution seems to have been accepted by many. Thus, the old manner of insuring that a wife remained a wife in the agnatic family is declining. At the same time, "gender equality" messages about the rights of widows to remain in their conjugal homes are respected in some Local Councils, and born-again Christian widows have mobilized support to remain.[10] The situation in contemporary Uganda is that gender is still key, but it does not absolutely determine where women can live and get access to resources. A range of possibilities exists for women as wives, widows, mothers, sisters, and daughters among all ethnic groups.

When their husband died, MamaGirl and MamaBoy stayed on in his family home, in the house he had built in the village from money earned working in town. Neither of the two women was formally inherited by his brothers, although there were rumors that the father of MamaBoy's last child, born after her return to her dead husband's home, was his brother. Presumably, MamaGirl's position was strong at first because of the money she received from her husband's employer and, perhaps, because her sister was married to one of the brothers, who had a good job in a nearby town. As a member of the LC3, she brought recognition to the home. Both of the women had borne children with their dead husband; although the children were girls without a claim to inherit land, the household was firmly established in the homestead's biggest house and it came to include the dead man's mother when the women started cooking together. In other instances, widows' claims to a household in the home of their dead husbands were based on the patrilineal entitlements of their sons. Recall Suzan (case III), also a widow, whose husband's paternal uncle tried to take the land her husband had left. Her argument was not so much that she had a right to it as that it was for her son. In the same way, Robinah thought it was necessary for her son to stay on his dead father's land in Kumi when she moved south to Tororo District.

These examples of widows retaining residence in the homes of their dead husbands are countered by the many examples of widows who returned to stay with their consanguineal relatives. Helen was married to a man in western Uganda who worked for the district administration. She did not get along with her co-wife until their husband began to sicken. They suspected that he had been bewitched because of envy, either by colleagues or by one of his male relatives. But after the husband's burial, his father told the co-wives that his son had died of AIDS. He also announced at the ceremony for choosing heirs that no one in the family should inherit the widows, but neither should they disturb them. They were welcome to stay unless they wished to go and marry elsewhere. Helen remarked that her father-in-law was an educated and enlightened man and that she still appreciates what he did. Yet when her two brothers in England heard that her six-month-old baby had died, she said, "They quarreled, asking what I am doing at my late husband's place—I should go with my children; they will look after me. So I left that place and came back home."

It is not only widows who leave husbands' homes to stay with their siblings or parents. Wives who have problems with their husbands or who are sickly frequently move to stay with a blood relative. Mary was a second wife to a man in Busoga, but when she began having frequent bouts of fever, she went to stay with her twin brother near Kampala, who drew on a network of their relatives in and around the city to help her get treatment. When Jenipher and Susan visited her, she was living in Mbuya Parish with her "cousin-sister" (her father's brother's daughter), that cousin-sister's husband, his sister, and their two children. Although it was cramped staying in one room, the family knew about the Reach Out Mbuya program because of another brother who had been treated there and wanted Mary to stay in the parish so she could benefit. A brother lived next door and owned the house where they were staying. Mary had broken off with her husband and emphasized that she now had very many relatives nearby. And when Ivan and his wife quarreled, she often went home to stay with her mother. On one occasion, an annoyed Ivan told Jenipher, "My mother-in-law is also not easy, because she says, 'I am looking after my daughter; let them also look after their son!' Can you imagine? So I don't know whether my wife will come back." The wife did return, but the comment highlights the importance of consanguineal ties for married women, especially when they have trouble. Not only did they seek support from their parents and siblings; they belittled or even broke conjugal links in doing so.

The lesson seems to be that women and men can make use of different arguments for activating kinship ties, consanguineal and affinal. But it is the actual performance of sharing and caring that realizes a relationship—that is, that makes it strong or weak. Living with ART involves just such enactments of "looking after" by feeding, supporting, accommodating, and providing money.

Who Can Help?

Family reconfiguration was driven largely by the extra needs for support and care necessitated by HIV illness and ART. Earlier in the epidemic, the terrible burden of nursing sick and dying family members weighed heavily on mothers, wives, sisters, and daughters.[11] Taking care of orphans was often the economic responsibility of uncles. Members of the first generation also needed nursing care at first. But later, as they gained some strength, that was less important than assistance with food, accommodation, and money. To the extent that kinship is a network of possibilities, those family members who have more resources, or particularly useful ones, are called on to help. Kinship politics are based on inequality, with some members having more money and education, better jobs, and more usefully located households.[12] They are in a better position to help people on treatment get on with their lives.

The reconfiguration of family was an ongoing process for James, a twenty-five-year-old university student. His parents had never married, and he grew up with his maternal grandparents. He met his father for the first time six years before he joined our study and had seen him only a couple of times since. After he finished secondary school, he went to Kampala and lived in the house of his mother's sister, where his mother was also staying. When the two sisters died, within a few years of each other, he continued to stay in the house with his younger brother, his maternal cousin Tito, Tito's wife, Lovisa, and their children. None of them were working, and Lovisa's mother was contributing to the support of the household. When James found out that he was

HIV-positive, he informed Tito, who, he assumed, told Lovisa as well as his brothers, who stayed in the house off and on. Considering that James had hardly any contact with his father, it was striking that he shifted to live with his father's brother shortly after Godfrey got to know him. Tito told Godfrey that he and his wife simply did not have the means to support James since they were not working and had other relatives staying with them. He also confided that James's father was a drunkard but that the father's brother who had taken him in was a good man who had some money and was understanding because he was on ART himself.

It was James's friend Kenneth who asked James's uncle and aunt to take him in. Kenneth told Godfrey that Tito neglected James and even discriminated against him by making him use a special plate and cup. He claimed there was a world of difference in the care James received in the more prosperous household of his father's brother, and, indeed, James's health did seem to improve. Yet before long, James moved back to Tito's house because he was well enough to resume his studies and needed to be near the university. Tito and his wife moved out, but some of Tito's other brothers remained and the household of bachelors managed somehow, partly because some of Tito's brothers were able to sell a house that had belonged to their dead mother. James struggled to scratch up tuition fees for himself and his younger brother, approaching aunts, uncles, and grandparents on both his mother's and his father's side.

James's family seemed to consist of a whole set of possible relations that could be activated but might lie dormant for long periods. As Edwards and Strathern showed, biology is always intertwined with other social considerations in galvanizing relationship.[13] James did not turn to his father with whom he had an immediate biological link. He managed to survive and even resume studying without any income of his own through appeals to the amity of kinship. When an aunt from Mombasa came to visit, she was moved to contribute some tuition. At another point, James was trying to raise money to pay for transportation to find his maternal grandfather in Mukono, who might help him. Apparently, all of these people knew that he was HIV-positive and in treatment, but they hardly ever talked about it. Their actions confirmed their relatedness to him in a way that might not have happened if living with ART had not moved him to seek them out.

In their analysis of English relatedness, Edwards and Strathern reported that their informants talked in rather hypothetical terms about whether they would help different relatives in need or whether they were "close" enough to hear whether particular kinds of relatives were having problems and to share confidences. For our Ugandan interlocutors, these matters were not at all hypothetical. It was the effort to get help so one could get on with life that provided occasions to practice kinship. And here, the issue of sharing confidences took on special significance.

Who Needs to Know?

The reconfiguration of families starts with the response to illness and continues through the process of testing, getting into, and staying in a treatment program. Throughout this process, different family members have different kinds of knowledge about the status and treatment of the sick person. It was very evident to us that "disclosure," as it is technically called, was not a simple matter of telling or not telling.[14] While some family members were explicitly informed in words about testing HIV-positive and getting into treatment, others guessed from symptoms or from what seemed implicit in conversation. Asked who knew about the situation, our interlocutors often said that they thought certain people knew even though they had not been told. Their thoughts about sharing and controlling information revealed much about the processes of reconfiguration over time.

At one extreme were people like MamaGirl and MamaBoy, who were receiving treatment in the HBAC program. Because field officers visited them once a week to bring medicine and check on them, the fact that they were on ART was general knowledge, not only in their households and families, but in their neighborhoods.[15] Ivan did not want to tell his mother, but she got to know because of HBAC. Being visited at home meant that other members of their household not only knew about their treatment but also had the opportunity to be tested and offered treatment themselves, as was the case for MamaBoy.

At the other extreme was a person like Grace, married with four children. When she developed symptoms such as frequent urination, painful spots on her feet, a rash, and boils, she went to her brother who worked at an NGO clinic. He tested her and found she had diabetes, but when her rash and boils did not respond to treatment for diabetes, he tested her for HIV. When he told her the results, he said, "This is going to be a secret between you and me." Still she decided to share the secret with her eldest daughter, who was twenty-eight, who in turn told the next eldest, her brother. The daughter knew a nurse at the Joint Clinical Research Centre (JCRC), whom she contacted about getting her mother on treatment. Grace never told her husband or her other two children, although both were in their twenties. They only knew that she was being treated for diabetes. Because she did not often fall sick, and because she was taking regular medication for diabetes, she seemed confident that other members of the household did not realize she was on ART. Since she had a fairly good job, she did not need to ask for financial help.

The pattern of selective disclosure was very common, in the sense that many people explicitly told only some members of the family, with the understanding that they would not talk about it with others. A person who needed help usually told the one who could provide it, as Grace told her brother, and as Bernard in a similar way confided in his sister, who had contact with a doctor. Thus families were reconfigured in terms of who knew and who helped. As Roscoe explained about telling his parents and siblings, "I had to be open to them. They had to know, because they look after me. They had to make contributions—even transportation that I was using to come to the hospital and back—they hired a vehicle. They helped." Robinah and Joyce were unusual in disclosing their status to all. But even this full disclosure has happened gradually, in stages and in more or less direct ways—telling some and letting others, such as the children, see that they are taking medicine, then talking about it much later.

Telling a sibling first, rather than a parent or child, was a pattern we often heard about. It was not unusual for people to link the sharing of knowledge with the help a sibling could provide. Hanifa had not told her cousin who lived with her and did not want David to visit her at home, because her cousin talked a lot. But she told her sister, who lived elsewhere in Kampala and provided important assistance. Jackson also claimed that he had only told his sister, who lived in Mbarara and was taking care of one of his children. The other children and the cousin who lived with him in Kampala had not been told. William, who had twelve siblings, said, "All my brothers know because they also help me financially." Major Charles explained the delicacy of communication. Ten of his siblings were still living; he had chosen to tell only one of them that he was HIV-positive and on ART because "he stays in the village, and I wanted him to be aware so that he can take care of my property and, in case I die, he can pass it on to my son." However, he also said he thought the others knew: "they don't tell you directly, but they usually talk: 'Afande [the officer] is sick.' When I get sick, they get so concerned, they tend to give very special attention; they attend to me differently. But I don't want to tell them directly." Major Charles was managing to buy medicine himself and even to care for four orphans of his late brother, so he did not need assistance except to carry out the very special task he had assigned to his village brother.

As for sharing with parents, some found it natural to inform them, especially if they were living with them or if they were sources of help. Young women such as Alice (case IV) and Jolly (case IX) had resourceful parents who provided money, advice, and other kinds of care. Norah was living with her husband, but when she developed a terrible cough and began to lose weight, her mother called her to take an HIV test. She moved in with her mother for a time and started paying for treatment at the Mbale branch of JCRC. She praised her mother as "a courageous woman" who had to support nine children after her husband died. She had already lost one daughter to AIDS and was caring for the orphans. She was helping another daughter who had started on ART and then "organized some money," as Norah put it, to help her start at the same clinic. Such mothers took the initiative to reconfigure households and families based on their knowledge of their children's serostatus and needs for treatment.

However, other people said they hesitated to tell their parents because it would upset them too much. Some told us that they thought their parents knew, although they had never raised the painful topic in conversation. It was not always possible to control the information. Herbert had lost all his brothers and sisters to AIDS. When he tested HIV-positive, he decided not to tell his mother, because he was sure she would commit suicide. "When our last born died, my mother sent for poison," he said. "She deceived her grandson that she was going to kill rats, and when they told me, I went and talked to her, and she revealed that she actually wanted to kill herself because she was not seeing why she is burying all her children and she is not dying." But later, Herbert's first wife, whom he disparaged by saying she "had never seen a blackboard" (meaning she was not educated and thoughtless), told the old woman, who collapsed when she heard that her son was HIV-positive. On the following visit, Herbert was still annoyed at his wife. "I am even worried all the time that she might die," he said, "but it seems she goes on getting used [to the situation]."

The sharing of knowledge is important because of what it means for relationships. It is not only a matter of imparting information; it is a basis for giving and receiving help. In fact, informing a relative that one is HIV-positive can be a way to ask for help and impose an obligation that might be avoided if the knowledge were left implicit, as Hanne Mogensen has shown.[16] But it is also a way to share intimacy and even to encourage someone else in the family who is sickly or tests positive. Hanifa had ten full siblings and told only one of her sisters. But she also had a stepsister who had lost several children. "One of her daughters was very ill, so I brought her to the AIDS Information Centre, and she tested positive," Hanifa said. "I took her to my home and tried to encourage her to start ARVs. She was always defiant, saying, 'I am going to die soon. Why should I bother?' Then I told her, 'I am also positive,' as a way to encourage her. Those two, and my husband, are the only people I have told."

The decision not to tell others is often explained in terms of the consequences for relationships. One justification is that old parents, like young children, must be shielded from worry. If they cannot help anyway, there is no need for them to know. Paul remarked that there was no reason to tell his parents, since they could not contribute anything toward his treatment and welfare and would only feel frustrated. When the sick person is a source of support for others, he or she may not want them to fret about the possible loss of help. Perhaps "strong" people also want to maintain their image as competent, virtuous, or trustworthy. Martha explained why she preferred to pay for her medicine from the JCRC and maintain discretion: "I am the bread earner in my family. Sometimes it is not necessary to tell family members, because when you are the caretaker like me, parading me before all my dependents and tell[ing] them about my health—I don't think it is right." For Martha, the issue was less about whether to enact a relationship by sharing a confidence than about maintaining a certain quality in the relationship she had with her dependents.

Together, these concerns about sharing knowledge with family members underscore our point that people differentiate and specify kinship when they confide in some and not others. It was evident, as well, that there were often practical reasons for doing so, in that those confidences might be the basis for sharing other, more substantial resources. In the process, some kinship links were strengthened, and others were left aside.

The Reevaluation of Relatives

The amity of kinship as an ideal and the sociality of family as a daily practice were challenged in learning to live with HIV and ART. The gendered dimensions of patrilineal belonging were brought into sharp relief as women sought support from their consanguineal families while trying to maintain rights in the families of husbands or partners. Sociality was a process as well as a practice, as appeals were made to different kin.

As a biogeneration, those on ART got a reprieve because of the newly accessible biotechnology, which included a new form of sociality in its requirement of therapeutic clientship. They were able to maintain clientship and survive because of pre-existing forms of sociality—in particular, the everyday family relations practiced within and between households. In the process, family ties were illuminated and revalued. Historical generation and genealogical generation shaped and reshaped each other.

In the reflections of our interlocutors about who needs to know and who can help, we heard their reevaluations of kin and relationships: this one talks too much; that one will ensure that my son inherits my village land. People considered the possibilities of calling different relationships into action. As they mobilized some relatives rather than others, they refigured family networks. In a sense, surviving AIDS put family relations to the test, strengthening some and bringing tension into others. It made interdependence more obvious and more differentiated.

Notes

1. Moore, *A Passion for Difference.*
2. Fortes, *Kinship and the Social Order.*
3. Meinert, *Hopes in Friction,* 119–35.
4. S. Whyte, *Questioning Misfortune,* 156.
5. McGrath et al., "AIDS and the Urban Family"; Seeley et al., "The Extended Family and Support for People with Aids in a Rural Population in South West Uganda"; Ankrah, "The Impact of HIV/AIDS on the Family and Other Significant Relationships."
6. S. Whyte and M. Whyte, "Children's Children"; Mogensen, "New Hopes and New Dilemmas"; Dilger, "My Relatives Are Running Away from Me!"; A. Wolf, "Orphans' Ties."
7. Carsten, "Introduction"; Carsten, "The Substance of Kinship and the Heat of the Hearth."
8. Edwards and Strathern, "Including Our Own."
9. Southall, "On Chastity in Africa."
10. Christiansen, "The New Wives of Christ."
11. Obbo, "Who Cares for the Carers?"; Kipp et al., "Family Caregivers in Rural Uganda."
12. Mogensen, "New Hopes and New Dilemmas," 62.
13. Edwards and Strathern, "Including Our Own."
14. Twebaze, "Medicines for Life," 167–211.
15. Apondi et al., "Home-Based Antiretroviral Care Is Associated with Positive Social Outcomes in a Prospective Cohort in Uganda."
16. Mogensen, "New Hopes and New Dilemmas."

CASE V

Alice

KEEPING A
GOOD MAN

Jenipher Twebaze and
Susan Reynolds Whyte

PARTNERS

(overleaf)

Advice on a controversial
billboard in Kampala.

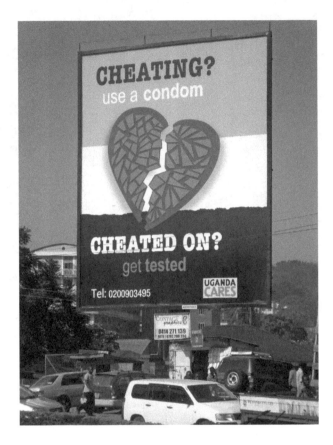

"No, he doesn't know anything, and one time he actually told me that we need to go for HIV testing since we intend to get married to each other, and I said it's OK." Already at the first meeting with Jenipher, Alice was thinking about whether and how to tell her boyfriend that she was HIV-positive and on treatment. Jenipher asked whether he had seen her medications and her papers lying about at home, but Alice thought he had not noticed. "My boyfriend is calm. He doesn't do those things of checking in my bag," she said. "He usually sees my files because they are spread all over, but he has never asked me what they are used for. He doesn't check anything, and he is patient, cool, and OK. I have no problem with him." Jenipher asked Alice whether she planned to tell him. She answered, "I don't know. My mom was encouraging me to tell him, and she was insisting that she is going to tell him herself." But why could she not tell him? "You see, I have been with him for one year now, and he is good to me. I don't want to lose him." Alice said they did not use condoms at all.

Alice was an attractive young woman of twenty-six, from a fairly prosperous family, who had earned a diploma in communications after completing senior secondary school. She had her own apparel shop in an eastern Ugandan town, where she and Jenipher had their first long conversation, having agreed that whenever a customer came, Jenipher would close her notebook and pretend to be a visitor. Between customers, Alice told Jenipher about her education and earlier love interests:

I first had a boyfriend in my second year of secondary school, but, you know, being young, you get boyfriends just to pass time. In the last year, I got one who later went to Masindi, and we never met again. I don't know where he went. Then I got another one in my vacation who went away. When I was doing my diploma in Kampala, I had a boyfriend. But you know the *bayaye* [toughs] of Kampala. He used to beat me up after finding me talking to other men. He was such a rough man that I reached an extent of reporting him to the uncle with whom I was staying. He called him and warned him that he was going to report him to police. One time, I was on my way home with my friends—the ones with whom I was studying. He called me on the phone, and I told him how far I had reached. He asked why I was walking back home. He said I should wait for him. I did that, and he came with another friend; they beat me until I could not say a word.

Then he put me in a taxi and dropped me off at home. They took me to hospital, where I spent two days, and after that I separated from him. He was a killer. I suffered with that man.

It was around this time that Alice started to fall sick on and off. She said she told her mother, who immediately speculated that it might be HIV and asked Alice to go for an HIV test. "You know, being a nurse, [my mother] doesn't like staying with health problems when you are not sure what you are suffering from. So I agreed," Alice said. "First of all, we went to an ordinary laboratory and found that I was HIV-positive. My mom was not content with the results, and she chose that we go to the JCRC [Joint Clinical Research Centre in Mbale]."

Alice said she did not feel bad when she got the news because she was told that acquired immunodeficiency syndrome (AIDS) was a disease like any other and could be treated. She appreciated her family's sympathy. "They all know about it, including my dad, because with mom he helps me pay for the drugs," Alice said. Yet despite her openness with her family, Alice preferred discretion with others: "I did not disclose to many people or my friends. You know, people may not be wishing you well, and they start pointing at you."

As Jenipher concluded the first conversation, Alice's mother arrived at the shop. She was happy to hear that Jenipher had come to talk about HIV issues and greeted her with a hug when she discovered they spoke the same local language. In an immediate display of trust, Alice's mother revealed a secret: "I hope she has told you her problem." Alice laughingly objected, "but mom." Jenipher ventured, "what is the problem? She doesn't swallow the drugs?" Alice's mother burst out, "She is pregnant!" In a low tone, she asked for advice about whether Alice needed special food or special medicine. Jenipher ran short of words but urged the women to inform the doctor about Alice's pregnancy and ask him for advice.

About three months later, Jenipher found Alice's boyfriend, Mike, tending the shop while Alice rested on the floor behind the counter. She was visibly expecting, and Mike said, smiling in a teasing and caring way, "I am trying to help, but as you can see, she can no longer carry anything. She is just lazy, but I think she needs to rest." The way he dealt with customers and prices made it clear that Mike was often at the shop. Although he worked in Kampala, he spent a lot of time with Alice. As Jenipher was leaving, Alice escorted her part of the way, leaving Mike in the shop and taking the opportunity to talk about the problem of disclosing to him. "You know, it was my mother who wanted me to tell him," Alice said, "but now we are OK, and you can see how

I am. How do I tell him? It can be disastrous. I will wait and have my child, then I will tell him that I was told we should go for HIV testing. That is when things will be revealed, and I will also pretend like I am learning about it for the first time."

Alice's pregnancy progressed, but still Jenipher observed that care was taken not to say anything about her HIV in front of Mike. When Jenipher saw Alice's mother before the next visit, she warned, "Please don't ask her about those things, because her boyfriend is there. Talk to her outside the house." When Jenipher met Alice herself at the gate, Alice whispered, "We are here, and my boyfriend is around. Please don't talk about my issues because my mother and I, we are trying to find a way to tell him. You see, he might wonder who you are, but I told him last time you came that you are just a friend."

At the next visit, Alice was only a month from her due date, looking healthy and sounding appreciative that Mike had taken leave from his job to care for her and help in the shop. As they sat talking, Alice got a phone call, and Jenipher heard her saying, "Yes, I took the juice, and I have talked with the doctor. I have also bought the milk bottles." It was her mother, more and more concerned about Alice's health. "My mom is so worried," she said. "She wants me to rest and wait for the day. Can you imagine? She talks to me like I'm a child and thinks I'm not going to look after the baby well. She told me that when I deliver, I will be staying at home with her the first two weeks." Talk turned to their impending shift to a larger house, and Mike said, with evident excitement and happiness, "The next time you will find us there with our baby." Jenipher got the impression that Mike genuinely cared for Alice.

But out of Mike's earshot, Alice confided, "My dear Jenipher, I don't know what to do. My health is very good and I have no problem. I even went to check my CD4, and they told me that it was above 600 and they told me that was very OK." Alice said she was still taking her medicine and she had been given Nevirapine to protect the child from getting the virus:

My worry is . . . how to tell him, because I was instructed that I should make sure that I do not breastfeed the baby. How will I explain to Mike why I am not breastfeeding? These days, everybody knows that if you do not breastfeed a baby, then you are sick. My mother was saying that we should tell him, since we might get problems after delivery. Even my father actually asked whether I have ever told my boyfriend that I am on drugs, but I said I have never. He kept quiet, but mommy told me that he wants us to inform him. I tell you, I am confused. But I know God who gave me this problem will help me get out of it. I pray every night, and I leave everything to God to handle.

Jenipher advised Alice to make an agreement with the counselor at the testing center to pretend that she had not yet been tested and to go for testing together with Mike. It was a very emotional visit, and Jenipher had a lot of thoughts afterward about whether she had given Alice the best advice.

Just before Jenipher's next visit, she received a text message that said, "Hope the Lord has kept you well. We, too, though we have been so quiet. Anyway, good news. I delivered a bouncing baby boy on 31 August [20]06 at 9.15 AM . . . and his name is Jesse. It was a successful operation by Dr. John. Thanks for your care and love that made this baby see the world. May God bless you abundantly and also take care of your needs just like you do to others. All will always be well with you. Keep smiling, Alice." When Jenipher found Alice at her mother's house with her new baby, Mike was in the shop, so she could speak freely. After describing the tribulations of her hospital stay, and the daunting caesarian section under partial anesthesia, she came to the denouement of her "long-time worry of disclosure" to her boyfriend:

Jenipher, I tell you what: God is good. I passed through it well, and he now knows. The advice you gave me worked so well, and we are living happily. I don't know what will happen next, but we are so far fine. When you left last time, I talked with my mother about the advice you gave me, and she bought the idea. So I went to the JCRC and discussed with one of the counselors, and my doctor also knew the whole situation. So I came and told Mike that I have been instructed to go with him for HIV testing and that they could not deliver me without knowing my status. He said, "I have always told you that they had to check you unless you were planning to deliver from the village." He then accepted, and we went. My dear, we were first counseled, and then they took the blood; we waited for about fifteen minutes, and they called us inside to tell us. The counselor asked us how we were planning to live in case we were HIV-positive or HIV-negative. First he asked Mike, who said that he would live positively or negatively, and he then asked me. I first kept quiet and said I would also live positively or negatively depending on whatever would come out. He started with me—that I was HIV-positive. I screamed, and Mike held me tight as I leaned on him. He then told Mike that he was HIV-negative. Mike stood up and said, "That is not possible. How come Alice is positive and I am negative?" My dear Jenipher, it was a difficult situation. I cried, "will my child survive?" Then, after some time, we settled down, and the counselor kept talking to me and said that we needed to test three times. So he told us to come back after three months [and] to start using condoms. . . . That is where we are.

Asked whether Mike had changed in his behavior toward her, Alice said he was the same and wondered why. Perhaps Mike was not surprised by the results, because he had seen the medicine at home. Alice said,

We are also wondering whether he saw anything, because I used to keep my drugs in the refrigerator, my files in the living room, and sometimes tins on the table in the bedroom. I would get drugs for a month, sometimes two months, so there would be many tins of drugs in the house. I would sometimes swallow tablets when he was looking at me, but he never asked me why I was taking them, and I also kept quiet. I don't know what will happen, but he is OK, though we have not met yet because of the situation I am in. But we were advised to use condoms.

At the following visit, Alice's mother greeted Jenipher effusively. "My daughter, you are welcome, and I want to tell you that my daughter loves you so much and has not seen anyone who likes her like you do," she said. Jenipher was overwhelmed and did not know how to answer. The mother later continued, "You know what, my daughter? You seem to be a well-behaved girl, and you should tell your mother that you found another mother here at our place. Or give me her phone number and I will tell her myself. I will also buy you something like a beautiful dress that will make you keep remembering to like my daughter."

During this visit, Alice and her mother were bantering about who knew how to look after the baby best. They both laughed, but the conversation turned serious concerning Alice's plans to have their son circumcised. Alice's mother pleaded with Jenipher, "Please convince my daughter Alice not to circumcise her son." Then turning to her daughter, she said, "Your father, brothers, and nephews are not circumcised. Is your husband circumcised? [Laughter] Surely, why do you want to circumcise this young sweet boy? Didn't I bear you as my children even if your father was not? Please don't. I hate it." In the end, Alice went ahead and had the baby circumcised. "These days, they are saying that circumcised men do not get problems," she said. "Why can't I do it for him when he is still young so he doesn't suffer the way I see men here suffering when they are older." (Alice appeared to be referring to a campaign that was under way for medical circumcision as a way to reduce the risk of

HIV infection, but she may also have had in mind the ritual circumcision of teenage boys by the Gisu people of eastern Uganda.) Mike later remarked that it did not matter to him whether the boy was circumcised or not, but he did not mind that Alice wanted it.

Despite the disagreement about circumcision, Alice's mother was pleased with the new little family and especially with Mike. "I tell you, my daughter has a good man, who is cool," she said. "He paid bridewealth, four million [shillings], and he is remaining with a two million [shilling] balance, because we asked him to bring six million [shillings] in total. [Bridewealth is a payment by the groom or his family to the bride's parents that confirms the marriage.] Alice and her husband are doing well. They bought a car, and their house is almost complete, I gave my daughter a house because I don't want my children to suffer. Then after that, they wed."

Alice also appreciated her partner:

We are fine. Mike buys food for me and the baby; as you know, the baby does not breastfeed, so Mike spends a lot of money on powdered milk. He also pays rent for the house and is planning to get the balance [of the bridewealth], two million [shillings], and is also preparing for a wedding. The problem is that we are living an expensive life—house, food, rent, car, baby. It is too much, but he tries. And you know, my mom wants me to eat well, so he buys the food, but mommy also buys me fruit and greens. My mom cares for me so well. We are planning to wed in a few months and then enter that house so we can save on the money we are spending on the [rented] house.

But the capstone of her happiness was that their baby seemed to be healthy. The joy on her face was unmistakable as Alice told Jenipher that her son had tested negative for HIV.

Jenipher hoped to meet Mike alone at some point to get his side of the story, but she was also worried about questions he might ask about her relationship with Alice. She never managed to see him alone, but on several occasions she noticed that he looked suspicious, as if he was wondering what their secrets were when he saw Jenipher and Alice talking quietly together.

At the last visit, Alice said that after all her worries about telling him, Mike was still supportive: "we have no problem. Sometimes Mike reminds me to swallow the pills, and I am OK with the medicine." He went with her for counseling but did not like the advice about safe sex. "I insist that we use condoms strictly, although sometimes Mike wants us to have 'live' [unprotected] sex," she said. "When we go for counseling, they give us more condoms, but Mike doesn't want them. He refuses. He wants live sex, but for me, I don't want to become pregnant again. It is still early for me given my condition."

When Jenipher explained that the study was coming to an end, Alice was upset. She was sad that her mother had not managed to buy the gift for Jenipher yet, but Jenipher assured her that she would still visit them when she was in town. After the completion of the study, Jenipher kept in touch so we know that Alice and Mike did have a wedding and that they had a second child before very long, but also that there were many conflicts after their wedding and that they separated on a couple of occasions. Alice's mother asked Jenipher to try to intervene. After their first separation, Jenipher helped Alice and Mike get back together. But then she went to Denmark for a long stay and does not know what happened after their second separation.

CHAPTER FIVE

Partners

Susan Reynolds Whyte,
Godfrey Etyang Siu, and
David Kyaddondo

Sexual partnership has long been a central concern in the literature on HIV in Africa. Sexual networking, the number of consecutive or concurrent sexual partners, and the use of condoms have been in focus because they are believed to determine the risk of infection.[1] Our study raised different issues. As Alice's case shows, the first generation confronts the implication of testing and treatment not only for sexual practices, but also for partnerships as long-term social relations. Alice delayed telling her boyfriend that she was HIV-positive and in treatment because she feared he would leave her. She saw her whole future, with hopes of marriage, in jeopardy. As the situation turned out, the relationship seems not to have been noticeably affected by Alice's "secret." But for other partners in our study, testing and treatment had farther-reaching implications. We argue that the management of HIV opens a new space for talking about partnerships, negotiating the expectations partners have of each other, and reflecting on previous sexual relations. Even the power dynamics between men and women shifted in some cases.

Education campaigns about AIDS and the advent of HIV testing and treatment came on to the Ugandan scene at a time when other influences were changing marriage relationships. Shanti Parikh suggests that Christian discourses on monogamy and development rhetoric about women's rights combined with the public health messages to make faithfulness to a spouse or cohabiting partner a mark of enlightened respectability. Concurrently, other factors, such as gender inequality, opportunity structures, and expectations about masculinity, supported a continuation of poly-partnering by married men (and, to a much lesser extent, women). Parikh's research in southeastern Uganda showed that women were less and less tolerant of their men's infidelity and spoke out critically, even if they did not leave their partners on those grounds.[2] In this chapter, we take Parikh's observations further to focus on the ways that testing and treatment provided opportunities for reflecting on and talking about partnerships in contemporary Uganda. We also found that women pointed critically at men's poly-partnerships. But more than that, both men and women reviewed their pasts and considered the present and future with partners in a new light.

Patterns of Partnership

The kinds of partnerships our informants formed, in the period we knew them and in their accounts of their pasts, covered a wide spectrum. Even a young woman like Alice had already experienced a whole range: from having "boyfriends just to pass time" to living with the man who fathered her child; having a formal, "customary" union confirmed by the payment of bridewealth; and having a wedding at a church.

Our interest here is in the more enduring relationships of marriage and cohabitation. Marriage is formalized by religious ceremonies and the payment of bridewealth. At the very minimum, the partners should be introduced to each other's families, a step that requires hospitality and some exchange of gifts. But because these social forms are expensive and demand the involvement of family members from both sides, it is extremely common for couples to live together, sometimes for many years, without undertaking the ceremonies. Cohabitation is recognized in most Ugandan settings as a kind of marriage, although it does not have the same legal or social status as formalized arrangements. The blurry lines of marriage are reflected in the very words for "my husband" and "my wife": in most Ugandan languages, they can also be translated as "my man" and "my woman." Even cohabitation is not always clear. Has the man provided accommodation for his woman/wife, as is generally expected in a marital arrangement? How often do the man and woman stay together? When we first met Alice, Mike was visiting her on weekends and staying at her place. Particularly when the man has another wife, with whom he stays part of the time, the question of cohabitation is moot. Just as it is not always clear whether someone is married, it may also be unclear whether someone is divorced. Even after her husband's death, MamaBoy claimed the status of wife, although he had rejected her in life.

Male dominance in marriage is commonly expected and accepted. This was very clearly expressed by our male informants from eastern and northern Uganda, in settings that were strongly patrilineal and where women had little opportunity to earn their own income. Men expected their wives to be sexually faithful; as Tom, the soldier, said, "Women are never shared." Women wanted their men to be faithful but did not necessarily expect it. Referring to the custom of paying bridewealth (often called "dowry" in Ugandan English), Dominic (case XI) declared stoutly, "I wanted to marry, and as you know, here in Bunyole we buy women." Dominic's confidence in his position as a husband once he had paid bridewealth was evident in an incident that occurred around the third time Jenipher visited him. He had quarreled with his wife because he felt she was not helping enough when his two sisters and mother were sick: "I told her that if she does not want to be part of the family, I would chase her away and marry another one."

Men's right to take multiple wives was recognized in Ugandan law and was a common part of most people's experience, either in their own marital lives or in the marital lives of their close family. Polygyny means that a man's extramarital affairs may be interpreted as courtship leading to marriage, so there is less general condemnation of them than of women's adulterous liaisons. But whether or not men had a "right" to such affairs, they tended to keep them secret from their wives because they almost invariably led to domestic conflict. Wives objected to their husbands' affairs and to the prospect of a co-wife. Often they eventually accepted the situation, sometimes because they wanted to keep their marriage and had little alternative. Because polygyny and men's sexual affairs were so widespread, wives were sometimes urged to calm down and accept the situation. When Grace found that the father of her children, whom she was supposed to marry, had another girlfriend, she was ready to drop him. But her mother persuaded her to stay. "I am your mother," she said. "You will go through the same challenges as I have gone through as a mother. And another thing: we do not want you to produce children here and there from different men. Since he is the father of your children, just calm down." Grace's mother thus voiced the "respectability" argument that Parikh suggests is associated with not confronting husbands' infidelity.[3]

However, some women refused to accept such advice. Hope and her husband were both university graduates, with good jobs at government ministries. When she was pregnant with their third child, they started quarrelling over his affairs. "I don't know what happens with these men. When they get money, it's as if they should not stay with their wife alone," Hope said. "My husband started getting girlfriends, and my friends used to tell me." She was furious when she caught him with another woman and went home and packed her things to leave with her children. But when she called her brother to come help her, he advised her to accept the situation. Hope did move out and established her own household (and later had a secret affair with a married man).

Whether or not a woman leaves depends very much on whether she has somewhere else to go. Many stay with their own parents or a sibling. Others have the means to support themselves. Jackie (case VI) compared her situation of dependence on the man she thought of as her husband with the situation of women with good jobs: "they don't have to beseech because they have their own money. When they want to leave their husbands, they don't have to go back to their parents—they go to stay in hotels."

Talking about Testing and Treatment

It is considered essential to the control of the HIV epidemic that people who test positive tell their sexual partners and encourage them to go for testing. "Disclosure" is thus framed as a public health measure at a societal level and as a way to protect the individual partner from infection or to help the partner seek early treatment if he or she is HIV-positive. However, such communication is problematic. A small study of Voluntary Counseling and Testing (VCT) and disclosure in Uganda found that half of married women and slightly more than half of married men revealed their test results to their spouses. They were far more likely to disclose if they tested negative than if they tested positive.[4] Our interlocutors more readily revealed their HIV-positive status to a sibling, parent, or friend than to a sexual partner. For reasons we will discuss, it is most difficult to reveal HIV-positive status to those who, from a health point of view, most need to know.

Talking seemed easiest in cases in which a person was seriously ill, even hospitalized. It was common for a partner—and maybe even the patient—to suspect HIV by this point. Taking the step to test was a necessary part of dealing with sickness; this was more like Routine Counseling and Testing than VCT. The drama of the test, with its implications about the past and the future, was overshadowed by the immediate life-threatening illness. The patient needed help there and then, and keeping the secret was pointless. Just as we saw that people revealed their HIV-positive status to family members who could assist them, so patients might tell their partners because they needed their support and help in sickness. Ivan's wife told him she had tested positive from her hospital bed, and he said he was not shocked; he had suspected since she had grown sickly and their children had died. James's partner cared for him while he was hospitalized and kept asking him whether he had AIDS.

Yet sometimes even very sick people refused to test or to tell their partners that they had tested positive. Several women recalled how their desperately ill husbands grew angry or sullen when the topic of testing was brought up. MamaGirl (case IV) never knew whether her husband had tested. When she asked him about it, he turned quiet or barked, "Who told you?" It was not until he died that she was tested. Goretti's husband similarly refused to be tested or to talk about it when he was very ill. But Goretti gathered courage and went to be tested by herself. When she returned and told her husband that she was HIV-positive, he would not discuss it except to say, "Let me die." Bernard not only tested but started paying for treatment without telling his wife. When his health improved, and his finances deteriorated, he dropped ART. Subsequently, he fell seriously ill, and his wife insisted they go for testing. When Phoebe talked to Bernard, he still had not told his wife that he had been in treatment once before.

Why did partners find it so difficult to talk about these matters? In our conversations with them, three major reasons emerged: fear of confronting one's own serostatus and mortality; fear of blame; and fear of losing the relationship. To be told that your partner is HIV-positive is to be struck with fear that you might be so, as well. Jolly (case IX) described her feelings of dread when her boyfriend, Boxer, told her that he had tested positive. The first generation by definition consists of many people who confronted these issues in the time before treatment became widely available. For them and their partners, testing positive was tantamount to a death sentence, as Jolly believed. A few of our interlocutors had first tested more recently and recounted how they discussed testing in light of possible treatment. One couple agreed that it was better to know so they could start treatment soon. But for others, even the knowledge that ART was available did not erase the fear. Several of our interlocutors said that their partners had either declined to test or had tested and never gone back for their results, even though they saw the effects of treatment in their partner. It seemed that some felt fine and wanted to postpone finding out about their serostatus until they fell ill.

The second reason that made people avoid or postpone discussing their status with their partners was fear of blame. Announcing that you are HIV-positive is to lay yourself open to accusations of sleeping around and endangering the life of your partner. Especially if the partner subsequently tests positive, quarrels and hard words ensue. Philip recounted that he had taken his three wives to test: two emerged composed from counseling and said they had tested HIV-negative but the third came out angry, shouting at him, "You are a womanizer. I told you to stop, and see, now you have killed me!" Several men recalled their wives' reactions with pain, and it seemed evident that they felt deep regret and, perhaps, guilt for infecting their partners. Jolly described how Boxer ran into her on the street years later and begged to talk to her. He fell on his knees and asked her pardon for infecting her. Jolly was stunned. "I felt like crying," she said. "I did not know what to tell him, and I think I have never felt like that in my life. Do you know—someone asking you to pardon him for killing you and spoiling your life and future? I looked at the man and I told him it was OK. He could not believe it."

Martha was convinced that her husband was HIV-positive. He refused to go with her to test, but she noticed how intently he listened to the health program "Capital Doctor" on the radio every Tuesday. Finally she went and tested alone, against his wishes. She did not tell him right away that she had tested positive. "I did not want people to think that I was the one who brought [the infection]" she said. If they had tested positive together, things would have appeared better; but as it was, she alone confirmed her status, and he later accused her of infidelity. She blamed him, too—for infecting her sister, with whom he had an affair and who later died of AIDS.

Fear of losing the relationship was the third impediment to talking about testing and treatment, so clearly evident in the case of Alice and her good man, Mike. Martha separated from her husband (although she continued to support his children, whom she had always treated as her own, having never given birth herself). Her partnership did in fact end after she started treatment, just as Alice feared that her relationship to Mike would. Yet Martha's description of their problems suggests that it was not only her testing and treatment that caused the split; in fact, her husband was even paying for her treatment for a time. Rather ART exacerbated other difficulties in their relationship. The refusal of Martha's husband to talk about testing and ART was one more knot in a web of conflicts about their house, her barrenness, and his children. Communication was abysmal at times. She recalled, "He developed a habit of drinking foolishly. He would sit in the living room up to morning without saying anything. I feared he would kill me."

Changes in the Quality of Relationships

Research among TASO clients in Jinja, done before ART became widely available, found that few who disclosed to their partners actually experienced negative outcomes, although fear of the consequences held others back.[5] Our study of the first generation provided more detailed pictures of how relationships were affected by testing and treatment. We found that some partnerships went through an initial rough period, followed by acceptance and support. Others were affected by a loss of trust and respect. Some seemed almost to have been strengthened by testing and ART. The effects depended partly on the serostatus of the partner. Of the forty-eight people we originally talked to, twenty-nine were in a partnership. Six of these did not know the serostatus of their partner. Seven of the remaining twenty-three said their partner was (still) HIV-negative; this included two polygynous men who had one HIV-positive and one or two HIV-negative wives. (Discordance among couples is a well-recognized phenomenon in Uganda, estimated to affect about 40 percent of HIV-positive people living in an established relationship.[6]) The remaining sixteen had partners who had tested HIV-positive, although they had not necessarily started on treatment. So it is important to bear in mind that partners could be in different situations regarding both serostatus and treatment.

Matayo and his wife, both health workers, tested at the same time. His wife was initially shocked that Matayo was HIV-positive, but she got over it, and they discussed their life and future together. "Madam is OK, and for us we are discordant," he said. "So we have learned to manage ourselves. The support from Madam is great. She knows and understands me, so we work together for the family. My wife told me, 'I will not leave you despite this situation, because you are my husband. We have to work hard for the future and for the children.'"

Where both partners were HIV-positive, there sometimes seemed to be a sense of commonality. They shared restricted knowledge. Ivan said that at first, he and his wife had decided to keep their HIV-positive status a secret between the two of them, although they later became very open about it. They were jointly exposed to the guidelines about "living positively," so they both knew the expectations and ideals. They also shared the routine of treatment, even if one was taking only Septrin while the other had already started on ARVs. They could remind each other about swallowing their tablets. However, quarrels still flared up between Ivan and his wife, as they did in many partnerships. Even relatively harmonious and well-established partnerships underwent periods of tension, as we saw in the year and a half that we followed people.

Changes in the quality of relationships can be seen in light of a broader undermining of men's authority. When the husband was weakened by HIV and on treatment, he needed the care of his wife. If she was also unwell, she might not be able or willing to provide all of the attention he wanted. If the husband believed he had infected his wife, he might feel that she had the moral high ground. Moreover, the whole process of testing and treatment recognized women as independent actors. Women were clients in their own right, even if they were so with the support of other people. The concern about mortal illness drove women to act against the wishes of their partners in some cases, as we have seen. Indeed, there is evidence that women seek help earlier than men and, as a consequence, have a lower mortality rate.[7] Those women who became active in Post-Test Clubs, drama groups, or other HIV-related activities gained experience and affirmation beyond the everyday domestic sphere.[8]

One of the clearest articulations of these issues came from John (case VII). His wife and child were both HIV-positive, and he believed he had infected his wife. Their relationship had always seemed strong and collaborative to Godfrey, but during the last visit, John put a different light on it. The immediate occasion for his reflections was that his wife's cousin, his classificatory sister-in-law, was leaving their household to marry. She had been very attentive to his needs while he was on treatment—in contrast to his wife, who seemed more concerned with the children than with him. John said that things had not been going well between them. His wife no longer showed any respect to him; she did not accept any correction or implied criticism, and her responses were harsh and rude. "She does not care much about doing even the simple things, like washing my clothes and ironing," John said. "If I try to ask her, she answers that I am bothering her with sickness all the time." Asked whether he thought she was acting that way because of his serostatus and treatment, John replied thoughtfully that it was not that she was trying to harass him because of his condition. Rather, he had changed in his relation to her. "Partly it is because ever since I started falling sick frequently, I decided not to be confrontational and to avoid any quarrels," he said. "As a result, my wife finds me more soft, because whenever she barks at anything I say, I only keep quiet and never respond back."

Men's authority can be undermined in another way, as well. The economic security that men are expected to provide becomes more problematic under long-term treatment with bouts of sickness and periods of weakness. Several men in treatment remarked that they were dependent on income generated by their wives because they were now unable to work. Women who did not get adequate financial support from their partners might be tempted to look elsewhere or to make greater efforts to generate income themselves. Of course, women in treatment may become more economically dependent on a partner. But most women in treatment had other sources of support within their own families or from their children.

Changes in the quality of partnerships following testing and treatment could also be seen in polygynous arrangements. While Martha left her husband to her co-wife, in other cases the rivalry of co-wives seemed to diminish in the face of the common challenges. MamaGirl and MamaBoy (case IV) came together after their husband died. As co-widows, they ran a household and were clients in the same treatment program. Herbert constantly compared his two wives, to the detriment of his first, "village" wife. But his educated wife, who was HIV-negative, encouraged him to care for his HIV-positive first wife. She also advised the first wife not to hassle their husband about bringing the disease. Through the time Jenipher visited Herbert, however, there was a period when even the educated wife was annoyed, because he was seeing another woman and conceived a child with her. But at the last visit, there was peace; the educated wife had moved to Herbert's village home, where she and the village wife were getting on all right.

The Meanings of Condoms

Counseling about safe sex was part of HIV testing and continuing care under ART. People were advised to abstain from sex or to use condoms, even if both partners were HIV-positive, to guard against reinfection with a different strain of the virus. (Although AIDS professionals knew that being on ART could reduce the viral load to the point at which there was little chance of transmitting HIV, this was never mentioned in educational sessions during the time of our study.) When couples were discordant, safe sex was strongly emphasized to protect the uninfected partner. Most of our interlocutors seemed to have been aware of this message, and some made a point of mentioning that they followed the advice. Being on ART focused attention on sexual practices and in some cases made them topics of discussion. Couples became aware of the influence each had over these matters.

According to Matayo, he and his wife, both health workers and discordant, were careful. "We agreed to live in the status we each are in and live positively," he said, "so we use condoms each time to protect each other, especially my wife." There were examples of both men and women insisting on safe sex.

Bernard said of his discordant wife, "She became reluctant to play sex with me; even up to now and I cannot force her." Hanifa said that in the past, she did not use condoms with her husband, a long-distance truck driver, but after she commenced ART, they had started to use them; she gets them free from TASO. The explanation Major Charles gave was somewhat unclear: "sex, I stopped, although when you have diabetes you become sexually weak. I told my wife, 'Now, you know I am sick. We should use condoms. And I have diabetes. I cannot have sex as much as I used to.' My wife has not yet tested, and what I do, I try to convince her that since I am sick we should use condoms." Whether because of abstinence, impotence, or condoms, he implied that he was following advice.

Using condoms was seen as an indication of education and enlightenment. Ivan made this clear through a story he told about his first counselor, a woman without tact or understanding. "People who are not educated are difficult, and you need to know how to approach them," he said. "A man [a neighbor and fellow client] was still sleeping with his wife live, without a condom. The wife discussed this with the counselor, complaining that her husband forced her to have live sex. When the counselor saw the man in the trading center, instead of talking to him nicely and privately, she quarreled with him: 'You! Why do you have live sex with your wife? Don't you know you are sick and need to use condoms? You will die!' The man answered back: 'I paid bridewealth for that woman. I don't see why I should use a condom. If you contributed at least a cow or hen to the bridewealth, come and stop me!'"

Herbert's first (and uneducated) wife was HIV-positive, while his other (favored and educated) wife was HIV-negative. He used a condom with the latter but said, "With the first wife, we meet live." On several occasions, sometimes when a friend or his other wife was present, he laughingly referred to his first wife's annoyance that he did not do "the work of the night" that a husband should do. Herbert claimed that his first wife would not accept condoms. "That woman is dense," he said. "I don't think she can accept a plastic sack (kavera). But I also don't have the energy now to do those things, because with this one [nodding at his second wife], we understand each other and do it few times, but that one may want every night, which I may not afford." During another visit, he confided, "That wife of mine in the village does not know condoms, and we are advised to use condoms. She might scream if she sees me putting on something to sleep with her." Herbert was no doubt exaggerating in an effort to amuse, but the point holds that unfamiliarity with condoms shows lack of sophistication.

In addition to enlightenment, the use of condoms was an indication of care and kindness for some. Jackie complained about her (HIV-positive) partner's sexual aggressiveness and his refusal to use condoms: "if I find another man and I remarry, I would wish to get a man who is understanding, and we can discuss and agree to use condoms." Jolly compared her current boyfriend to her previous boyfriend, Boxer: "I love him because . . . he can humble himself, and we negotiate, but Boxer could beat me even for requesting to use a condom." Jolly was concerned about infecting her present boyfriend—or, as she put it, about "killing someone innocent." Later, when her boyfriend tested negative and she wanted to bear his child, she thought about the danger to which she might expose him.

Much as our interlocutors showed their awareness of the warning against unprotected sex, it was evident that not all heeded it in practice for various reasons, as we shall see in chapter 6. Testing and ART served to problematize sexuality, to cast sexual relations in another light and make them objects of concern. Condoms took on meanings of care, responsibility, virtue, and enlightened modernity.

Reviewing the Past, Imagining the Future

Just as testing and ART impelled people to consider their current sexual partnerships differently, they also moved most to rethink past relationships. In asking our interlocutors to tell us about their lives, we did not pointedly inquire about how they became infected. Yet nearly everyone mentioned this. While some said they were not sure where they got the virus, many named a particular partner. Suspicion was often based on whether the partner was sick or had died or had had a child who died. Some people put two and two together several years after a partner had passed away. It was only when they or another sexual partner of the dead spouse fell ill that the realization hit them. Harriet said that her three co-wives had not known the cause of their husband's death. "He suffered from malaria for three days and passed away on the fourth," she said. But two years later, one of Harriet's co-wives fell ill, and when Harriet herself was hospitalized, she told one of her co-wives, "Our man died of this virus. Don't attribute his death to any other sickness or to witchcraft."

Several of our female interlocutors recalled their husbands' promiscuity. Harriet said, "Whenever we would complain about his many women, he would say, 'Are you the ones to stop me from loving women? It's a man who has authority; it's not women who have authority in the home.' We wives had nothing to say." Jessica had similar reflections. When she married her husband, he already had six wives, and they were all living together in a big house with a bedroom for each. She did not realize then what kind of life he was living. "Truck drivers! They are really promiscuous. They are killing us so much," she said. "Wherever they go, they just find a woman and crash with her. He really had wives, that one. He even had more outside. He would bring children for us to take care of. When he died, he left sixty-four living children and seventeen graves of children. He was sixty-eight years old." Women tended to blame the behavior of their men; Saddam (case II) was an exception. Although he admitted that he was "running" two women besides his wife, he claimed that he had been driven to this course of action by his wife's infidelity.

More striking even than the review of partners' sexual behavior was the sometimes regretful and sometimes fatalistic consideration of one's own past sexual life. Men in the Army talked about soldiering as almost inevitably involving many women. "I used to have girlfriends, very many," said Tom. "You know the nature of our work. You are transferred all the time, and for us men, it may be difficult to avoid women when you don't have your wife nearby." Philip contrasted his present positive life with his past: "I used to be a sex maniac, a womanizer, to love many women." Youth was remembered as a time of carefree pleasure. Benjamin recalled, "Those days as young people at school, we used to take life in a simple way. One would see himself as great and wanted to have every woman around. You just don't see beyond enjoying life."

It was not only men who mused on their careless pasts. Norah remembered, "After secondary school I went to stay with my sister in another town. I got boyfriends. Maybe this is where I got the problem." Jolly was the most reflective and regretful of all. "You know those days when you have men disturbing you and telling you that you are beautiful," she said. "But I also had conceit. I was feeling great, but now. . . . You know, when you are young and beautiful, everybody saying you are beautiful, you are just vulnerable to many men." Expanding on how she let herself be deceived by men who had other girlfriends at the same time, and how she even stopped using condoms after testing negative, she kept repeating that she had been naive.

The way that testing and ART can open a space for discussion between partners and reflections on the nature of partnership is further evident in people's imaginations of the future. While some single people, such as Robinah (case I) and MamaGirl (case IV), said they had been advised not to initiate new relationships, others who got a second chance to live with ART looked for partners with whom they might share that life. Finding someone who was also HIV-positive provided a basis for discussion and understanding.

This pattern of "sero-sorting" is also reported from other research on life with ART in eastern Uganda.[9] During the time we carried out our study, the lonely hearts columns in the national newspapers frequently had advertisements like these:

> Ugandan female aged 34 who is outgoing and very friendly, with a good job but HIV positive and on ARVs, seeks intelligent, HIV positive man on ARVs with a stable job. (*Daily Monitor*, 20 October 2005)

> Guy, 39, HIV-positive businessman and a resident of Kampala, seeks HIV-positive lady for a serious relationship leading to marriage, and to have a child. (*New Vision*, 6 January 2007)

> An HIV+ single mother of one, employed with stable income is seeking a male companion who is HIV+ and a single father. Northern and eastern tribes are encouraged. Adulterous men are advised not to bother. (*Daily Monitor*, 17 November 2005)

The assumption was that an HIV-positive partner would understand the requirements of positive living and that there would be less worry about infecting each other.

Several of the single women among our interlocutors voiced this view. Cathy, a young widow who seemed bitter and unhappy when Phoebe first met her, changed her life during the time Phoebe knew her. She remarried and soon conceived a child. "He is also on ARVs; he is infected like me," she said about her new husband. "I had to get someone who is HIV-positive, because it would be very unfair to have a relationship with someone who is HIV-negative." After recounting how her former boyfriend Boxer fell on his knees and begged forgiveness for infecting her, Jolly went on to say that he had wanted to resume their relationship: "he said he still loved me and that he was looking for me so that I [would] go for testing, and if I am positive, we should live a positive life and, if possible, have children, and if not, we live together until we die." His proposal to her appeared to be based on the idea that they should have a common future with their common virus.

The second chances that ART facilitated meant that people weighed possibilities of partnership. As Janet Seeley and colleagues found in a similar study, some did not want to squander the precious time they had won on difficult, potentially disappointing new relationships, preferring to concentrate on their children and livelihoods. For others, the continuation and renewal of previous partnerships or the formation of new ones instantiated their "rebirth" and their hope for a better life.[10]

Second Thoughts on Partnerships

Testing and treatment problematized partnerships; they invited discussion of matters that mostly had been implicit. Making those matters explicit was often painful and threatening, as we saw from the many examples of how difficult it was to talk and negotiate not just about sex but also about gender relations. Emphasizing faithfulness and safe sex had an influence beyond sexual practices. Women, some of whom had already been encouraged by charismatic Christianity and pro-women discourses, could feel more justified in complaining about men's sexual affairs and poly-partnering. The discourse on fidelity and loving carefully supported ideals about modern partnerships that often were not being met. Where they occurred, willingness to talk and showing concern about sexual practices have become elements in a more companionate form of partnership, something that many women appreciated and for which many of them hoped.

The first generation lived in a time when Yoweri Museveni's National Resistance Movement government promoted women's rights to political representation and donors supported women's economic, social, and educational "empowerment." In many ways, it seems, the response to the AIDS epidemic supported efforts to strengthen women's position by problematizing gender relations at the intimate level.

Notes

1. Thornton, *Unimagined Community*; Epstein, *The Invisible Cure*, 54–62.
2. Parikh, "Going Public."
3. Parikh, "Going Public."
4. Nsabagasani and Yoder, *Social Dynamics of VCT and Disclosure in Uganda*, 36.
5. King et al., "Processes and Outcomes of HIV Serostatus Disclosure to Sexual Partners among People Living with HIV in Uganda," 240.
6. Bunnell et al. "HIV Transmission Risk Behavior among HIV-Infected Adults in Uganda."
7. Alibhai et al., "Gender-Related Mortality for HIV-Infected Patients on Highly Active Antiretroviral Therapy (HAART) in Rural Uganda."
8. Russell and Seeley, "The Transition to Living with HIV as a Chronic Condition in Rural Uganda."
9. Seeley et al., "Sex after ART," 710–11.
10. Seeley et al., "Sex after ART."

CASE VI

Jackie

CHILDREN WITHOUT
GRANDPARENTS

David Kyaddondo and
Susan Reynolds Whyte

CHILDREN

(overleaf)

Girls with hopes for the future
playing bride and groom.

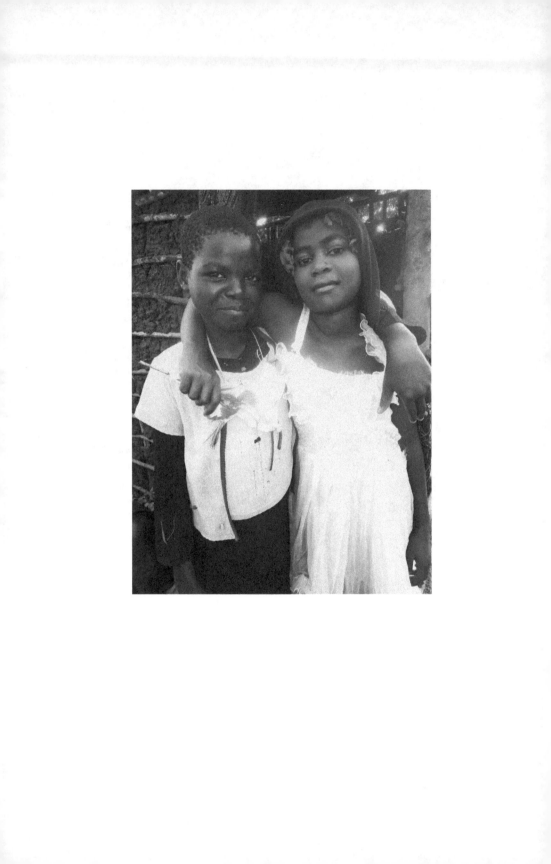

"I have children, but they don't have grandparents. Yet both his parents are still living, and he has two brothers and three sisters," said Jackie, complaining again about the father of her children. "He has never taken me to his parents, and he has never gone to see my parents, either. . . . My future is not clear, he doesn't want me to talk about issues concerning my life. I ask him, why don't you build a house for me? At least if he took the children to the village to show them to their grandparents. But now, if anything happens to me, I don't know—for example, if I die."

Jackie lived in rented rooms in Kampala with her three daughters, one from her first husband and two from her current partner. During the year and a half that David followed Jackie, her relationship with her partner was stormy. He refused to formalize their relationship and acknowledge their children. Her fears about the future were confirmed the last time David talked to Jackie. Her children's father had died, leaving the situation of the children still unsettled.

Jackie was in her mid-thirties when David met her, the fifth born in a family of eleven children, of whom two had died of acquired immunodeficiency syndrome (AIDS). She had to drop out of senior secondary school because her parents could not afford the fees, and an older sister brought her to Kampala in 1994, promising to help her continue her education. "Instead, she took me to her bar, where I was working as a slave," Jackie said. "She was not paying me." When Martin, one of the regular customers, approached her and said he was looking for a wife, she accepted. "I did not like this man, and I had wanted to continue with school," she said, "but I thought, instead of suffering, let me get married." Their marriage was not legally registered, but they had a wedding ceremony with a reception and lived together as man and wife, and Jackie soon gave birth to a daughter.

When Martin lost his job, Jackie found one as a receptionist in a hotel and became the provider for the household. At work, Jackie met Joseph, who had a job that paid well, and he began to woo her. At first, she discouraged him. "I never thought I could ever love him; he was short and thin and was not attractive at all," she said. "My Martin was tall and good-looking. But one day, Martin beat me terribly, suspecting that I had cheated on him. He gave me these scars. [She showed David her hands.] I started wishing that Joseph would say something to me so I could punish this man who beat me." By that time, Joseph had almost given up, but Jackie now took the initiative. "I went to his office pretending I wanted to borrow 60,000 shillings [about $37] from him." As she narrated this, Jackie smiled shyly. "It was like a spark, he lit up and even doubled the amount I had asked for. He gave me 120,000 shillings, saying, 'Go and solve your problems, but you don't have to repay it.' That is how it started." Joseph had money, and he was persistent.

Joseph was also married, but all three of the children born to him and his wife had died. Jackie and Joseph kept their affair secret for some years, remaining with their spouses. But Joseph's wife became suspicious and confronted Jackie, saying that she would never have a share of their property. The wife added, "Do you know what killed our children?" Apparently, she wanted to tell Jackie that Joseph was infected with the human immunodeficiency virus (HIV).

Martin was sickly and had developed the belt (*kisippi*) of herpes zoster; it was Jackie who encouraged him to get tested. He was HIV-positive and started on antiretroviral medicine (ARVs) in 2001. Jackie's second child began to sicken at the age of nine months, with intermittent fever and pus from the ears. "It was the child who showed me that I was sick," she said. Jackie tested HIV-positive but because she did not feel unwell, she kept the information to herself. She was still living with Martin, who believed that the child was his. She never disabused him of this but did tell David that Joseph was the child's father. Even people at their workplace remarked that the child resembled him. Although Joseph sometimes denied Jackie's status as a wife, he took responsibility for the little girl, giving Jackie money to have her tested at a private laboratory. She was HIV-positive and diagnosed with tuberculosis. Medicine for TB is supposed to be free, but Joseph bought it privately because he wanted to keep the child's sickness a secret. While still on treatment, the child got burned and spent two months at a private hospital, again at Joseph's expense. Finally Joseph convinced Jackie to leave Martin and rented a house for her.

When David contacted Jackie for the first follow-up meeting, she suggested that they meet in a bar. David would have preferred to visit Jackie at her house and felt uncomfortable about sitting at a bar with her but understood that she feared Joseph would become suspicious if he heard that a man had been visiting her at home. For the next meeting, David suggested they use Jackie's workplace instead.

Jackie was exceedingly forthright with David about her relationships with her partners—about how they mistreated her and how she deceived them. Although Martin used to beat her, leaving him for Joseph did not bring her happiness. "He refused [to use] condoms right from the start," she said. "But sometimes he would tell me lies that he has put it on, but would tear it at the tip." She said he used to force her to have sex, even while she was menstruating. She could not cry out because the neighbors would hear, and it would be shameful. Moreover, he was the father of her child.

When Jackie got pregnant again, the doctor recommended that she start ARVs. "I remember that time I had a high viral load of about 60,000,[1] and the doctor said it could easily infect the baby," she said. "But when I started medicine, it reduced. I was checked after delivery, and it was less than 400. During pregnancy, my CD4 had dropped to 300, but after delivery it rose to 800." The baby received Nevirapine, and Jackie got medicine to stop the flow of milk in her breasts. She bottle-fed the baby, as recommended, and the child was indeed protected from HIV infection. It was an expensive delivery, at 800,000 shillings [about $462], because she had special care from a consultant. Joseph met these costs and others.

Jackie started on ARVs in 2003, before they were widely available for free. It was Joseph who paid, again secretly, because he did not want people to know that she was on treatment and that he was supporting her. The cost at first was 60,000 shillings per month, but prices fell to 30,000 shillings, and then to 10,000 shillings. Jackie managed to get her second child, Joseph's daughter, started on free ARVs. "The doctor helped me and put her on the The Regional Antiretroviral Therapy (TREAT) program as an orphan," she said. "I claimed that she was the child of my sister who had died." Later, in August 2004, Jackie also was switched to free antiretroviral therapy (ART) as a "widow caring for an orphaned child."

Jackie's relation to Joseph did not improve when Joseph's official wife left Kampala for their rural home. He became more elusive and no longer took her on trips, as he once did. While he paid the rent for her house, bought food, and often slept at Jackie's place, Joseph maintained his own residence and took care that he not be seen as living with her. Jackie complained that he never ate lunch at her place. "He does not even brush his teeth from my home in the morning," she said. "He comes at around 8 PM and leaves early in the morning for his apartment. Even the clothes, it's me who washes them, but he takes them away to his house, where he dresses before going to work. He keeps everything away from me. All of his documents and papers are at his home, and I have never seen them."

Although some of Jackie's relatives knew that Joseph was the father of her children, Joseph never took steps to be introduced to them—or to give them gifts or pay bridewealth, as an in-law should. Once, when Jackie's father visited her and found Joseph at her home, Joseph did not give her father money for transportation—a form of respect and recognition. Jackie was under pressure from her parents and other relatives who said, "That man has money, why is he hiding you?" Jackie's father was especially critical. Once when he came to see her and found Joseph there, he asked him, "You are with my daughter, but when are you coming to see us officially? What if something happens to her? What will you do?" Jackie's father encouraged her to leave Joseph, saying that he treated her like a loose woman (*malaya*) and was just using her to have children.

Jackie knew the location of Joseph's rural home because in the early days of their relationship he had taken her there and showed her around his farm. But he never introduced her to his family, and they spent the night at a hotel in the nearby town. One time she took matters in her own hands. "I picked my children [up] and went by myself to his parents," she recounted. "But they said they cannot accept me as their daughter-in-law when I have not been introduced by their son. When he learned that I had gone to his parents, he got so annoyed and stopped giving me financial support for some time, until later when he came and told me that I should never do it again."

Jackie's complaints about Joseph were legion. It was not only that he did not acknowledge her as a wife. He was not a loving father. He did not play with his children, as she recalled Martin used to. Although Martin was poor, they were always openly together. He used to mind the children and play with them. "I would tease him by putting the child on his back, and he would feel shy and we would laugh together," she said. (Traditionally, it is women, never men, who carry children on their backs.) "But this one is so tough that you can't do it, he will rebuff you." In the time David followed Jackie, she often considered leaving Joseph but always decided against it because of the financial support he gave her. Yet money was one of the constant bones of contention. Jackie thought Joseph should pay the children's school fees—or, at least, provide her with some income-generating project so she could supplement her salary at the hotel.

Six months after David first met Jackie, she said she had made a big change in her life: she had been saved and become very active with prayers and church services. "I used to suffer a lot, and I always felt like doing some things, because of the behavior of my husband," she said. "I was having sleepless nights. Whenever he was away, I would be imagining that he is sleeping with another woman. It is the demons that bring all this anger and jealousy. I always felt like getting another man, to revenge against him. Sometimes I went to my friends and found men who would buy me beer." Members of her church advised her to leave Joseph because he was married. Jackie often talked about demons, including the demons of prostitution and adultery, and about the black magic that even she had used to ensure control over her lover. She said that Joseph thought her salvation was simply a ploy to break off with him. He had stopped coming to her house, but she felt torn about leaving the sinful relationship. "I fasted for days and prayed to God to give me answers to the many questions I had," she said. "How will I survive? He pays the rent; he buys the food. What will I do when he goes away?"

As always, Joseph returned. One evening, he bought four pounds of meat and sent it to Jackie's place with a message that he was coming. Jackie cooked the meat but went to church afterward, and Joseph arrived before Jackie returned. She found him in her house and unhappy, and he accused her of going out with the pastors. After dinner he went to bed, and Jackie started praying with her children. She recounted the conversation they had later that night:

> He asked me why I got saved. I told him about my problems. "You put me out of the life I was leading. Maybe I didn't have HIV, and you infected me. Poor me, I bore you children. You rented a house for me, but you always come like a guest. You leave in the night because you don't want to be seen. I gave birth to your children, but you refused to take me to your home; you refused to build me a house; you refused to support the children in school. Your wife is sending demons—I get demons every night, things that want to strangle me. . . . Now I have to put my life in Jesus."

Joseph promised to buy her a plot of land and build a house. He added that he would keep coming to her place because he was paying for the house. Jackie said that she conceded then, adding that perhaps these were God's plans. They resumed sexual relations. "It was difficult to refuse," she said. "You can't make an alarm because of the children, and they know he is their father. But I prayed to God that he does not give me his demons. You know you can get someone's demons by sleeping with him."

When she talked about what she wanted Joseph to do for her, building a house was always very prominent. She sometimes gave David examples of how other men built houses for their partners. Certainly, one of the obligations of a husband is to build a house for his wife. (The Luganda term for an independent woman, *nakyeyombekedde*, means "she who builds her own house.") But it was not just that construction would make her a wife; a house seemed to represent future security for her and the children.

At the next visit, Jackie was shifting house—not to one Joseph had built but to one she had rented near her church. She intended not to tell Joseph where she was moving and even showed David a text message in which Joseph complained that she was refusing to take him to her new place even though he was the father of her children and helped her financially. "You are a counselor," she said to David. "Tell me what I should do. What should I tell him? I have told you almost everything about my life; you should help me out now." But David did not know what advice to give, and Jackie's plan did not hold. When David next talked to her, she said that Joseph had come to her new place and raped her. Yet she stayed with him. "I wish I had somewhere to hide to get away from this man," she said. "I would wish to get another man who is understanding, and we can discuss and agree to use condoms. But young men would like to have children."

Jackie often talked about her dreams, to which she attached great significance. "I have been dreaming about [Joseph] as a dog, catching me and forcing me into sex," she said. "And those are the same things he has done to me. These days I dream he has many wives he is hiding from me. For God gave me a vision. What I dream usually comes true." In September, she said that she was having scary dreams about her co-wife: "I learned that our husband had died, and I went for burial at their home, and the wife was chasing me with a bottle of acid."

David last saw Jackie in August 2007. She gave him the startling news that Joseph had died the week before. He had fallen sick, vomiting blood, and been admitted to the hospital. "The day before he died, he asked me to take the children to see him," she said. "He spent the whole day playing with his children in the corridor of the hospital." Joseph's body was transported to his rural home for burial, and Jackie attended. She explained that her colleagues provided security at the burial ceremony, because Joseph's widow, whom she called her co-wife, had vowed to beat her up if she came. But as it turned out, the wife's rivalry with Jackie was overshadowed by other surprises: at the burial, another woman presented herself as Joseph's wife and the mother of his two daughters; a third woman, who was tall and frail, revealed that she had borne three children with him over ten years; and a fourth woman, whom he had befriended more recently, arrived with a baby who was seven months old. It turned out that Joseph's colleagues had nicknamed him "*Empaya* sharp" (an *empaya* is a male goat).

Jackie said she had tried to make a list of the property Joseph had left in Kampala and went to the Uganda Association of Women Lawyers to seek advice on how to make a legal claim to the property and ensure future assistance for the children. But Joseph's relatives warned her not to litigate and planned a meeting to discuss how to handle the property and care for the children. At Jackie and Joseph's workplace, some of the money collected for the family was given to her—a recognition of their relationship. She worried about how to manage without Joseph's financial assistance and felt that she had lost respect.

Still, Jackie found some consolation in her children. "My children resemble their father's sisters and their grandparents, and at least I have the children to think about," she said. "I wonder how the wife without children is coping. That's why she is always angry." Yet Jackie was also relieved that she had not had more children with Joseph. She thought she had conceived again some months before he died, but by "a blessing from God," she miscarried. "Since he died, I have not dreamed of him," she said. "I think he went to heaven. I asked him to accept God when he was sick in the hospital." Laughing, Jackie added, "My daughter one day asked me, 'My dad died, and now my father is Jesus, but Jesus doesn't come to see me. Has he got a car?'"

After our study ended, David learned that Jackie had remarried and had another child.

Note

1. The viral load is a measure of the level of HIV in the blood. The goal of treatment is to bring it down to 40-75 copies per unit, which is considered "undetectable."

CHAPTER SIX

Children

Susan Reynolds Whyte,
David Kyaddondo, and
Lotte Meinert

Jackie's story, like that of Alice (case IV), is about partners and the place that children have in relations between adults. Having a child with someone changes the relationship to that person; it also transforms and expands other ties—or, at least, it should. Jackie's recurrent concern was that, although Joseph recognized the children they had together, the children had no proper relationship with Joseph's parents and siblings. It was only after his death that she seemed on the way to gaining acknowledgment for herself and her children—those children who resembled their paternal grandparents and father's sisters, as she noted in the last conversation. As in so many of the other stories we came to know, children were central in the unfolding situations of people on ART.

Three interconnected points help us to understand the significance of children for those on ART. First, having children is valued as an essential part of personhood. Historically, children have been considered wealth; prayers to the ancestors in eastern Uganda included a plea for fertility, "Give us births. Give us male and female. Let us deliver two by two so that we may always hold twin ceremonies here."[1] Parenthood is so necessary to personhood that it is difficult to gain respect as a full man or woman without offspring.

Second, children are about social relations; they create kinship and strengthen (and disturb) existing relationships. This is not to deny that they are agents in themselves, with their own perspectives and intentions. But like adults, they are enmeshed in social relationships; they can constitute links, and those connections are essential in life with HIV and its treatment.

Third, children introduce a time perspective into social life and social relations. This is true partly because of the obvious fact that young children grow and change so markedly. Perhaps even more important is the way that children make people imagine the future. "Children are the future" is a rather tired cliché but useful nonetheless in alerting us to the ways people on ART think about children and time.

Before the advent of ART, HIV was associated with the loss of small children born to infected parents and with the terrible increase in orphans who were left behind when their parents died.[2] Philip, a father of twenty-one children, recalled his mother's questions when she heard he was HIV-positive: "what about all these children? What will happen when you are no longer here?" For the first generation, treatment brought new hope in relation to having and caring for children. They could bear children with greater confidence that both child and parents would survive, with children assuming their central place in relations to affinal and consanguineal kin. The concern with children's futures, which was such a wrenching worry for those who never got the second chance, became something to continue struggling with for those on ART. The future was still uncertain, but at least our interlocutors could prepare for a future in which they might still take part.

The Wealth of Children

Wealth is measured in people as well as in land, livestock, and money—a value that promotes a pro-natal ethos.[3] It is often said that people want many children when children's labor is important for subsistence and when children provide insurance for old age. But the desire for children goes far beyond these practical matters. A woman who has given birth to many children is highly respected, and a man who is able to look after a large family is esteemed.[4] This is related to the fact that children are potential links between adults. In the long run, children expand people's social existence by staying with other relatives, by making friends, and, in time, by marrying and creating links to other families. In the short run, having a child can strengthen the relation to a sexual partner or spouse: Jackie could make financial and other demands on Joseph as the father of her children, and she accepted his sexual demands partly because his children might overhear her objections. People were quite conscious of how children reinforce relations between partners. Jolly (case

IX), who longed for a child of her own, was supporting her boyfriend's child. When she went to Europe, she left the child with her relatives and sent money for fees at an expensive school. Asked why she was spending for a child that was not hers, Jolly said that she loved children, but she also did not want to lose her relationship with her boyfriend.

In the patrilineal and virilocal societies of Uganda, children belong to their father's clan, and ideally they and their mother should live with the father's family. Although the lives of many parents and children do fit this ideal, the reality is more complicated, as our forty-eight life stories and twenty-three extended cases richly demonstrate. Separation, divorce, death of spouse, and remarriage were frequent. Having children out of wedlock was equally common. This means that many adults have children by different partners; where and to whom children belong is a matter of negotiation, as Jackie's story shows so well.[5] The expansion of sociality through children becomes a more problematic and open-ended set of possibilities. We emphasize this because many of the people we spoke to had children by different partners and cared for children who were not their biological offspring.

Jackie's eldest child, who was nine when David first met her mother, remained with her and not with her father, Martin, when Jackie left him. It was common for young children to stay with their mothers after divorce; even older children, especially if they were girls, often remained with their mothers for years. As we have already seen, there was a greater concern that boys should keep to the paternal home to claim their entitlement to a share of their fathers' land. But in all cases, those children whose parents had married—or, at least, lived together in a union recognized by others—were more clearly affiliated to their fathers' families. In chapter 5, we pointed out that it is not always clear whether partners can be considered married. This is an issue for the children as much as for the partners themselves.

Children who were born of short-term relationships were present in the stories of both men and women. Their situations varied, in part depending on cultural practices, and in part depending on more individual arrangements. Loyce, a thirty-year-old market seller, spoke from a mother's point of view. She had dropped out of primary school because her family could not pay the fees and conceived when she was only fifteen years old. She went to live with the father of her child, but he turned out to have many wives, and she left him three months after delivering in 1991 and moved in with her mother. The first husband used to call her to bring the child to visit him; he was sick and died two years later, but it was not until she was diagnosed as HIV-positive in 2005 that it occurred to her what might have caused his death. In 1995, she gave birth to a baby girl. About that child's father, she said, "He just disappeared, and I didn't know where his home was or where he came from." In 2000, she had a baby boy and stayed two years with the child's father before separating and moving back in with her mother, who was also caring for three children of her own, from whose father she was separated. So Loyce's children, from three different fathers, grew up together with their mother and grandmother, having little or no contact with their patrilateral families. Children not claimed or supported by fathers often lived in such matrifocal households consisting of mothers and daughters or of sisters, as with Robinah and Joyce (case I).

Men also talked about having children with women they never married. Dominic (case XI) had children with his wife, but he also had six other children from six different women; all were staying with him and his mother. James, the twenty-five-year-old university student we met in chapter 4, who himself grew up without knowing his father's family, had three children with three different women. Tom, a forty-four-year-old soldier, had divorced his first wife but kept their three children, whom his second wife was looking after. What the second wife did not know was that he also had three other children with women he had never married. "I got one boy from a police lady, one boy from a student, and a boy from another student," he said. All were staying with their mothers or mothers' families, a situation he explained by citing "culture": "you know, in our culture, if you are not married to a girl, her parents can never allow you to take the children." Thus, while some men had their "outside" children staying with them, others had no intention of letting them grow up in their homes. Most men spoke as if they had some sense of obligation toward children living with their mothers, but because of short resources, convenience, and the perspective of being HIV-positive, they often left the worries and expenses to others. Some did not want their wives to quarrel because of money being channeled outside the household when there was not even enough for the "inside" children.

Having children meant more than having one's own biological children. Many of our interlocutors included in their households children who had lost one or both parents, usually to AIDS. These were often orphans left by deceased siblings, as in the case of Robinah and Joyce, or by in-laws who had died, as in the case of MamaGirl and MamaBoy (case IV). But they also included children of living relatives. Suzan (case III) kept the daughter of her dead daughter and also her brother's daughter's daughter, whose mother was alive but married elsewhere. Others supported the children of family members, living or dead, even if they did not stay under the same roof. Herbert, a fifty-year-old shopkeeper, declared that he was looking after thirty children, of whom nineteen were his own. Caring for the child of a relative is not merely an expression of the amity of kinship. It is the very practice that creates and re-creates kinship ties.

ART and the Desire for Children

This is the background against which we must understand the dispositions of people on ART towards childbearing. Like all those who tested HIV-positive, those on ART had been counseled to avoid pregnancy and to use condoms if they engaged in sex. By 2006, some treatment programs (such as Reach Out Mbuya) were tempering the anti-natal message by telling individual clients that if they wanted a child, they should wait until they had been on ART for some time and had discussed whether their health was strong enough with their doctor. But generally people were advised not to have children, and there was growing concern among AIDS professionals that so many HIV-positive people were ignoring this guideline. Even Joyce, Robinah's sister, spoke critically about the many women in her Post-Test Club who were getting pregnant—mostly widows, she said, who were having affairs with married men whose status was not known.

A minority of our informants declared that they wanted no more children and were using condoms. Matayo, a health worker in his early forties, said that he had only two children because he knew that other children, left by his brothers who died, depended on him. Major Charles had seven children (one from the wife who died, two from his current wife, and three from different women). He talked about the cost of educating children in addition to buying ARVs and diabetes medicine and concluded with advice to the researcher: "for you still having children, don't produce many—perhaps it should be only three." Those who wanted to limit their families expressed more concern about the problems of supporting many children than the health risks of unprotected sex and pregnancy. In a sense, they, too, were confirming the significance of children, using the logic that they would concentrate on the children they had.

Several were explicit about their desire for a child, especially those who had none or only one. The wish to have children when you are HIV-positive was largely ignored by Ugandan HIV/AIDS policy at the time and even considered immoral. Yet it was a very important desire for many.[6] Rachel (case X), still young at twenty-six and the mother of an HIV-positive five-year-old, said that she wanted another child, but the doctor at Reach Out had advised her to wait. John (case VII), whose first wife had died, said he had wanted to protect his new partner, who was a secondary school student and had no children. When he insisted on using condoms, she became concerned and asked, "Won't I have children?" Jolly was obsessed with her wish for a child and brought up the topic at every visit. "The only problem I have is people asking me why I don't have a child, and that disturbs me a lot," she said. "I think I am growing old." When she finally got the courage to tell her boyfriend that she was HIV-positive, they went for testing and found that her boyfriend was negative. Jolly was perturbed: she very much wanted to have his child but was afraid of infecting him. She confided that she wanted to ask "the million-dollar question" of whether he would accept having a child with her. She talked to her doctor, who said she should wait until her CD4 count exceeded 900 before getting pregnant. She feared raising the issue with her boyfriend; her counselor suggested that she bring him so they could discuss it together. She had heard about in vitro fertilization and even got her sister living abroad to agree to pay for it. However, by the last visit Jolly still had not discussed the matter with her boyfriend. She seemed to have decided that if he did not want to make a baby via unprotected sex, she would try to get pregnant using in vitro fertilization.

It was not only young women who expressed a wish for children. Gregory, a forty-year-old rural brickmaker, had two wives. The first was HIV-positive; together, they had five living children (four girls and a boy). He also had a child with a woman he had never married. Still, he wanted to have another child with his second wife, who had borne him two sons, of whom one had died. When she learned that he was HIV-positive, he said, "She quarreled with me and she told me that I am not going to have any other son, although I wanted to have a second child with her, and up to now we are using condoms. She said to me, 'If you want to sleep with me, you must use condoms.'" Moses, a construction worker, said he had tested positive together with his wife, who was sickly after the birth of their first child. After both mother and baby died, he stayed alone for three years and came to Kampala. "When I worked and got some money, I felt like I should really have a kid," he said. "But I wondered whether I should marry another woman or just find someone and have a kid." He found a partner who conceived knowing that he was HIV-positive; she tested negative, gave birth to a girl, then had a boy two years later. Moses said that he did not want more children because of the expense of educating them while he was also paying for his own ARVs.

While some men and women said explicitly that they wanted children, others just had them, without talking about whether they were planned.

Given the low use of contraception in Uganda, pregnancy is not necessarily the result of a conscious decision. Where a partner had not disclosed his or her HIV-positive status, as in the example of Alice, conception "just happened" before marriage, as is so often the case. Of the twenty-three people we followed, at least eight had conceived or fathered children after they had tested positive. Some of the pregnancies and births occurred during the eighteen months over which we visited people. In some cases, such as those of Alice and Cathy, the baby seemed to be the confirmation of a new and, they hoped, lasting relationship. In other cases, such as those of Dominic and John, married or cohabiting partners who already had children together simply had another baby. Finally there were those cases—such as those of Herbert, James, and MamaBoy—in which babies were born to HIV-positive parents who did not live together or see each other regularly.

Treatment held out the prospect of a more normal life, and that meant a life with children, something that had seemed less possible before starting treatment. In fact, having children seemed to be a confirmation of the second chance that ART promised for life with other people and life with a future. Quantitative research confirms the association of ART, the desire for children, and higher incidence of pregnancy. A study in western Uganda found that women on ART had stronger fertility desires than HIV-positive women who had not started ART.[7] Better health and the anticipation of living long enough to raise the children made having them seem possible and feasible. A study among clients of Home-Based AIDS Care in eastern Uganda and another in seven African countries found that the incidence of pregnancy increased once women started on ART.[8] Not only did better health make having children feasible, but the healthy babies facilitated by the Prevention of Mother-to-Child Transmission of HIV (PMTCT) program confirmed that the parents were indeed in good health themselves.

Positive Children

Uganda's mortality rate for children younger than five was 137 per 1,000 live births in 2006.[9] Thus, the loss of children was a tragedy that many Ugandans had experienced themselves or in their families. But for the people in our study, the death of children had a particular significance. It was widely understood that an HIV-positive mother could transmit the virus to her baby—so much so that the death of a baby could be grounds for suspecting the serostatus of the mother and, by implication, of the father. Sometimes it was only years later that people reinterpreted the loss of a child, speculating whether they had already been HIV-positive at the time and treating the death as evidence that fit together with other indications. Robinah's sister Joyce said she "started wondering about HIV and AIDS" after the last of her four children died. Sometimes a child's death was the sign that motivated parents to be tested for HIV.

Jessica said that she and her surviving co-wife wondered about the deaths of three other co-wives. "How come they are all dying? Even the kids they are producing are getting finished," she said. "I told my co-wife, 'Don't you realize that our husband is sick?'" When Helen's brothers heard that her baby died, after she had also lost her husband, they sent a message that she should be taken to Kampala for HIV testing. Norah's five-year-old had recently been tested and found HIV-positive; that made Norah think that the baby who followed, and who had died, might well have been infected, too. Jolly mentioned that her lover had angered her by having a child with another woman during their affair. Then, four months later, he told her that the baby had fallen sick and died. Jolly was worried and asked him what could have killed the child. He replied that he wanted to be tested for HIV.

The PMTCT program started in Uganda in 2000 and was gradually rolled out to most public antenatal clinics. Under PMTCT, pregnant women were tested for HIV; if they were found positive, Nevirapine was offered to minimize the risk of transmission to the child, and the women were given advice about breastfeeding, since HIV can also be transmitted in mother's milk. Experts reckon that the chance of transmission falls sharply for mothers who adhere to the PMTCT regime. The first generation of people on ART seem to have used PMTCT in connection with pregnancies that occurred after about 2003. Whether because they sought out PMTCT or because antenatal services and the monitoring of ART programs identified pregnant HIV-positive women, the mothers in our study received Nevirapine for themselves and their newborns and either did not breastfeed or breastfed exclusively and weaned abruptly at six months, as advised. But many had not received PMTCT for earlier pregnancies and lost children, cared for HIV-positive children, or lived in uncertainty because they had never had their children tested.

The most difficult part of PMTCT was bottle-feeding a new baby. It was expensive to buy substitute milk, and it attracted unwanted attention in a country in which breastfeeding was almost universal. John's wife had been found to be HIV-positive when she was pregnant with their first child, who also contracted the virus. John confided his worries that the little girl was sickly and needed money for treatment. She was admitted to the hospital nutrition unit when she was a year old, and just at that time, his wife went into labor with their second child. At Godfrey's last visit, John was hopeful that the new baby might be free of the virus. His wife had been following the doctor's advice not to breastfeed, which she had not been able to do with the previous child because the couple did not have the money at the time to buy infant formula or cow's milk. Both Alice and Cathy, a well-educated client of Reach Out Mbuya, gave birth during the time we followed them, and both were bottle-feeding their babies, with the awkwardness that this entailed where breastfeeding is the norm.[10] In fact, once while Jenipher was visiting Alice at her shop, a stranger asked her why she was giving her baby a bottle instead of breastfeeding. Alice brushed off the question, saying she did not have enough breast milk, but it annoyed her.

Jackie, Suzan, John, and Rachel were all caring for HIV-positive children. Except for Jackie's daughter, the children attended clinics other than those at which their parents were clients, which presented logistical problems. But it was remarkable, and perhaps characteristic for the first generation, that their youngest children had been tested and enrolled in treatment programs. Although in some cases the parents did not tell the children why they were being given medicine, they were socializing the children to the same regime of medication and regular checkups that they had adopted (see chapter 10). There could even be reciprocity in maintaining the discipline, as Suzan explained: "my daughter takes her medicine because she used to see me taking mine. Sometimes she even reminds me to take mine before I sleep."

Talking to children about being HIV-positive was a matter of timing and depended partly on how old the child was. With the exception of Suzan's daughter, the children who were HIV-positive were mostly still young, and their parents had not yet told them why they needed to take medicine. At five, Jackie's daughter asked why she, but not the other children, had to take tablets. Jackie thought her daughter was too young to know about being HIV-positive, so she reminded her that she always used to have terrible ear infections; her daughter seemed content with the explanation and took the medicine. Explaining to a child that he or she is HIV-positive would usually entail revealing one's own status, and Jackie had not told any of her children.

The ART programs made people aware that it was important to test their children. Several, like MamaGirl and Cathy, recounted their relief when their offspring tested negative. But for others, knowledge of their own status and the possibility that they might have transmitted the virus to their children created worry and uncertainty. They did not want to test the children but were deeply troubled if they were often sick. Mark, who knew that his wife was HIV-positive but had not told her, said that he feared for his youngest child but was waiting for time to tell whether the child was HIV-positive. Philip, a former teacher from northern Uganda, had three current wives who together had ten children. All of his wives had been tested, and only one was HIV-positive. His children had not been tested, but he thought they were all right, except for the youngest, who was two. "She seems to be somehow sickly, on and off," he said. "Maybe she has contracted [HIV]. But her mother is OK. She tested again recently and she is [HIV-negative]. But maybe because I was careless about leaving razor blades lying around, maybe she could have contracted it like that." Knowing that he was HIV-positive filled Philip with worry about his sickly child, even though the child's mother had twice tested negative. Having their own blood tested was difficult for most of our interlocutors, and hearing about a partner's results was painful, but taking children for tests and learning about their status seemed almost insurmountable for many.

Even though many parents did not tell their children explicitly that they were HIV-positive until they reached twelve or thirteen, other studies suggest that children suspect there is something they are not supposed to know or talk about.[11] Myra Bluebond-Langner noticed the practice of "mutual pretense" in relationships between dying children and their parents in the United States as an intergenerational form of coping with serious illness.[12] We also saw that, even though HIV status was not disclosed to children in explicit ways, a family feeling of careful tacit mutual understanding of the situation often existed.

The Intergenerational Contract

As we have said, children highlight the time perspective in social relations. They do so through an expectation of reciprocity and mutuality that is imagined to extend over the intertwined lifetimes of parents and children. Such reciprocity is captured in the idea of the "intergenerational contract"—the implicit understanding that children who have been cared for will give care to their parents in return, in the present and, especially, in the future when the parents grow old. There is a moral weight in this expectation evident as often in disappointment about failures as in the satisfaction of realization. Parents who died young or were too ill, poor, or irresponsible could not support their children. And children who were chronically ill, went astray, or did not manage to establish themselves financially or socially remained a burden rather than a support.

The implicit assumption that parents would care for their children was one of the reasons that many parents hesitated to tell their children about their HIV-positive status, explaining that the children would worry too much. As Matayo, a health worker, said, "I don't want to give them psychological torture." Herbert explained, "I keep my drugs in a cupboard so my children don't see. . . . [T]hey might get shocked that they are going to be left alone if they get to know about it." That children do think about death when they are told about HIV was reflected in the question posed by Jessica's daughter to her mother when she finally told the girl that she was sick: "is it the same disease that killed my two aunties?" Older children could better understand their parents' illness. Philip first told his four oldest children that he was HIV-positive; he eventually also told the younger ones but still had not told those who were younger than five. Yet there were people in our study who had not revealed their status even to their adult children.

When people on ART talked about their children, it was very often about their worries. Being ill, not being able to work, having to spend money on treatment (whether for ARVs or other medicine, transportation, or tests) meant that they had less money to care for their children. The worst problem was fees for children in secondary school, the largest recurring expense for most parents. As MamaGirl said, sometimes it was "just a gamble." You never knew whether there would be money for the next term. Those without funds depended on relatives to help with the fees, unless they were among the rare lucky ones, like Philip, who had found nongovernmental organizations to provide school fees. When children fell sick, money was needed for treatment. Even the everyday expenses of food, clothing, and shelter were beyond reach at some points. Robinah and her children were completely dependent on Robinah's sister Joyce for a time. Joyce was HIV-positive herself but managed to support two other orphans who stayed with them. People who earned a salary very often had orphans in their care, since children were placed with those who had the most resources.

Once they reached five or six, however, children were also able to help with domestic matters. It was a rare home in which there was no child to send on errands, wash up, serve food, and keep the house while adults were out. In some cases, relatives sent a child to stay with a person on ART if there was no other child in the home to help. Sometimes when Phoebe visited Jessica, she found Jessica's youngest daughter, who was fourteen, at home. The girl had been attending school in Kampala and living with her older sister but had been sent to stay with her mother in the village to help. It seemed clear that assisting her mother had higher priority than attending class. Once the daughter told Phoebe that her mother had asked her to stay home from school to do chores because she had a headache. Dorothy, a civil servant, talked with gratitude about how her parents had sent her younger sister to help her, nodding at the schoolgirl, whom she had called to bring her water.

People also worried about the relationships their children formed as teenagers. Sometimes we found our informants distraught about daughters who had gotten pregnant while at school or sons who were responsible for a pregnancy. The pregnancy of Robinah's two teenage daughters upset Joyce deeply and created so much tension between the two sisters that it affected their health. Amid all of his other troubles, John was disturbed by his fourteen-year-old daughter's sexual affair and the ensuing defilement case.[13] This unfolded during a period when John was not well; at one point, he left his sickbed when called urgently about the case. He had to borrow money, deal with the police, and negotiate with the family of the twenty-eight-year-old "defiler." John lamented, "I have been struggling to do something for the children before I die, but you can see how my girl's future is ruined now. I don't even know, and I am worried he might have infected my girl."

Herbert despaired of his son and the trouble he brought by impregnating a schoolgirl. The girl's father threatened to bring a defilement case if Herbert did not pay 3 million shillings as bridewealth. While Herbert and his wife were desperately thinking about what to do, Herbert got word from the hospital that the girl was in a serious condition after attempting an abortion. "Remember, we have not paid the money," he said. "The girl is going to die. I saw my life coming to an end and all because of this irresponsible son." For Herbert, like so many others, worries about children at times overshadowed concerns about his own illness and treatment.

The hope always was that struggles and worries would one day be counterbalanced by an adult child's loving care. Esther's account of her illness was intertwined with references to her daughters. Four of her children had died, and she had separated from her husband and struggled alone to pay school fees for the remaining three. When a man impregnated her thirteen-year-old daughter and then hid her at his home, she traced the girl and brought her back with her new baby. She was disappointed when her daughter refused to return to school, took up with another man, and moved to Kampala. To make matters worse, Esther's youngest daughter also got pregnant and had to leave school. Yet Esther spoke gratefully about her daughters. As she and Jenipher talked, her grandson—the one she had rescued from the man who hid her daughter—wandered in and out. She had cared for him for ten years and had even managed to pay his fees to attend nursery school. His mother's second partner turned out to be a model son-in-law, who built a small permanent house for her. That daughter, who had been such a troublesome teenager, and her second partner now helped the whole family—not only Esther but also Esther's other children, and even some of Esther's brothers and their children.

The dream that children would grow up, get jobs, and support their parents was widespread. Grace spoke indulgently about the promises of her children, who said, "Mom, you work so hard. We want you to retire, and then we will look after you." But the dream was marked by its failure as often as by its fulfillment. Herbert and his second wife were grieving the death of Herbert's grown daughter during Jenipher's third visit. She was an orphan for whom he had cared since she was three years old. She had studied, married, gotten a job as a nurse, and begun to send money to help Herbert with the expenses of his many other children. "It was terrible," he said. "We lost someone who had started looking after us and our children." The dream was punctured not only by the loss of adult children but also by their failure to find work or prosper enough to help their parents. In Uganda, as in other parts of Africa, the intergenerational contract is often "inverted," with parents continuing to support grown children and children's children.[14] But the ideal remains nonetheless.

Children *Are* the Second Chances

As more and more people got on to ART, it became clear that the advice to have no more children was being ignored not only by those who had none or one but also by those who already had several. Once people gained strength on the medicine, they could get on with their lives and find new partners or reconfirm existing partnerships. The rollout of PMTCT, which slightly preceded the spread of ART, gave hope of having an HIV-negative child.

So much of the discourse about HIV is about relationships with sexual partners, yet in many ways relationships with children are the most intense and problematic. Children are about the future that is restored to those who did not die as they expected. On the one hand, children are their parents' future, their extension in time, their legacy. "Children are our resurrection," one friend, a practicing Catholic, once said. On the other hand, children have their own future for which the older generations must prepare them. People wanted the life that medicine gave them so they could have (more) children, see them grow, and continue to care for them. The prospects of a child were imagined as linked to family prospects, too, given the ideal of kinship amity and the obligation to help parents and siblings. To talk about children and the future is not to ignore the "present-ness" of children; their company, their help, and their troublesome needs were at the heart of everyday life. But like Jackie, most of those we talked to linked the uncertainties of the future to children.

Children are the strongest concrete embodiment of second chances. With the reprieve of ART, people were relieved that their children would not become orphans—at least not double orphans and at least not right away. Having (more) children confirmed the new life in the strong sense of conversion and confidence in the treatment. It meant affirming new relationships and believing in a future. Yet children instantiated chanciness. Parents worried about whether their children also would become orphans. They worried about children's food, clothing, medical expenses, and education, often without the support of a spouse and co-parent and in circumstances in which their own ability to work was impaired. Their second thoughts sometimes led them to concentrate on the children they had rather than on having more.

What ART has given to parents and children is time: time to care for and worry about one another in the present and in a possible, if still uncertain, future. Instead of intense compressed periods of nursing a dying child or parent, people on ART had to deal with all of the problems of long-term support in a situation of insufficient resources. The dependence among generations, in the present as well as in the future, was a contingency with many imponderables. The second chances that ART provided for the future relationship between the generations were warmly welcomed but at the same time fraught with insecurities and doubts.

Notes

1. S. Whyte, *Questioning Misfortune*, 55.
2. Hunter, "Orphans as a Window on the AIDS Epidemic in Sub-Saharan Africa."
3. Guyer, "Wealth in People and Self-Realization in Equatorial Africa"; Johnson-Hanks, *Uncertain Honor*.
4. Meinert, *Hopes in Friction*, 29.
5. See Roby et al., "Changing Patterns of Family Care in Uganda."
6. Folmann, "Motherhood, Moralities and HIV."
7. Maier et al., "Antiretroviral Therapy Is Associated with Increased Fertility Desire."
8. Homsy et al., "Reproductive Intentions and Outcomes among Women on Antiretroviral Therapy in Rural Uganda"; Myer et al., "Impact of Antiretroviral Therapy on Incidence of Pregnancy among HIV-Infected Women in Sub-Saharan Africa."
9. Uganda Bureau of Statistics, *Uganda Demographic and Health Survey 2006*.
10. Leshabari et al., "Difficult Choices."

11. Bikaako-Kajura et al., "Disclosure of HIV Status and Adherence to Daily Drug Regimens among HIV-Infected Children in Uganda."

12. Bluebond-Langner, *The Private Worlds of Dying Children*.

13. Defilement, defined as sexual intercourse with a girl younger than eighteen, is a crime in Uganda that is punishable by life imprisonment.

14. Roth, "Shameful!"

CASE VII

John

WORKING
CONTINGENCIES

Godfrey Etyang Siu and
Susan Reynolds Whyte

WORK

(overleaf)

Loading trucks with
used clothes for trade
in local markets.

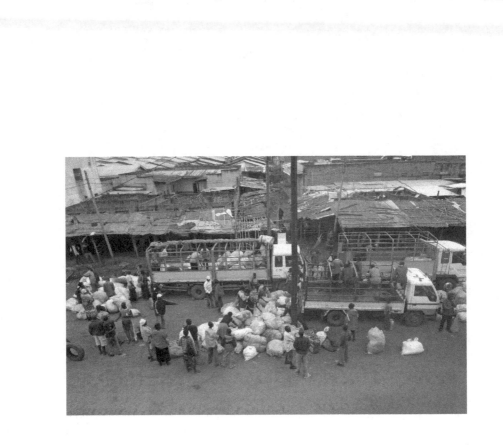

"My employer, the Uganda Railways Corporation, used to notice my poor health," John told us. "All the time I was ill, sometimes for long, and sometimes I even failed and got stuck somewhere on my journeys. They saw that I was affecting their work, and the board sat to discuss plans to lay me off. The decision to stop me was to be made, but I can tell you, God is good. That very day, the government announced that workers should not be laid off due to poor health. So rather than dismiss me, the personnel officer called me and said, 'You have been coming to my office because of your sickness, so get this form and fill it [out]. We are going to start paying for your treatment.' I had not expected this kind of news. I was overwhelmed and knelt down before the lady and said, 'Madam I don't know how to thank you. You have saved me.'"

Since he started receiving treatment in 2002, John had been paying out of his own pocket. Twice he had tried in vain to get into a free program at Mulago National Referral Hospital. So until the lucky day that company policy changed, John struggled. "Every end of the month, when my salary came, I headed toward the JCRC [Joint Clinical Research Centre] with cash for drugs," he said. "It was very difficult since my salary was not that big. I did not know what to do, but I had to continue to buy these drugs, so I had to look for the money using all means, sometimes asking for an advance on my salary."

From the time Godfrey met John in January 2006 until the last visit in May 2007, his life and treatment were closely intertwined with his employment. At first he seemed to be one of the most fortunate of all those we followed in that his treatment in the premier fee-for-service program at the JCRC was covered by his employer. But his luck shifted, revealing the precariousness of employment and the efforts required to balance work, illness, treatment, and family.

Godfrey and John soon developed a relationship based on the kind of sharing that is expected of brothers. When they found out that John's wife knew Godfrey's wife and her family (they were from the same ward), John remarked, "You see, you are indeed my real brother. You are very close to me." The gifts John offered were in kind—tea or soda—but Godfrey's gifts were often money. John's and Godfrey's wives gave birth to their second children around the same time, and they shared the joy of their babies—as well as the grief and challenges in John's life.

John lived in a four-room house owned by the Uganda Railways Corporation together with his three oldest children, who attended the nearby school. His wife had returned to their up-country home with the youngest child.

Mother and baby were both HIV-positive; the child was often sick, and they came regularly for checkups at the Kampala hospital where she had delivered and where they belonged to the HIV program.

Achieving a salaried job and a residence in Kampala had not been easy. John was born into a poor family, the fourth of six children. Although he was admitted to a reputable secondary school, he had no money and no one to sponsor him, so he decided to go to Jinja, where he had brothers working for the railway and where he might find a cheaper school. He worked hard doing odd jobs and managed to pay his own fees. He was even able to rent a small room so he could live on his own—whereupon various relatives turned up to stay with him. He did well enough on his exams to continue to senior secondary school, but there still was no money for fees. So he decided to get a job.

Through his connections to the railways, he was taken on by the corporation. He started as a porter and held that position for five years. First he was posted to Pakwach in northwestern Uganda, then to Tororo and, later, to Kampala. Although his salary was modest, he recalled that the job raised family expectations of support. "You know, I had to take care of everybody— relatives everywhere," he said. By that time, he had a wife and children who stayed with him in Pakwach, in the north. His parents were living in central Uganda; his brothers and their families in Jinja; and other relatives at his father's ancestral home in eastern Uganda, where John had rights to land. All needed help from his small salary. When he finally got a promotion, he was taken to Jinja for a year's course in train driving and management, followed by another year in Kenya. Finally he was posted back to Jinja and then to Kampala as a supervisor of the train crew. That was where Godfrey found him in 2006, thirteen years after he started working for the railway as a porter.

At that time, John was forty years old and had been married three times. His first wife died after bearing three children, of whom the second also died. He struggled to look after the two remaining small ones, but when he was called to go for the upgrading course in Kenya, he needed someone to keep them and hired a maid whom his cousin's wife had found for him. She became his second wife, and they had a child together, but that marriage broke down because of her mental instability. Before long another young woman, whose school fees he had been paying, moved in to help with the children while completing her studies. She became his third wife and soon conceived his fifth child.

John had not told his children that he was infected, but his apparent weakness, his slimness, and the spots on his skin were read and understood by other adults. He noted that his colleagues had changed in their attitude toward him. "They don't seem to value me and relate with me as they used to," he said. "They just pretend, and of course it can't be as it would be normally." He thought his poor health was affecting teamwork, as others feared he might not do his share. Some people were either reluctant to accept joint assignments that involved him or seemed to be thinking, "With this one, you have to be cautious."

John said that his work schedule had remained the same—tight on some occasions and involving long journeys in which he spent several days away from home. He had managed somehow except for one occasion on which he developed a fever as he was driving the train back from Kenya. He felt so weak that he could not drive and communicated to the office, which sent someone to help him.

People at his workplace became very concerned about his health. Shortly before departing on a trip to Bungoma, Kenya, his luggage was stolen at the train station. He lost his drugs and his good warm jacket suitable for this kind of journey. When news of the theft came to his boss's attention, the boss said, "No, I can't allow you to travel if you don't have your drugs with you."

At the first meeting, John was hoping that the government would keep him in employment so he could continue to receive medicine and keep his children in their Kampala school. His worry was that Uganda Railways was being privatized and some workers would be laid off. When Godfrey met John again four months later, John was in the process of relocating to the village, though not because of the privatization. He had been interdicted from his job (suspended pending investigations) because of an accident for which he was being held responsible. He was put on half-pay, barred from service, and asked to report regularly to the manager. "It was a very painful and sad moment for me as I started thinking about many things," he told Godfrey. "I tried pleading for mercy, but it didn't help. I had to go. Brother, I immediately organized to shift to the village. The problem was that I had to leave the children behind, since they were studying."

John worried about how the interdiction would affect his treatment but feared even to ask. When he went to pick up his next supply of medicine, he acted as if nothing had happened. "The JCRC might fear that I am already dismissed and [that] they won't be paid," he said, "so I will continue coming until they stop me. I am not going to reveal that I am interdicted."

Beyond the concerns about treatment, John was trying to manage on half-pay. He said,

> I am earning half-salary, but when they make the deductions, I am left with nothing. For example, in addition to the compulsory deductions, I

am still paying 140,000 shillings for this house. [The company rents out the houses to employees at a subsidized rate.] If you subtract all these, I remain with 18,000. Worse still, I don't get it here in Kampala. My salary is always posted to Jinja, where I used to work. Now if you include the cost of collecting that money there, it means I have nothing remaining. . . . All people are worried, especially my brothers. I used to help them, including some of their in-laws [relatives of their wives], when there was a problem. But now all this assistance is ending. My brothers are also worried about my life. They knew I was surviving because of Uganda Railways, so they have been worried since I lost the job.

There was another concern, and John was sure he would not survive it: the impending privatization of the corporation.

My biggest worry is that the job is over. My interdiction coincided with the privatization of the railways corporation and immediately I was interdicted, I knew I stand no chance of being retained since there was already a communication that privatization will affect many people—they will be laid off. So how can they retain a man with a bad record? The new management will come and the first thing they will look out for is people who have a problem of some sort. So for me I know I stand no chance. Brother, this accident happened at the worst time for it spoilt any chance of me remaining since they are going to reduce workers from two thousand to only six hundred.

In the meantime, John was cultivating land at his village home to make ends meet. His wife unsuccessfully tried some business, such as selling shoes in the local markets. John had earlier bought a milling machine to generate some income. The venture might have succeeded had it not been for other new entrants who rushed into the same business, along with poor management of the milling machine by John's brothers. In the end, the business lost.

John talked about life being "a gamble." On this occasion, he had had to come to Kampala with hardly any money in his pocket. He traveled by goods train, helped by his workmates, because he had no money to pay for transportation. Eating in Kampala was hit or miss—mostly tea and the ubiquitous cheap chapatis (flat bread—the Ugandan version is fried in oil). He had left his wife in the village with only 3,000 shillings, yet their child was sick and needed treatment. Moreover, she had to buy cow's milk because HIV-positive mothers are not supposed to breastfeed. John did not know when he would have to vacate his company house and was trying to find a cheap place for his children to stay so they could continue their education in Kampala.

When Godfrey met John again at the end of June, he, together with hundreds of others, had just been called for an interview with the new management. He was convinced that this was just a formality to justify their dismissal. In fact, one of the panelists, a South African woman, whispered that even if they were being interviewed, there were no jobs for them and their positions had been eliminated. John's only hope was to invest his termination package well so he and his family could survive. John was determined to use the money wisely and planned to consult Godfrey rather than his own brothers, whom he dismissed as simple villagers.

Worst of all, John had been told the day before that the JCRC was terminating his treatment. When he went to pick up his medicine, he told the receptionist, as always, that he was from Uganda Railways Corporation and had come on the basis of the usual arrangement. She snapped back, "Oh, so you are the people. Give me your identity card." He knew that the end had come; it was obvious that the corporation had withdrawn its sponsorship. As the receptionist took the card to an office, John was overcome with worry. Eventually, the receptionist returned and told him that he would be given his medicine for free for the last time, unless the JCRC heard otherwise from the Uganda Railways. When John asked what he should do next, the dispenser told him to start paying for the medicine himself, but also noted that his drug combination was expensive, at 200,000 shillings per month and was not available from any free program. When he heard this, John concluded that he would just have to return to the village and wait to die, because he could not afford the medicine. As a last effort, John went to his manager at work, but the man brushed all hope away. "He just told me to forget it," John said. "He was in the same boat [losing the privilege of corporate-sponsored treatment]. How can we expect to be paid for when the corporation is collapsing?"

Godfrey was worried about John, so he called him in August. The situation was looking a little better. His brother working for Uganda Railways in Jinja had agreed to contribute 100,000 shillings toward his medicines when the last free ones ran out. Moreover, and surprisingly, the company's new management had indicated that John might be among the few employees retained. He had been called for assessment, which included medical tests. He disclosed his serostatus and treatment, yet this did not seem to disqualify him. However, nothing would be certain until the end of the year, when the new management took over. John would be allowed to keep his company house in Kampala but was still desperate about getting his medication.

By the end of September, John had run out of medicine. Unable to depend on his brother for more money, he had gone to beg for help from the JCRC. The center agreed to put him on a waiting list, but he could not wait, so he went to another hospital, which agreed to give him a supply for a few days but asked him to get a referral. When he went back for the letter, the doctor announced that the JCRC had decided to give him free treatment.

Two months later, John was given a job by the new management of the railway company, with a new title and a doubled salary. He remained in his house, although he had been told to leave because staff houses were to be sold under privatization. Nothing had been communicated about medical care under the new company. He hoped to continue on free treatment from the JCRC, although it was requiring him to bring in a letter of termination to show that he was unemployed.

Three months after his new job began, he had reason to be grateful for the management's health policy. He worked normally in January and February, but began to feel sharp chest pains in March. The railway staff clinic referred him to Nsambya Hospital when he said he was on ART. He was admitted for four days, but when he heard the cost, he asked to be discharged, assuming that he would have to cover it. He did not realize that his stay was covered by his employers' insurance. The doctors transferred him to the general ward, to the dissatisfaction of the railways staff doctor who came to check on him and then transferred him to another hospital, where he was treated for three weeks.

When he started feeling better, he demanded to be discharged so he could get back to work. He did not want a bad record of absenteeism and health problems, especially since he was still on job probation. Although he was allowed to leave on those grounds, one of the doctors at the hospital warned that he would soon be back because he was not yet cured. He immediately started to work, but three days later he had so much pain that he cried like a child and had to be rushed back to the hospital. This time, he improved within a few days and again returned to work.

He found the work demanding. Supervising the train crew meant being with them constantly when on duty—sometimes even for twenty-four hours without rest. John realized that some of his colleagues were becoming unfriendly and were trying to avoid him. Some felt he was too ill to work. Others were known to talk behind his back, asking why he did not quit since he was in such a state. He heard that some even feared making long trips with him, but they did not tell him openly. They said that moving with such a person was dangerous because he might collapse and die in their arms. This made John sad, and he explained that it was the reason he wanted to be present at work rather than talked about as a person who spends most of the time in hospital. He said he tried to show that he was not as weak as some of his colleagues thought, but his appearance belied him. He had lost so much weight that everybody who knew him was becoming worried, especially those at his workplace.

At Godfrey's last visit in May 2007, John was feeling much stronger. He was happy to be working with more stability. The previous few weeks had been good because he had managed to go to work without taking sick days. However, John decried the working conditions. "It is my work which is affecting my health now," he said. He was often on the move, traveling between Kampala and Tororo. The major problem was that the train journey could be started any time, night or day, and sometimes he was away for two or three days at a time. Eating became a big problem: the work hours were awkward; the trains stopped at remote places where one could not obtain food; they traveled all day and hardly found time to eat a meal. John concluded that when he was on duty, he lived the life of a soldier.

CHAPTER SEVEN

Work

Susan Reynolds Whyte,
Godfrey Etyang Siu, and
Phoebe Kajubi

All of the people we followed were concerned with the relationship among illness, treatment, and the ability to work. Working was important for many psychological, social, and economic reasons. Some mentioned that being occupied helped to take their minds off their illnesses. "It is good to do something, and you don't just sit there," as Ivan explained, "because you become redundant, and it is not good. Now, like us, you start thinking about your health problems, and you may end up falling sick again and again." An active female farmer remarked, "A certain doctor advised me to stay busy so that I don't allow my mind to think about death. I actually don't have time to think about it. I take my drugs and do my work." But work was far more than a distraction from concerns about health. To be able to work, produce, and provide are fundamental for one's value as a person. Social worth lies in making a contribution through helping others and not being only a burden to them. People often said that HIV made them feel "useless," indicating that weakness was not only an individual bodily experience but also a social condition that inhibited them from contributing in their families and workplaces. Antiretroviral therapy gave them a second chance to work again and thus to be "useful," though not always with the capacity they once had.[1] The first generation on ART was differentiated in terms of work situations. Illness and treatment presented different problems accordingly, each with particular uncertainties and contingencies. But for everyone, the second chance to work caused people to reflect on their changing strength. Because of the projectification of the response to AIDS, HIV actually became a qualification for some kinds of work.

On the Kenyan coast in the 1970s, David Parkin noticed the greater value attached to monthly wage labor than to casual labor and small business ventures, even when the latter yielded a higher income. He explained this in terms of the greater control over one's destiny that a regular income made possible, along with the ability to plan accordingly.[2] Casual labor, trade, and artisanal work were less dependable and had that chancy aspect that Ugandans refer to as "gambling." The idea of work as an endeavor to control present and future circumstances is helpful for understanding the concerns of the first generation. Steven Russell and Janet Seeley recognized the importance of work in providing a sense of control for people on ART who were learning to live with HIV as a chronic condition: "narratives of work . . . were people's 'quests' to regain control, create order, reduce dependence on others, and to feel 'normal' again."[3] For our interlocutors, too, ART was a reprieve from "uselessness" and a chance to resume the efforts to control family destiny. But these efforts were not guaranteed to succeed. The difficulties of maintaining control, the unreliability of bodies, and the contingencies of cash needs all made the second chance to work uncertain.

Kinds of Work

In rough terms, work can be divided into endeavors that directly generate money, such as regular employment or business, and those that generate other value, such as subsistence agriculture or domestic work. Of people who are working to earn cash, we can distinguish those on a regular salary, the wage earners, from those who are "self-employed" and whose income may vary from week to week. The Ugandan Census of 2002 reported that 16 percent of the labor force were wage and salaried workers, while 43 percent were self-employed and 41 percent were unpaid family workers.[4] The first generation in general consisted mainly of people without a fixed income. But salaried workers are disproportionately represented among our interlocutors because we tried to include people who were paying for their medicine. That meant a higher representation of those with more resources, mainly members of the salariat: nineteen of the original forty-eight and eight of the twenty-three we followed over time were on salary. Industry, business, and commercial agriculture are not strongly developed in Uganda, so most salaries come from government jobs. Teachers, soldiers, health workers, police, and local officials are typical wage earners.

In Ugandan English, "working class" refers not to those who do manual labor but to those who are fortunate enough to have relatively permanent jobs. It also implies a certain amount of cultural capital, in the form of education and sophistication, and more middle-class aspirations. Several of our first forty-eight informants would definitely fit this description—for example: Hope, the financial manager with a master's degree in business administration; Benjamin, an official with the Uganda Revenue Authority; and Jackson, the university lecturer. Of the twenty-three we came to know better, Grace, a head teacher, and Matayo, the lab technician, could have been called "working class." "Working class" is an attribution made by others more than it is a clear and fixed category. From a rural farmer's perspective, policemen, office messengers, and people like John might be considered working class because of their regular wages and institutional affiliations.

But it is not only an individual's salary that counts. Family resources and parents' occupations confer a courtesy status. Alice (case V) and Jolly (case IX) might well have been placed in the working class by virtue of their backgrounds; although they only ran modest small businesses, they had support from families with education and good cash flows.

Some people in public service (teachers, health workers, soldiers) worked for institutions that provided housing for their staffs, as did the Uganda Railways Corporation. For them, work constituted a neighborhood and a framework for their households, as well as an occupation when they were on duty. (John lived in the same railway housing estate that the anthropologist Ralph Grillo had studied forty years earlier, and many of the patterns Grillo described were still recognizable in John's situation.[5]) Only a few of our working-class interlocutors had jobs that covered their treatment expenses at some point.

According to the 2002 census, the largest categories of the labor force were self-employed and unpaid family workers. In reality, most people do both kinds of work. Nearly everyone, including the salariat, engaged in some kind of small business or trading, at least sporadically, and most people living in rural areas did some subsistence farming. What distinguishes self-employment is that it generates cash and often requires a small amount of working capital. It covers a huge range of enterprises, from distilling alcohol or making bricks to trading in used clothes or keeping a small shop. It includes people who do construction, tailoring, or hairdressing for customers who pay by the job.

The Ugandan population is predominantly (about 85 percent) rural, and most people have land for agriculture, producing for their own needs and selling some crops for cash. Both men and women farm, with women often doing much of the routine work. Only five of the twenty-three people we followed described themselves as peasants (half of our informants were contacted through urban treatment centers), but almost all of the rural people—along with the self-employed and salaried—did some cultivation. By and large, farmers were growing their own food and trying to earn cash through trading or small business. According to the season, digging, weeding, harvesting, and processing crops demand strength, or they require help from others. Falling sick during planting season is no good; rural health centers experience a drop in patients' attendance when the rain starts, not because of better health, but because people cannot afford to take time away from their fields. In many parts of the country, cultivating and weeding are done by hand. Agricultural work is strenuous, and those who can afford it hire day labor in the most intensive work periods.

Like agriculture, domestic work is demanding. Cooking, washing clothes, minding children, sweeping, and all of the other chores of daily maintenance are unending. In rural areas, people must also fetch water and firewood. Most of these tasks fall to women and children. For the first generation, unpaid family labor also included caring for the sick by cleaning and feeding them, helping them to the toilet, and staying nearby in case they need help. Caregivers had to stay with those who were admitted to hospitals, and someone had to bring them food, because the hospitals do not provide meals. One of the benefits of ART was that household members who had devoted time to caring for the sick person were able to resume their other work as recovery progressed.[6]

The Security and Insecurities of Salaried Jobs

Like Parkin's interlocutors, and for the same reasons, members of the first generation attributed the greatest value to salaried work. Because most of the ART pioneers were paying for treatment, a regular income was even more important. Employed people could collect their wages at the end of the month and use them to pay for the next refill of medicine.[7] But the control that Parkin emphasized was never complete, and the security of a regular job was often tinged with worries. Belonging to a workplace in some ways was like belonging to a family. Although expectations of amity and solidarity were often realized, they were sometimes overshadowed by misgiving and rivalry.

Perhaps the single greatest advantage for the salariat section of the first generation was relative job security, despite illness. This meant that many continued to receive their salaries even though ill health prevented them from working regularly. Juma, who crossed the border to get treatment in Uganda, asserted that stigmatization was great in Kenya, where he lived and worked, and that many people lost their jobs when their employers found out they were HIV-positive. He thought that he would have been fired had a friend not pleaded for him with his boss. But our Ugandan interlocutors were not primarily concerned about being fired because they were HIV-positive. John's threatened dismissal was not due to his serostatus; in fact, he was rehired by the new management, who had full knowledge of his health record.

Members of the salariat benefited from amendments made to the Ugandan Employment Act in 2006, which protect employees when they fall ill, regardless of the diagnosis, and guarantee full salary for a total of thirty days' sick leave for those on contract. After that period, keeping a job depends on specific policy and contract terms. Government employees, a large proportion of the salariat, have long enjoyed considerable job security (which is one reason that "retrenchment" under structural adjustment was seen as such an infringement of their rights). Absenteeism is not uncommon among civil servants; teachers and health workers take time off for family and other reasons and sometimes report late for new postings. This pattern, which makes public services inefficient, allowed people weakened by HIV and the side effects of ART to stay home and still collect their salaries even beyond the statutory thirty days' sick leave. Toleration on this point was widespread; employees covered for one another in a kind of family solidarity.

As they did in families, people formed alliances in their workplaces, telling some and not others about their health status. They usually informed their immediate superiors about their illness and treatment to explain absences from work and to request lighter duties. Elizabeth, a health worker at a private facility, had not told her colleagues about her HIV status but shared with her pastor's wife, who advised her to tell her boss "because the workload would be too much for [her]." The soldiers to whom we spoke had told their superior officers and achieved some leniency in their assignments. Like Saddam (case II), they were assigned to barracks near medical facilities and were not sent on the most demanding missions.

Some of our interlocutors also spoke to colleagues about their status, and we heard examples of friendship and assistance, such as when Joyce's fellow teachers took over her class when she felt unwell (case I). Goretti, a nursing assistant, told all of her co-workers that she was HIV-positive and sang their praises for being supportive. She worked as a counselor in the weekly HIV clinic, turning her positive status into a platform for helping others and, in the process, receiving encouragement from her colleagues. Yet this was not typical. Margaret Kyakuwa found that even nurses who counsel clients to be open about their status often do not want their patients and fellow health workers to know that they are HIV-positive.[8]

The acceptance and toleration of HIV illness that characterized many workplaces did not mean complete openness. Most people told a few close colleagues, but beyond that point, they felt that workmates might not be genuinely sympathetic. Concern about "rumor mongering" and "backbiting" reflected uncertainty about the dispositions of others. As Godfrey Siu and his colleagues found in their study of men in rural eastern Uganda, disclosing to employers and fellow employees risked reducing job offers, as many feared working with people who were known to be ill. Not only does this affect earnings, but it also undermines one's identity as a hard worker.[9] Some people were very careful about keeping their secret and were convinced that no one knew except their boss. Others had not actually told their colleagues but thought they suspected. Jackie (case VI) explained that she thought other members of the staff where she worked were aware, though she had not told them. "They talk," she said. "When one tells one, they tell others. In the beginning I used to be angered by the talk; sometimes I reacted and quarreled. But now it is OK. Even those who were talking, some checked themselves and found they are positive, so they also stopped."

People worried that HIV status could play into the workplace politics on which their prospects depended. They did not want to be thought of as less competent or dependable colleagues because of their illness and need for treatment. They did not want their every mistake or absence to be attributed to their serostatus. They were very sensitive to being overlooked when chances arose for further education or promotion. Major Charles said that while his superior officers accepted that he should not be transferred to remote places far from treatment sources, still they discriminated against him. "For example, they don't take me for courses, and it affects my promotion, which affects my job," he said. "When you go for a course, there is some money added to your salary, and the chances of promotion are high." Julia, a nurse, thought that her younger colleagues watched for her slightest mistakes and that she was rarely offered further training. Benjamin, a civil servant, did not want to ask for more leave, although his feet were so swollen as a side effect of the medicine he was taking that he could not wear shoes. He feared not dismissal but, if he kept making excuses and missing work, that he "might be transferred, and it can be to a place where people don't understand and where there are no health services."

Many of our interlocutors told stories about what they saw as corruption, malicious manipulation, and envy in workplaces. These, together with gossip, affect everyone in a work organization, but our interlocutors connected them to their vulnerable situations. Dorothy, the prison officer, spoke warmly about some of her fellow staff members, who encouraged her as she endured the painful side effects of the drug Triomune. But she was also convinced that other colleagues wished her ill. First, she was supposed to be transferred, which she attributed to the fact that her bosses wanted to give her job to people from their own tribe. When that threat passed, she was designated to go for training for three months at Luzira Prison, far from her home. She worried about how intensive it was going to be. "I hope it is not real Army training," she said. "I don't think I can manage that, . . . and they do not know that I am sick. I am also worried about how I will be getting my drugs because they cannot give them to someone else. You have to pick them up yourself." When Jenipher asked Dorothy why she did not simply tell the authorities that she was on medication, she replied, "There are many people who want our jobs, and some are those who wanted me transferred from here. In fact, when they heard that I was going for further training, they were not happy about it. That is why I have to go."

Dorothy found confirmation of her mistrust when she discovered that she had been reported dead and struck off the payroll. "I went to our salary office to complain about not receiving my salary, only to be told that they knew I had passed away," she said. "I was very shocked and . . . could not believe someone could just go to the office and do that to me." The soldiers Tom and Saddam also found that their names had been deleted from the pay list because someone reported them sick and not active in the Army. Both men and Dorothy managed to get reinstated, but at considerable cost in terms of paperwork, going from office to office, and living without their salaries for months. Saddam was convinced that malice and corruption were to blame. Such problems were experienced by others in employment, but people on ART, who were especially dependent on regular income, were more deeply affected.

The Contingencies of Self-Employment and Farming

For those who were self-employed, there was no income during the time they could not work. Unless they could get assistance from "unpaid family labor" or were involved in an enterprise where someone else could step in to help, they did not earn if they could not work. Worse still they were even more vulnerable than others to dangers of losing their working capital. Their assets may have been depleted before they started on ART because of their poor health and, often, the sickness and death of others in the home. They needed resources for treatment beyond their ART, for transportation, and perhaps to buy extra food. Unexpected expenses and pressure to help family members consume the capital of many people who are trying to manage small enterprises. Those on ART felt such problems more keenly.[10]

Global health initiatives have focused on alleviating the bodily effects of HIV. To the extent they have been successful, they have allowed people to worry about supporting themselves and their families. Well-being is not just improved health; it depends on money. As Vincent said, "My main problem is not health but economy. I had to sell land in order to pay bridewealth, and now I must rent land from others. Plus, I had to borrow capital for my business of making bricks." Hanifa, who gave up her Rwanda trade, said, "What affects me mainly is lack of money. When I am broke, I feel so bad."

The shopkeeper Herbert was especially careful about conserving his resources—"stingy," his wife said—and was unwilling to spend money on good food because it would deplete the capital for his shop. Jessica had lost weight the second time Phoebe visited her. She explained that she had no money to buy the *matooke* (cooking plaintains), tomatoes, and groundnuts for her business of selling cooked food. She had even asked her health worker for a loan so she could restart the business and earn enough to buy maize flour and sugar for the porridge she craved.

Even cooperation was a source of problems for many of our interlocutors, because money brought disagreements. Ivan was trading in veterinary drugs until one of his friends, to whom he had entrusted 400,000 shillings [about $231] to purchase medicine in Nairobi, disappeared with the money. "I tell you, people are terrible, and when it comes to money, people are unpredictable, like weather," he said. "I advise you never to trust anybody with money, even if he or she is your close relative." That was advice that two other interlocutors wished they had followed. Dominic (case XI), who was in business with his brother, became convinced that his brother was not only cheating him but also trying to do him in. Herbert regretted bitterly that he had brought one of his sons to work in his shop during a period in which he was not feeling well. The young man neither banked the income nor used it to restock the shop. Such problems could touch anyone trying to do business, but those who were trying to control their disease, as well as their economic situation, felt that they were more affected. As Ivan put it, "People have frustrated me, even with this disease. When you are poor, not eating well, all the time worried about what follows next, you go very fast."

While those on salary were concerned about workplace politics, those with their own small businesses might be expected to worry about their images in the eyes of their customers. But we did not hear of any examples in which small businesses suffered because of prejudice. Some independent business-people drew a larger lesson from rare incidents of discrimination. Jessica sold cooked food in a trading center, where her illness was well known. She talked about a time when six people from one family, also businesspeople, refused to eat inside her house, where there were chairs for customers. "We can't eat from an AIDS home," she quoted them as saying. "Bring the plates of food outside." She continued:

> I felt like I should not give them my food but then thought I wanted the money. There are also chairs outside for people to eat. They did not have to say that they can't eat from an AIDS house. They should have just kept quiet about it and sat outside to eat. I gave them the food, and they ate, but do you know what happened to them? You know, it's not only AIDS that kills. The next day, all of them perished in a car accident. I was not happy about it, but [I was annoyed] by the way they said my house was not good just because I have AIDS.

For Jessica, this incident stood out not only because of the fate that befell prejudiced people, but also because the prejudice was unusual.

Reconsidering Strength

Once people improved on ART and got over the initial side effects of the medicine, another problem appeared: overexertion could be exhausting and make people fall sick again, as John worried. Finding the balance and figuring out what kind of work was compatible with life on ART were recurring themes in our conversations.

Poor men reconsidered strenuous jobs they had once done. Dominic, who had been herding cows, told his boss that he could no longer spend the whole day far from home, under the hot sun. He first asked to graze the animals close by so he could go home to rest, but he then stopped herding and estab-lished a butchery, which he could run with his brother's help. Hassan (case VIII) felt he was no longer strong enough to work in a factory, although his former boss offered to take him back. Nor could he join his wife, who worked smoking fish at a fish landing site. "I used to do such work for three years be-fore I fell sick, but no more," he said, "because the fire, heat, and smoke would be dangerous to my health." Several months later, we found Hassan feeling stronger and working practically outside his own door, cleaning and repairing shoes and mending the big tarpaulins used to cover the beds of trucks.

In his study of construction workers on ART in Milan, Matteo Carlo Alcano showed how concerned they were about their diminished physical strength.[11] They explained to him that they had to do manual labor but often felt weak from the illness and treatment. While our informants had similar concerns about their strength, like Dominic and Hassan they tried to find other ways to earn money that were less strenuous or that they could do with other people's assistance. Ivan did not have enough energy to do all of the work of brickmaking himself. Although he had to hire casual labor, which was troublesome and cut into his profits, at least he was earning an income. Those running small businesses and doing casual labor could adjust their workloads to some extent. Suzan (case III), who sold cooked food, said she once would have walked to several markets in a day, but that was now too exhausting. In-stead, she chose one market 4 kilometers from her home and went very early in the morning, when truck drivers came to eat. Even that was tiring, though, so she was thinking about switching to trading in used clothes, buying them at the Owino market when she went to Kampala to fetch her medications and selling them at home in Lira.

Bodily frailty is not only a problem for those who do physically strenuous work. When Joyce, a teacher, started taking ARVs, her hand became numb. "At one time during the school term, the numbness became too much," she said. "I couldn't write, and yet I cannot do without writing, given the nature of my work. This worries me so much because I need to provide for my family and myself."

Domestic chores and family cultivation cannot easily be exchanged for other work. They can be shared and reduced but not avoided. When Suzan's son went away to school, she had to manage both the farming and the house-work herself. She reduced the size of her farm and, on her doctor's advice, carried only 10–15 liters of water at a time rather than the usual 20 liters. Many people mentioned that other members of their households took on heavier work when they were feeling weak.

People who worked strenuous jobs or long hours, such as John, were concerned that the exertion would affect their health. Robinah (case I), who miraculously came back from the edge of the grave, grew strong on ARVs and took over much of the domestic and agricultural work in the household; she also distilled *waragi* (gin) to earn cash. But her sister Joyce wanted to find a project that was less labor-intensive for Robinah, fearing that the heavy work would break her down. "Sometimes I just plead with her not to dig so much," Joyce said. Although Robinah was proud that she could make such an important contribution to the household and relieve her sister, who was also sick, she worried: "when I see my friends deteriorating, I worry about my own health. It is because they have overworked themselves that their health is not so good."

Noah had been a casual laborer but had given up the heavy work. "I no longer have strength for heavy work," he said. "For me, it seems I overworked in those days. We could carry very heavy loads, including iron bars [weighing] 70 kilograms plus. So I feel I can't work now. I have failed to make money in my life, so it is no longer an issue, since I am old. I don't have any other hope to earn money, so I avoid being too active, trying too hard. I fear breaking down my body since rebuilding it to this state is very difficult." Like the others, Noah had come to see his body as vulnerable, needing protection from the exertions that earlier had been a given condition of life.

In a study of artisanal gold miners in eastern Uganda and their uptake of ART, Siu and his colleagues found the same pattern of concern that the strenuous work might exhaust the gains made from treatment. Not only did the men themselves reflect on this danger, but their workmates remarked that they should do lighter work. While the HIV-positive men appreciated the sympathy, they also felt that their masculinity was being undermined because they were not as strong as they once had been.[12]

HIV as a Qualification

The first generation was a biogeneration in that the response to the AIDS epidemic was a defining event—a magnetic field that oriented the consciousness and subjectivity of its members, regardless of whether they sought treatment. The plethora of projects that mushroomed in Uganda introduced a new element in livelihood struggles. They made HIV a qualification for obtaining assets for agriculture and small business enterprises. Some treatment programs, such as Reach Out Mbuya, also offered microcredit schemes to clients. Nongovernmental organizations appeared that targeted HIV-positive people with support in the form of seeds or domestic animals, much like the resources Joyce guided to the members of the Post-Test Club she led. While the reach and comprehensiveness of such livelihood projects was nowhere near sufficient for the needs of people in treatment, their existence was an innovation of which many people were aware.

Treatment and welfare projects offered work more directly, as well. Writing about nearby Kisumu in western Kenya, where AIDS research and ART projects have come to dominate the city's economy, Ruth Prince discusses how an HIV identity can accrue moral and economic value. While people sometimes want to hide their serostatus, in other situations it can be used to make claims: "people move between these different registers of invisibility and visibility, as they search for ways to make a living."[13] Among the first generation in Uganda, the same concerns were evident. While people wanted to control information about their serostatus and treatment in some work situations, they were ready to use it in others. In trying to improve their own livelihood circumstances as volunteers, expert clients, or members of support groups, they also changed the consciousness and disposition of a whole generation.

The GIPA Principle (Greater Involvement of People with HIV and AIDS) called for the participation of HIV-positive people at all levels of policy making, administration, and implementation of AIDS activities. It has been widely realized in the recruitment of "expert clients" as assistants in clinical and outreach work and as peer counselors for others who are HIV-positive or in treatment. Expert clients provide some relief for hard-pressed health workers who are struggling with the enormous workload of treating so many people, although there are also tensions between professionals and volunteers over competence and responsibility.[14] But what GIPA meant for the clients themselves was that HIV became a qualification for getting work.

The way to a wage often went through volunteering. Starting as a volunteer meant one was not paid a salary, but at least there were opportunities to receive allowances for lunch, transportation, and attending workshops. And by volunteering, people achieved recognition and positioned themselves in case proper salaried jobs opened up. The chances were best for those who were better educated. Jolly said with delight during Jenipher's final visit that her program had chosen her to be a peer counselor. "They looked for people who had some level of education and could speak English," she said. "We shall be starting training in two weeks' time." As is often the case, Jolly was taken on as a volunteer but said she hoped transportation would be provided. Ivan's wife had quit her volunteer job as a nursery school teacher because it offered neither pay nor prospects. A colleague tried to persuade her to come back: "I want us this time to teach and we do not request for any money because Plan International thought that for us we just want money without teaching. So let us not pull out, we will teach those children until they realize that we need to be paid." In other words, the colleague was acknowledging that they were supposed to be volunteers, but voicing the widely held hope that volunteering would lead to a salary.

Volunteering is not new in the health sector. The history of village health workers—community distributors of contraceptives and antimalarial medication, vaccination assistants in immunization campaigns, trained traditional birth attendants and traditional healers—is a story of volunteer work. While the sponsors of such donor-funded programs expected people to give their time for the good of the community, those who volunteered were interested in the small allowances and other benefits (such as rubber boots, T-shirts, medical equipment). They hoped to parlay their training and experience into an income. After the projects closed, some opened drugshops and small clinics and some were taken on as paid nursing aides at local government health centers. At the very least, they were often recruited for the next project, with whatever allowances it might bring. For HIV-positive volunteers, the transition from one project or assignment to another is also common. Experience and training workshops accumulate and enhance qualifications for the next job. The difference between earlier health volunteering and the current wave of "expert clients" is that a diagnosis is a prerequisite for positioning oneself.

The First Generation at Work

Getting back to work, with all that means about usefulness and attempts to reassert some measure of control over one's own and one's family's destiny, was an essential part of the second chance. Ugandans seemed generally supportive of attempts by people on ART to work. Legislation and common practice ensured the right to miss work without losing one's job for members of the salariat. Supervisors and colleagues were sensitive to needs to adjust the workload of people on treatment. It was unusual for customers to discriminate against traders and small entrepreneurs because they were known to be HIV-positive or in treatment.

Still, the second chance to work was not exactly a reassertion of normality or a continuation of life as it was before. Because few people regained the strength they once had, and because their work had already been disrupted before they started treatment, they were more concerned by the contingency and uncertainty that everyone feels to some extent. Their worries differed according to their occupational locations. The fortunate ones on salary feared that their prospects for promotion were impaired and that their colleagues were too ready to blame their disease for shortcomings in their work. Those who were self-employed earned no income when they could not work. Reliance on others for help involved disillusion as well as affirmation. Farmers and entrepreneurs easily lost essential assets and necessary capital.

Thus, members of the first generation came to have second thoughts about work. They saw the need to make adjustments where they could, and they worried about overworking renewed bodies. A person on ART should not overexert himself or herself by engaging in very strenuous labor. Efforts and work situations that had been taken for granted were being reconsidered, not only by those whose lives had been saved, but also by their families and workmates.

Notes

1. Kaler et al., "'Living by the Hoe' in the Age of Treatment," 7–9.

2. Parkin, "The Categorization of Work," 318.

3. Russell and Seeley, "The Transition to Living with HIV as a Chronic Condition in Rural Uganda," 376.

4. Uganda Bureau of Statistics, *The 2002 Uganda Population and Housing Census*, 27.

5. Grillo, *African Railwaymen*.

6. Kaler et al., "'Living by the Hoe' in the Age of Treatment."

7. In principle, some employers paid for ART for their most valued employees when prices began to fall, as was the case for John. However, relatively few were covered by such arrangements; of the nineteen people with salaried jobs we originally interviewed, just two had their treatment fees paid for by their employer.

8. Kyakuwa, "Ethnographic Experiences of HIV-Positive Nurses in Managing Stigma at a Clinic in Rural Uganda."

9. Siu et al., "How a Masculine Work Ethic and Economic Circumstances Affect Uptake of HIV Treatment."

10. Russell et al., "Coming Back from the Dead."

11. Alcano, "Living and Working in Spite of Antiretroviral Therapies."

12. Siu et al., "How a Masculine Work Ethic and Economic Circumstances Affect Uptake of HIV Treatment."

13. Prince, "HIV and the Moral Economy of Survival in an East African City," 548.

14. Kyakuwa, "Ethnographic Experiences of HIV-Positive Nurses in Managing Stigma at a Clinic in Rural Uganda."

CASE VIII

Hassan

SOFT FOOD AND
TOWN LIFE

Phoebe Kajubi and
Susan Reynolds Whyte

FOOD
(overleaf)
Oily snacks for sale
in a small town.

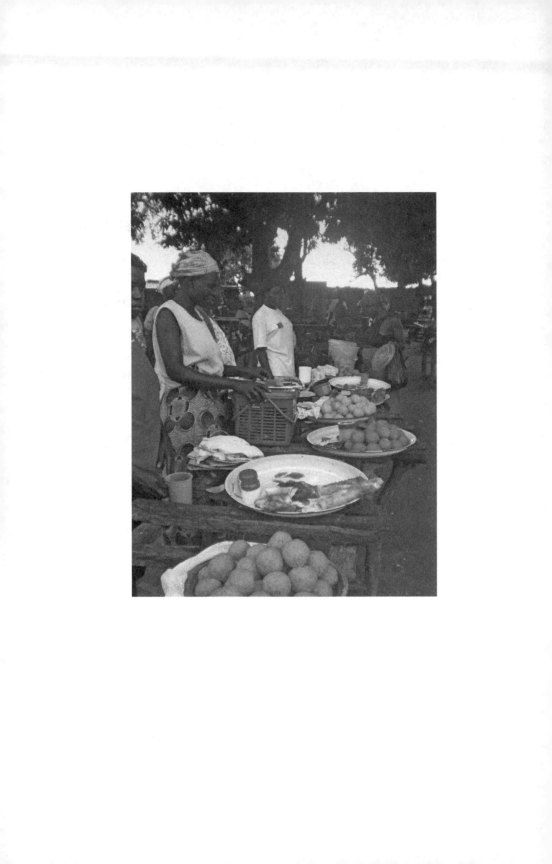

"This illness has been too bad on me. I was in Butaleja without proper help. My wife is in Kampala, and my mother is old," said Hassan. "So sometimes my brothers' wives used to assist me. They would cook some food for me, but as you know, the conditions here in the village are bad. Most times, I would eat food that is not good enough for my health." Hassan had come to the hospital on this day in December 2005 to get his monthly refill of antiretroviral medicine (ARVs). One glance revealed that he had been seriously ill. He looked weak, and his ash-gray skin was marked with black spots. He had a runny nose, and he kept sneezing; his constant coughing seemed painful. He was dressed in black pants and a white shirt that looked too big, making his loss of weight very obvious.

Nevertheless, Hassan walked with confidence and appeared to be excited about meeting Phoebe and Godfrey. "For me, I don't fear to tell you people about what I am going through," he said, "because I know you may help me in future, even in Kampala when I go back." Hassan viewed the interview as an opportunity to share his experiences and establish friendships and contacts. He wanted to keep in touch and wrote their names and telephone numbers on a piece of paper. "You know with this disease, you have to be open," he said. "You die fast and so badly if you hide. However, my only worry is always what to eat. Even now, I haven't had breakfast. Otherwise, [I have] no other worries health-wise." He spoke freely and laughed occasionally, but at times he looked sad and worried as he told his story:

> I was born in Butaleja in 1963, one of my mother's ten children. I went to primary school in Butaleja and attended secondary school in Tororo. But I dropped out in 1981 due to lack of school fees and went to work in the rice fields in Doho. I got married in 1996 and had two children with my first wife. We separated, and I moved to Kampala in 2002, where I met my second wife; we had a child in the same year. I now have three children with her. The two children I had with my first wife live with my sister and are studying in primary school in Tororo.

Hassan talked about his job in Kampala working for a fruit drink company. "I worked in the factory boiling water and making mixtures, packaging, loading the boxes of juices and doing other manual labor," he said. "My employer was very hardworking and shrewd in business." Hassan lamented the financial consequences of his sickness: "I used to earn 70,000 shillings [about $28] a month, but now I can't work. I am just in treatment. Recently, my former employer met me in Tororo and asked me whether I will go back to work, and I just told him that I cannot work anymore."

The turning point in Hassan's life came when he developed a terrible fever and had to spend a week in the hospital. When he realized he was not improving, he asked his wife to take him back to his home district, where he could be treated at Busolwe Hospital by health workers he knew. He sent his wife back to Kampala with a promise to join her later. Hassan had planned to do some cultivation before returning to Kampala. He planted rice, but his farming was constantly interrupted by periods of hospitalization. He said,

> I was so sick, on and off, and consumed so many drugs. I had developed wounds in the mouth and skin rashes, so I thought it was wise to test my blood. I thought testing was the only solution. So I came here to see the health worker—you know, he is a good man. He told me that I would be tested, and World Vision tested me for HIV and found me to be positive. They referred me to TASO [The AIDS Support Organization] Tororo to be checked again there. They also found that I was infected. I went back home and said, "I have nothing to do since I am now infected." You see, with this disease, once you are infected, you have nothing else to do. When I learned that I was sick, I decided not to hide, or else I would just die. So I decided to get the drugs in order to have life. I have nothing to fear with this disease, because I know that once it has come, it has come.

Hassan told his father, mother, brothers, and sisters. "They were not shocked or surprised," he said. "For us, we take it just like that because we know that this disease is like *musuja* [fever or malaria]."

While Hassan was very sick, in and out of the hospital, his mother and sisters-in-law looked after him at his father's rural home in Butaleja. "At home, my mother continued to take care of me, but she is old," Hassan said. "I told her, 'Mom, you are too old. Don't bother yourself with me.' But my sisters-in-law also used to help me." He started receiving Septrin (cotrimoxazole) from TASO in July 2005 and ARVs from his local hospital in the same year. Plagued by skin rashes, he occasionally received ointment for relief. For about two weeks, he suffered side effects such as nausea, vomiting, and painful headaches from the medicine. "I know why all these sicknesses happened," he said. "I was not having a proper diet. I was alone in the house, although my sisters-in-law tried to look after me. There was no adequate food; feeding was so poor—no tea for breakfast, and even when it was there, it was black and sometimes it would lack sugar." It was around this time that Hassan decided to move to his father's house in Tororo town to stay with his lame sister. She earned money frying chips on the verandah in the evenings and welcomed him by saying, "You come and we stay here. We shall eat whatever we find."

Hassan said that when he moved to Tororo, his health improved, and he gained twenty pounds. He stopped having coughs, malaria, and diarrhea and only suffered from backaches and occasional muscle pains. "Since I went to my sister's place, feeding has improved," he said. "At least in town, there is better life; you can find what to drink. There is food, and there is a possibility of changing diet, but in the village where I was, there is no adequate or good food."

Hassan's wife used to urge him to return to Kampala, where she was still living with the children. But Hassan put her off by claiming that he did not have money for transportation. He did not want to disclose his serostatus to her when he was far away and was not sure how she would react. "I had two children before we got married, and she also had two," he said. "I want her to take the test, and it's up to her to decide what to do when I reveal to her that I am sick."

In addition, Hassan was frustrated with the lack of promised material support from TASO. "We have been made to fill out forms several times, but nothing comes," he said. "They are complicated. At some point, you hear that the forms have to be taken to Kampala; that they have not yet been signed; and so on. Now there are these so-called counselors; they are tricky and are not straightforward. Recently I talked to my counselor about blankets I had heard about, but there was no truth [to the story]. So I have given up now."

Hassan explained that he gets encouragement from reading about the history of the disease. In the 1970s and 1980s, it was "a mysterious disease," he said, and it destroyed many lives because hardly anything was known about it. "At least for the current generation, we are fortunate that the disease is known; we have organizations like TASO that help us, give us support, and you get the chance to know the problem you have." Hassan recalled how near to death he was before he started AIDS treatment. "I was really a gone man," he said. "This disease caused tremendous pain all over my body. I was so weak and had no strength at all. But now I am OK." He was proud of the improvement in his health. "When people see me now, they can't believe [it]. They ask, 'Are you the same Hassan, or is this another person?'" Hassan's health worker confirmed that he was enthusiastic about the treatment that saved his life. He even tried to recruit others. He had brought two men to hospital whom he suspected were HIV-positive. Unfortunately, Busolwe Hospital had no testing kits at the time, but Hassan persisted and took one man to Tororo for testing and the other to Mbale.

Phoebe and Godfrey's first long conversation with Hassan ended on a positive note. He praised the staff working at the AIDS clinic, some of whom he had known for years because they came from the same village in Butaleja. While he was living in Tororo town, Hassan had access to free treatment for other illnesses (coughs, fevers) from the Tororo Municipal Health Facility. The problem was the distance of 30 kilometers to the hospital in Busolwe, where he had to pick up his monthly refill of ARVs. "I just stand at the roadside and request a lift from any vehicle heading to Busolwe, be it a private or commercial vehicle," he said. "I talk to them and explain my problem, and I do the same when I am returning to Tororo." As for the ARVs, he was devoted to them. He kept them on top of a high wall where nobody, not even rats, could reach them. Wherever he went, he carried his bag with some medicine. Hassan vowed never to leave Tororo as long as he was in treatment to ensure continuity.

Four months after the first interview with Hassan, Phoebe returned to visit him at his father's house in Tororo. She hardly recognized him. Hassan was neatly dressed in a cream shirt, jeans, and black shoes without socks. His head was shaved, and he looked clean and smart. Most of all, he looked healthy—heavier and stronger. He seemed proud of the positive change in his appearance, and Phoebe marveled at his great improvement. He was very open with her, and she felt they were already friends and would continue to deepen their friendship.

There had been important changes in Hassan's life. His elderly mother had died, and his wife had come for the burial. She was also amazed by how good he looked, asking, "What are you feeding on? What has made you fat?" He replied that he was "feeding on" medicine and it had improved his life greatly. Thus, it was at his mother's funeral in February 2006 that he disclosed his serostatus to his wife and advised her to go for an HIV test. She had left Kampala and was living with her parents in their lakeside village in Mukono District. Their youngest child had been hospitalized for three weeks, and his wife had been unwell. Hassan was worried and wanted to check on his family but could not afford transportation.

Hassan's sister, who invited him to stay in Tororo and eat town food, had gone back to their father's village in Butaleja when their mother died. There she was caring for the orphaned children of their sister, along with Hassan's two children. She continued earning money by selling food but had switched from chips to boiled cow heads, a meal enjoyed by many people in Butaleja.

Hassan's younger brother and sister had come to stay with him in Tororo and study at the town's primary school. He commented that they were too old to be in the primary grades. As Phoebe sat talking with the siblings in their room, Hassan's brother was ironing his uniform and other clothes on the bed using a charcoal flat iron. A teenage boy, also a relative, walked in and out of the room, checking for something in a schoolbag that was hanging on the wall.

The building was formerly owned by Indians. Hassan's father had bought it in the early 1970s when President Idi Amin expelled Asians from Uganda. It had two front rooms facing the street that were rented out to a shop and a bar for 200,000 shillings each. In the rear of the house, where Hassan stayed, were four rental rooms that each brought in 40,000–50,000 shillings in rent. His father used the income to pay university tuition for two of Hassan's siblings and to pay school fees for other brothers and sisters. Hassan paid no rent, but also had no money. He was desperate to get a job.

In the following months, Hassan was well but somewhat withdrawn. He made it clear to Phoebe that he preferred cash to the sugar and soap she brought as gifts. She wondered whether he was still interested in being part of the study because she had so little to offer compared with AIDS organizations such as TASO. Hassan still longed to visit his family in Mukono District and to see his son, who had been discharged from the hospital, but lacked money for transportation. His wife had tested HIV-positive and started receiving ARVs from Mulago Hospital. She was working with her sister and mother smoking fish at the lakeshore.

Then things started looking up. Hassan was totally different the next time Phoebe visited him. He welcomed her warmly and was the same open, friendly person she had met at the beginning of the study. He and another man had gone into business repairing shoes. They worked on the verandah in front of his father's building, where his sister used to sell chips. One day Phoebe found Hassan sewing a big tarpaulin used to cover loads on trucks. "I am so strong that I even run," he said. "I wake up in the morning and bathe in cold water, and I no longer feel feverish. I feel so good. I have never been down with sickness, even malaria. I repair shoes and polish them and mend tarpaulins and can earn 3,000 shillings a day."

Since December 2005, he had been getting about one hundred pounds of maize meal and a four liter jerrican of cooking oil from TASO every month. "The food has helped me so much to care for my kids in Butaleja," he said. "When my wife came for my mother's burial in February, she took fifty-five pounds of meal and two bottles of cooking oil back for herself and the other children." In Tororo, Hassan shared food with his younger sister, brother, and niece. They used the meal from TASO to make porridge; in addition, their father sent them maize meal, beans, and millet flour from their rural home every two weeks.

Concerning feeding, he said, "We were told that when one is on ARVs, we must eat well of foods like maize porridge, beans, greens, cabbages, passion fruit—things that are within our means. They instructed that we must eat first before swallowing any medicine." Although the food rations from TASO were stopped after nine months, Hassan was able to eat three times a day with the money he earned repairing shoes and the food provided by his father. In the morning, he drank milk tea and ate two *mandazi* (fried buns) or chapatis before swallowing the tablets. For lunch, he ate beans and *posho* (maize meal). In the evening, he had milk tea and two chapatis for supper, after which he took his evening dose of medicine and went to sleep.

He still had plans to check on his wife and children, especially the youngest, who was sickly. The eldest child was in a free government primary school, and the second born was in a private nursery school, for which his wife paid 5,000 shillings (about $3) a month. (His father paid school fees for his other children in Butaleja.) He owned a boat with his wife, and she wanted him to contribute money so she could buy fishing nets and hire the boat out to fishermen. He wanted to see how her work was going and how she was getting medicine from Mulago. He thought he might be able to get a referral letter from his health worker to get ARVs from the health center near his wife's village or from Mulago Hospital. He said that it was not transportation that had hindered him from traveling to see his wife and children; he just did not feel strong enough to go.

He was laughing and smiling during the entire visit. "I am so strong now that I can even run," he repeated. Phoebe gave him 5,000 shillings when she left and thanked him for a very enjoyable afternoon. She mused about the change in his mood—maybe it helped that he was working and making a bit of money, along with seeing improvements in his health.

The next time Phoebe visited, Hassan told her that he had suffered a bout of malaria but had not been seriously sick. He attributed the fact that he was still alive and growing stronger to his health worker, Mwangale, who checked on him often. (Mwangale came to Tororo regularly because his family lived there.) When Hassan talked about Mwangale, he gave the impression that they were very close friends and confidants. He said that he saw Mwangale when he passed going to and from work and when he brought him medicine. "I have known Mwangale all my life," Hassan said. "It's not this disease that brought us together. I knew him before that. Mwangale's father used to own that building next to my father's."

During a period in which Phoebe was out of the country, Jenipher stopped by to have her shoe repaired and took the opportunity to catch up on Hassan's news. His plans to visit his family had finally materialized. He had discouraged his wife from coming to spend the Christmas holidays with him because transportation fees always doubled then. But he stayed with his family for two months at the beginning of 2007. Thereafter, his wife brought the children to Tororo during the school break, and Hassan gave her money to take them back to school. When his siblings and niece went back to the village for holidays, he managed to cook for himself and do household chores. Asked about his health, he said, "I am OK and taking my drugs well, with no problem. Don't you see me? I am very healthy, and I don't fall sick, not even with malaria fever. I eat well and drink a lot. I don't even think about AIDS because I realized that thinking about it affects me negatively and sometimes makes me fall sick." His CD4 count had never been taken. "For me I don't know whether we need to test for CD4. It is costly, but when I get my drugs, then why should I go for that? I weighed myself about two weeks ago, and I was almost 160 pounds, which made me feel encouraged to continue with my medicine."

CHAPTER EIGHT

Food

Michael Whyte and
Susan Reynolds Whyte

Hassan's account of his situation begins with a point that many of our inter-locutors made one way or another: the importance of food for people on ART. He was well aware that his health depended on eating well, a message that has been central to AIDS education for years. But it is also clear that eating prop-erly is a matter not merely of following nutritional advice but also of depen-dence and interdependence. Like about a quarter of our original forty-eight interlocutors, Hassan received food aid for a period from an organization of which he was a client. He relied on his sisters-in-law, father, sisters, and niece to provide and prepare food. His repeated emphasis on the superiority of "town life" reminds us that the social value of food is not just about quantity and sharing, but also about the quality and appeal of food. What to eat, where to eat, whom to feed, and how to share food are all thoroughly social matters.

Scholarly work on food security and AIDS has mainly emphasized two themes. One is the impact of the epidemic on food production, income, and household livelihoods.[1] The other is the problem of hunger for people on ART, both what it means for adherence and what it means for people's sense of rights and justice.[2] Our approach takes a different tack. We review Ugandan patterns of eating and how they were changing during the lives of the first generation. This provides the context for understanding the sociality of food access and eating within the daily life of Ugandans. We show how members of the first generation dealt with hunger and how the sharing of food pointed up solidarity and its opposite. Social relations were enacted and assessed through the medium of food and eating, and conflicts over cultural or economic resources emerged in social transactions over food—a point captured in Arjun Appadurai's term "gastropolitics."[3] This holds for people who are ill and short on food and money, as it does for others. Our assumption is that the special needs of those in treatment must be seen within more general patterns of eating and that the shifts associated with HIV nutritional awareness might be part of wider changes that were occurring in the country in the years of the first generation.

Eat a Balanced Diet

Attention to diet and nutrition have been a part of AIDS education in Uganda for a generation. Before effective medicines were available, messages about eating as well as possible were a major component of the management of AIDS. One of the main principles of "positive living" was eating a sufficient and balanced diet. That meant eating from three food groups: body-building foods (groundnuts, beans, eggs, milk, meat, fish); energy-giving foods (cassava, maize flour, plantains, rice, millet, potatoes); and protective foods (fruit and vegetables). The AIDS Control Program advised that one could choose inexpensive local foods and still eat from each group at every meal.[4] The concept of food groups was taught in school and sometimes as part of general health education for mothers and children, so it was not new. But with the advent of AIDS it took on clinical significance as part of the package that would allow people to live longer.

The AIDS Support Organization was a pioneer in supporting nutrition for HIV-positive people. From 2002 on, it combined food relief for them and up to five members of their households with instruction in hygiene, nutrition, and food preparation. Although it provided mainly maize and soybean meal and vegetable oil, TASO reported that its clients were able to eat a more varied diet, presumably because the money they would have spent on meal and cooking oil could be spent on other food items.[5]

The advent of ART cemented the link between diet and management of HIV. Guidelines from the Ministry of Health encouraged people on ART to eat a sufficient amount—actually, to increase the amount of food and frequency of meals. For many, eating enough was a daily concern because their appetites returned in force once they were established in treatment. When they were sick, they did not feel like eating, and most had lost weight. Once they began to feel better, they were hungry and regained their lost pounds. This common experience, also reported from tuberculosis treatment programs, gives rise to the widespread perception that "the drugs give appetite"—or, as William put it, "the tablets ask for food all the time." Jackie (case VI) said that when she started on ARVs, her daughter began taking food from her friends in class. Especially during the first months on ART, people wanted maize or millet porridge because it was cheap, easy to prepare, filling, and recommended by health workers as nutritious (particularly millet porridge). William, a construction worker, said he woke up to eat in the middle of the night and always had a thermos of millet porridge with him. But later his appetite normalized somewhat, and now he does not even want millet porridge.

In addition to eating plenty, people on ART need to eat a varied, balanced diet that includes items from the three food groups. Many of our interlocutors mentioned advice they had been given by health workers about how to eat well, and they often repeated the phrase "a balanced diet." But what exactly is a balanced diet? When people recalled more specifically what had been recommended as good food for those on ART, they named vegetables, fruits, eggs, milk, and starch staples. Porridge was good, especially when pounded groundnuts or sesame were added. They recounted the advice:

> They tell us to eat maize meal, sweet potatoes, cassava, millet, greens like *dodo* [a leafy vegetable like spinach], cabbages, eggplants, *mukene* [small dried fish], eggs, milk, and porridge.

> I was told to eat papaya, guavas, *dodo* or other greens, eggs, and milk.

> You don't have to eat meat. You can eat things like avocados, eggs, greens. Some greens have like blood in them.

> I was told to take good drinks like milk, millet porridge, passion fruit juice.

> I am advised to take a lot of energy-giving foods, fruits, and a lot of greens. I am supposed to have fruit juice before breakfast.

Eating a balanced diet seems to mean eating a variety of food items. Diversity always includes comestibles that must be purchased, even though the principle is that readily available local food is sufficient.

There is one more dimension that ART added to the relation between food and treatment: health workers told people to take their medicine with food, every day, always. The first combination therapies comprised many different ARV pills. The JCRC, an early provider of ARVs, explained in a pamphlet titled

"Basic Facts about ART": "Some ART drugs must be taken when the stomach is empty, but others only after eating some food."[6] However, for our interlocutors, most of whom were taking Triomune in the morning and the evening, the requirement was simple: take your medicine with food at twelve-hour intervals.

Other studies have shown that many Ugandans with HIV, including those on ART, have difficulty following these guidelines. Interviews with 133 women in Jinja living with HIV (of whom 18 percent were on ART) revealed that while nearly all had been trained in nutrition and thought it was important to consume a balanced diet, only 22 percent had eaten at least three meals on the previous day. Just 52 percent could correctly define good nutrition, and only 40 percent were regarded as having eaten an adequately varied diet on the previous day. Those receiving food aid were the most likely to consume three meals and to have eaten a diversified diet.[7] Another, more qualitative interview study with forty-seven people attending AIDS treatment programs in Mbarara and Kampala explored the ways in which food insecurity was a barrier to sustained ART adherence. The researchers defined food insecurity as "the limited or uncertain availability of nutritionally adequate, safe foods or the inability to acquire personally acceptable foods in socially acceptable ways." Under these terms, a large proportion of their respondents were considered food insecure, whether or not they adhered to their medicine. Many ate only once or twice a day, and even more were not able to eat the kinds of food they wanted, such as fish, chicken, or meat. Having to buy food competed with other needs, and the requirement to eat a balanced diet was onerous to the extent that some people hesitated even to start ART. Since ARVs increased appetite, and many people reported side effects if they took their tablets without food, some said they skipped doses if they had nothing to eat. Interestingly, the examples people gave of missing their medication because they lacked something to eat concerned the morning dose, a point not discussed by the researchers.[8]

While our interlocutors also were keen on following the advice to take their medicine with food, quite a few remarked that they just took the tablets with water when they had nothing to eat. The majority also reported that they could not afford to buy the varieties of food items they would have liked to eat, but that is true of most Ugandans. The medical advice merely put their poverty into sharper relief. It was clear that eating patterns changed over time, as people returned to better health, the seasons changed, and household economies shifted. Most of all, it was evident that the relation between food and

ART needs to be understood against the background of Ugandan concepts and values around food and the sociality of eating within and beyond the immediate household.

Commodification in Eating Patterns

While the nutritionists recommend that a meal be composed of items from three food groups, most Ugandans consider a proper meal as consisting of elements from two categories. In both rural eastern Uganda and in town, a meal consists of "food" and "vegetables." "Food" and "veg" are the common Ugandan English glosses marking the widespread linguistic contrast between a starchy staple and a sauce into which one dips a portion of the staple. It is the "foods"—starchy and bulky—that are considered the principal and essential component of the meal and the basis for sound nutrition.

"Foods" may include stiff porridge made from ground millet, sorghum, or maize, as well as boiled potatoes or boiled cassava, steamed plantain bananas, or boiled rice. Uganda differs from Kenya, Tanzania, and the countries of southern Africa, where maize porridge is almost universally served; rural and urban Ugandans prefer to vary "foods" whenever possible.[9] "Vegetables" can be simple boiled greens or beans or more elaborate dishes made on a base of cowpeas, sesame, or groundnuts to which mushrooms, smoked fish, and other delicacies may be added. "Veg" as a category also includes fish, chicken, or meat; these are particularly prized and ideally served to special guests. But many families go for months without eating these dishes because they are expensive (with the exception of the small dried fish called *mukene*). This form of meal is repeated once or twice a day, every day, especially in the countryside.

In addition to proper meals, people take porridge (which is drunk) and tea with "escorts" (groundnuts, eggs, roasted maize, cassava, or plantain), and they eat snacks such as fruit, grilled or fried meat and chicken (*muchomo*), or the starchy items sold in trading centers, markets, and town streets. These include the chapatis and chips that figured in Hassan's account, fried buns (*mandazi*), fried cassava pieces, and a host of other oily, tasty "bites."

Subsistence farming remains important in this predominantly rural country, and home-grown food and veg are valued for consumption and as gifts. Yet the commodification of food is evident in several ways that are relevant for people on ART. Even the rural informants who grew much of their own food and veg had to buy some items that they produced in insufficient amounts or not at all. Obviously, this included items that are only produced commercially, such as cooking oil, salt, sugar, and tea leaves. But nowadays, money is also needed for milk and eggs, which many rural homes used to produce themselves. Most homes served sweetened milk tea when we first lived in eastern Uganda in 1970; now "dry tea," without milk (and sometimes without sugar), is most common. Rural diets are strongly seasonal, with hungry periods before the harvest and times when some items are in short supply. Seasonality can be countered with cash, but many do not have money to spend on staples or veg that are out of season.

For people living in urban and semi-urban areas, proper meals consist of purchased ingredients (though many get some food supplies from rural relatives, as Hassan did). They are also confronted with a wide array of prepared food for sale. When Hassan complains, "In the village where I was, there is no adequate or good food," he is not speaking about hunger but, rather, about choice and availability. Hassan had spent years in the Kampala region and at a lakeside fishing community. In both contexts, commodity foods are part and parcel of modern life.[10] For Hassan, village food, like village social life, represents if not failure, then at least an unappealing lifestyle. Although he joined his ART program in the countryside, he quickly took up residence in a nearby town. There he was able to "consume chapatis and drink tea with milk at any time"; his niece prepared "Ugandan food" (beans and *posho*), a meal that conforms to the food-plus-veg structure, although maize and beans are not traditional in his rural homeland. With this diet, Hassan marks his "urban" identification and his ability, despite his HIV, to continue a "modern" lifestyle.

Commodity foods, like Hassan's beloved chapatis and other snacks, have been enjoyed for generations. What is new is the elaboration of choices, which is clearly linked to increasing urbanization and the number of consumers. Informal economies have expanded greatly, and there are more Ugandans subsisting wholly or partly on cash incomes in cities and towns, and even in rural trading centers. Not only snacks but also plates of food and veg (ready-to-eat cooked meals) are available, even in rural trading centers.[11] Commodity cooked food was relevant to our interlocutors as producers and as consumers. As producers, some women earned cash by selling prepared food; as consumers, our interlocutors appreciated the convenience and economy of "fast food." For people like John (case VII), who traveled and worked at odd times, chapatis were a cheap and easy way to fill the stomach, although he pointed out that they were not a meal. James said that while he was living a bachelor life with his male cousins, snacks sometimes substituted for a meal. Street food is also survival food, a significant part of the daily diet of the urban and peri-urban poor.[12]

When rural people talk about the tasty fare that epitomizes eating well, they seem to have in mind food items that have to be bought: milk and sugar for tea, meat, chicken, fresh or smoked fish, and eggs. In eastern Uganda, people sometimes speak of "soft food," which seems to mean matooke (cooking plantains) and Irish potatoes rather than the standard millet and maize porridge. Cooking oil adds to the taste of veg and makes a meal—or a snack—more satisfying. Newer vegs such as cabbage, tomatoes, eggplants, carrots, and onions are not so commonly grown and must be purchased. Chapatis, buns, and bread made from wheat flour are welcome, even if they are not really food. Passion fruit juice is widely considered ideal for sick people, and many of our interlocutors mentioned that they wanted to be able to drink it. But few people grow passion fruit, and even if one does, sugar is needed to make the juice. Once when David gave Hanifa cash for transportation, she smiled and said, "Now I have got passion fruit." All in all, eating a "balanced diet" or eating a varied diet with some tasty items requires money. As Elizabeth, a nurse, summed it up, "I would want to eat a balanced diet, but money was not there because of paying rent and children's school fees."

The advice to take ARVs with food at twelve-hour intervals seems to assume that people eat breakfast at 7 or 8 AM and dinner twelve hours later. Yet in rural Uganda, and even in towns, many people go to work on an empty stomach and take porridge or tea at ten or eleven. Having breakfast earlier requires making an extra effort, including lighting a fire, and breaking the routine. It also requires the ingredients. Cold leftover food from the night before is often eaten along with tea or porridge, but both of those beverages should be sweetened with sugar. (The maize and soybean meal provided as food aid was appreciated for porridge because the soy made it a bit sweet.) MamaGirl (case IV) explained the problems she and her co-wife had with breakfast after their food aid was stopped: "we could not afford having breakfast every day. These days, we try to have millet porridge and at times tea, though not always. I can say the whole experience of trying to provide breakfast for the family is not easy. At least for other meals like lunch and supper, you look around and you will have something. The problem with breakfast is that you have to buy things like sugar and at times some accompaniment. Yet in our situation we do not have the money." Even taking the evening dose with food could be a problem, because dinner is not necessarily served at regular times in most Ugandan households. One informant said she saved leftovers from lunch to eat with her evening medicine, because dinner usually came very late.

In this situation, being able to eat enough, to eat a "balanced diet," and to eat at the right time depends on other people, not only on oneself. Making a special effort for the person on ART shows care and concern; not doing so may be taken as evidence of neglect.[13] The sociality and morality that characterizes the production, preparation, and sharing of food in general is brought into sharp focus with the advent of ART.

Gastropolitics

For our first generation, meals and the quest for food were practical contexts for expressing solidarity and belonging—and for marking individual desires and conflicts. We heard about, and observed, the everyday practice of sharing resources in today's Uganda, where providing food and eating together are both an entitlement and an expression of personal concern and attention, and sharing is both a value and a tactic.[14] Sharing food is about caring, as both practice and metaphor. Our ART clients had experienced different degrees of illness and need; many were very ill before and at the outset of treatment, when they were almost totally dependent on others to provide and prepare meals. Even later, during recovery, eating and feeding are about care as well as calories and quality as well as quantity, where quality stands for love and concern.

Several of our interlocutors said that family members in other households provided special or soft food for them because they were on treatment. Dominic (case XI) was living on the produce cultivated by his wife. "We have millet, maize, sweet potatoes, groundnuts and greens," he said. "But I want to eat special things like matooke, rice, meat, and juice that I cannot afford. Sometimes my father gives me some little money when he has it." Harriet, a forty-five-year-old widow, underlined the concern of her brothers and children. They had brought her from her rural home to the small town of Busolwe so they could look after her. Like Hassan, she appreciated the greater variety of edibles in the more urban setting. Where she used to eat mainly millet, sweet potatoes, greens, and beans in the village, she could partake of "softer" food such as matooke and rice and more interesting vegs such as fish, cabbage, and tomatoes, all of which could be bought in Busolwe. She said that her brothers and children gave her money and sugar. "I just see them bringing passion fruit and pineapples," she said. "When they give me some little money, I use it to buy passion fruit juice. They have taken good care of me." Two of our interlocutors, Alice (case V) and Jolly (case IX), were fortunate to have parents with the wherewithal to ensure that they ate very well. Jolly thanked God that her parents were working abroad and sent her money by Western Union every week so she could buy good food, including such special items as eggs, powdered milk, and liver. Few had these luxuries, but the underlying point holds more generally that comestible gifts were taken as indications of affection.

The daily household routines of acquiring, preparing, and sharing food were complicated. Although it is ideally based on gender and age complementarity, the household can be an arena for conflict as well as cooperation. This is especially the case when cultivation or production fails, when food stocks are poorly managed, and when cash inputs are lacking. Such conflicts are even more fraught when the domestic group itself has been stressed by migration, illness, or death. Then food-supply issues may come to express underlying conflicts about gender roles and kinship entitlements, amity, and enmity. As we followed people for a year and a half, we saw the play of gastropolitics as the everyday tensions of household relations were worked through in the idiom of food.

The ideal of sharing within the household was the measure against which people praised and criticized one another. Yet sharing meant that it was difficult for one person to eat special food alone, unless, like Hassan, he or she bought a ready-made snack on the street. Women on ART who were caring for children were explicit about this. Joyce (case I) explained, "Providing for the family is my responsibility, and sometimes we don't have enough, yet we are supposed to eat well. So when I don't have money, I do without breakfast, or when there is little money, you have to sacrifice. You can't eat good things alone. You can't eat when the children are there watching or when the sister is watching. Sometimes I have managed to get an egg, but how can I eat it alone? So I can't buy an egg for me alone. I feel bad to buy things for myself alone."

A special diet for someone on ART requires a kind of individualization that goes against the requirement to share food and, especially, to feed children. Like Joyce, MamaGirl had reflected on this problem. "Regarding special care for me?" she said, "Nothing really. In these circumstances, you can't achieve it. How can you prioritize yourself with so many young children around? I find it difficult, and people here, including my mother-in-law, would not take it lightly that I am preparing special meals for myself alone. I would appear to be selfish." But she also pointed out that one person in the family saw her as an individual with unique needs: "my niece, the daughter of my late brother-in-law, sometimes tries to be sensitive to my needs. Whenever she returns for the school holidays, she tries to ensure that I don't sacrifice everything for the children. She talks to me about it and knows that I require things like fruit, enough drink and food for my health. She sometimes tries on her own to prepare some juice for me, and pumpkins. This girl is the only person in this home whom I have seen directly concerned about special feeding for me. The rest take it for granted."

Men on ART were sensitive to their wives' attentiveness as expressed in food preparation. In the home of Ivan, a rural trader, gastropolitics were played out among his sister, mother, and wife. He claimed that his mother, who had a house in the same compound, was difficult and neither gave nor received food from them. He praised his sister, who used to stay in the home, as the only person who supported him by providing something to eat in the morning when he had to swallow his ARVs. Both his sister and his mother criticized his wife harshly for not feeding him properly, but Ivan was more circumspect about his HIV-positive wife. During Jenipher's last visit, he said, "I admit I am not looking well. I don't eat well, and sometimes I don't eat because my wife is busy and sometimes she is not around and it's only my sister who tries to prepare food for me. But I have my mother here, who is also a problem. Life is very difficult. No juice, no porridge, bad food. Where would I get things to give me energy?"

Gastropolitics involve relations among households, as well as within them. When close relatives have houses in the same compound, they sometimes share food as one household, and at other times they maintain separate arrangements. As we saw in the case of MamaGirl and MamaBoy, widows living in the homestead of their deceased husband, conflicts with their brothers-in-law were often phrased in terms of food. (MamaGirl remembered as a gesture of reconciliation that one brother-in-law had bought her a soda and cake when he met her at the trading center.) They sometimes shared meals with their mother-in-law, and when their kitchen collapsed, they began to cook in hers and thus merged the two households. This exacerbated tensions with the old woman's sons, because they thought the co-widows were eating their mother's food. Their example also reminds us that people on ART are not just dependent on others to provide and cook food; as they gain strength, they also cultivate, cook, and affirm relationships by sharing food.

Food Aid for People on ART

Nine of the twenty-three people we followed closely received food aid for at least some time after they started on ART. They mentioned five different organizations that supplied food: TASO, Uganda Red Cross, World Vision, Plan International, and World Food Program. The rations and amounts were slightly different and even seemed to vary within a single program over time. But basically, the rations consisted of some combination of maize meal, soy flour or soybeans, rice, cooking oil, and sugar. Reach Out Mbuya also gave out beans or peas. Everyone who received food aid contributed it to the common household pot. Hassan even sent some to his children who were being cared for by his sister in the village and gave TASO meal and oil to his wife to take back for the children who were staying with her. MamaGirl remarked that the TASO food had to be shared with many orphans at home. It was for everyone in the entire family so a hundred pounds of maize meal could not last until the end of the month. She liked it for morning porridge and dreaded the day when the food aid would come to an end.

No one—probably not even the suppliers of food aid—considered it wrong that food items were shared within a household. In fact, some programs determined the amounts they gave according to the number of mouths in the household. It was widely recognized that people do not eat alone and that those who feed a sick person need to eat, as well. Moreover, those who are sick need to feed their children. A few of our interlocutors mentioned that some recipients sold a portion of their food aid; Cathy, a university-educated widow in Kampala, was planning to buy soy flour from other clients when her own entitlement ended. Given the general commodification of food and the constant shortage of cash, it did not seem unreasonable to her that some clients might be in less need of food than of money—for example, to buy veg. What did offend was the one case we came across of appropriating an entitlement and not allowing the legitimate client to benefit from food aid at all. Dominic's stepmother had asked for his TASO card, promising to fetch his food rations for him. But she never brought anything and never returned the card in all the time Jenipher followed Dominic. When he mentioned this to his health worker, who told the stepmother to return the card, the stepmother sent Dominic beans, maize meal, and sugar ("Maybe as a bribe so I would not report her," he said) but still did not return the card. What really bothered Dominic was that although his stepmother had wrongly acquired another card from a friend who was registering people for TASO, she continued to cheat her own stepson out of his food aid.

When free items are distributed to particular target groups, it is often the case that everyone wants some, because, as people say, "We are all poor here." Ivan, the rural trader and leading member of the local Post-Test Club, laughed as he explained how difficult it was to deal with food distribution. The NGO Plan International usually cooked food for the children of Post-Test Club members on Thursdays. "But my friend, you need to be there on Thursday," Ivan said. "My God! Every member brings all the children from the family, even from the whole clan. Even old people want to eat, though the food is supposed to be only for the children. But I talked to one of the people in the Plan office on how best they could supply this food. Otherwise, it was going to bring problems. People hate you, saying you do not want them to eat, even people you expect to understand. But what I have seen—on things related to food, no one is a gentleman."

The striking thing, however, was that most food distributions did proceed in an organized manner.[15] Order was imposed. Indeed, Ivan's point was that he had suggested a way to organize the chaos, even though he expected some people to hate him for restricting access to the food. Although there were a few cheaters, like Dominic's stepmother, the greatest proportion of food aid by far did benefit the people who were entitled to it and the households on which they were dependent. Everyone who received the aid appreciated it, although they pointed out that it was not enough. Nor did the items provided constitute a meal, since there was no veg (except in the rare cases in which beans were supplied). The food aid was a supplement that was especially valued for the maize or soybean meal that enabled hungry people to drink porridge.

In the early 1990s, when AIDS programs were largely limited to "material support" of one kind or another, programs for HIV-positive people often included food and other items like blankets and mosquito nets. Counselors as well as clients spoke about this kind of support in terms of an implicit contract: people "cannot test and receive nothing," they told us.[16] However, the advent of ART programs has changed the nature of the "contract." Whereas simply being HIV-positive was a sufficient ticket to food support at the time when it was understood as a ticket to the grave, entitlements these days depend on more biologically nuanced criteria. Food aid is initially offered to those whose CD4 counts or clinical signs qualify them to start on ART. As people gain weight and strength, and as their CD4 counts increase, they lose food entitlements, regardless of their social and economic situations. Our interlocutors seemed to accept the reasonableness of these assessments of the individual body, even though, as we have seen, they did not consume the food aid alone, and their households might still be in need. Several explained that food aid was for the weak, and their health was now much better than that of clients just starting on ART.

Many programs take a narrowly biological view of people suffering from HIV; for the most part, food aid is offered more as an adjunct to medical treatment than as a contribution to easing general subsistence problems. Researchers point out that families perceive food aid in a broader economic and political context, focusing on the insufficiency of food rations, the competition for food, and feelings of injustice that clients experience, given this medicial approach to survival. Frontline health workers experience dilemmas, knowing the difficulties of feeding a family in conditions of dire poverty.[17] Concerns about insufficient food aid are particularly keen for those initiating ART and for people in urban settings, where all food must be purchased. Taking the perspective of everyday sociality puts food aid in another light. The rations allow the clients to contribute to their households and families, which sustain and must be sustained every day, even after food aid comes to an end.

Eating Well

The messages about eating properly while on ART focus on the biological individual at the expense of a broader understanding of food and eating as elements of social relationships. Yet access to food, and to a variety of foodstuffs, is an integral aspect of sociality. The virtue of giving food and sharing food ensured that people who were weak received something to eat, even when they were unable to produce or cook themselves. The emphasis on sharing also made it difficult for people in large and poor households to have the special feeding recommended for those on ART. There was a tension between individual needs and the commonality of household eating. Yet it seems that the ART messages may have contributed some new terms to the vocabulary of food and eating. Some people did insist on the individualization of eating. To make a special effort for the dietary needs of someone on ART was a way to show a particular individual recognition and care. It also said something about the enlightened nature of the one who engaged in such recognition.

The dietary advice that has been so central in the response to AIDS came at a time in Ugandan history when food was increasingly becoming a commodity. More and more, comestibles were being purchased, whether as ingredients for home-cooked meals or as prepared snacks or ready-made meals sold by the plate. The commodification of food was especially pronounced in urban areas, of course, but it had become widespread in rural regions, too, as fewer households were able to produce most of their own food. Money to buy food items allowed greater choice. Eating a balanced diet, in the sense of eating a varied diet, came to be associated with buying power and with a more urban kind of life. People on ART were advised to eat well for their health, but eating well was conflated with eating "soft" food, more cosmopolitan food items, the diverse commodities that money can buy. In the long run, the focus on healthy eating in connection with ART probably contributes to a more general awareness of diet that is evident in the emerging consciousness about "lifestyle diseases."[18] It has also contributed to the growing conviction that you cannot eat well without money.

The food aid that is so important an entitlement of clientship in treatment programs and certain NGO activities was greatly valued. Taking a longer-term historical perspective, these foods, delivered by trucks in sacks, drums, and boxes, are visible imports, packaged and produced elsewhere. The food items and distribution mechanisms strengthen the trend toward the commoditization of food that was already in process. From the point of view of individuals and families, food aid provided a welcome supplement during a brief period when a recovering patient experienced the most intense hunger pangs. It was never sufficient to make a proper meal, and it certainly was not enough to sustain a person, much less a household. That required sociality beyond relations to a clinic or to an NGO.

Notes

1. De Waal and Whiteside, "New Variant Famine"; Barnett and Blaikie, *AIDS in Africa*; Barnett and Whiteside, *AIDS in the Twenty-First Century*, 238–61; Baro and Deubel, "Persistent Hunger."

2. Hardon et al., "Hunger, Waiting Time and Transport Costs"; Weiser et al., "Food Insecurity as a Barrier to Sustained Antiretroviral Therapy Adherence in Uganda"; Kalofonos, "All I Eat Is ARVs."

3. Appadurai, "Gastro-Politics in Hindu South Asia," 495.

4. AIDS Control Program et al., *Living with AIDS in the Community*, 38.

5. H. W. K. Muzoora, A. G. Coutinho, and A. Mugume, "Mitigation of HIV/AIDS through Nutrition: The Taso-Uganda Experience," poster exhibition at the Fifteenth International AIDS Conference, Bangkok, July 11 to July 16, 2004.

6. Joint Clinical Research Centre, "Basic Facts about Antiretroviral Therapy (ART)," 15.

7. Bukusuba et al., "Nutritional Knowledge, Attitudes and Practices of Women Living with HIV in Eastern Uganda."

8. Weiser et al., "Food Insecurity as a Barrier to Sustained Antiretroviral Therapy Adherence in Uganda," 2.

9. M. Whyte, "Social and Cultural Contexts of Food Production in Uganda and Kenya."

10. Beuving, "Playing Pool along the Shores of Lake Victoria."

11. M. Whyte and Kyaddondo, "We Are Not Eating Our Own Food Here."

12. Elizabeth Namazzi, "Living on Sh1,000 a Day in Kampala," *New Vision*, October 13, 2007.

13. Meinert et al., "Faces of Globalization," 107–11.

14. Appadurai, "Gastro-Politics in Hindu South Asia"; Holtzman, "Politics and Gastropolitics."

15. S. Whyte et al., "Health Workers Entangled."

16. M. Whyte, "Talking about AIDS."

17. Kalofonos, "All I Eat Is ARVs"; Prince, "HIV and the Moral Economy of Survival in an East African City."

18. S. Whyte, "The Publics of the New Public Health."

CASE IX

Jolly

APPEARANCES AND
NUMBERS

Jenipher Twebaze and
Susan Reynolds Whyte

BODIES

(overleaf)

ART clients are weighed
at each clinic visit.

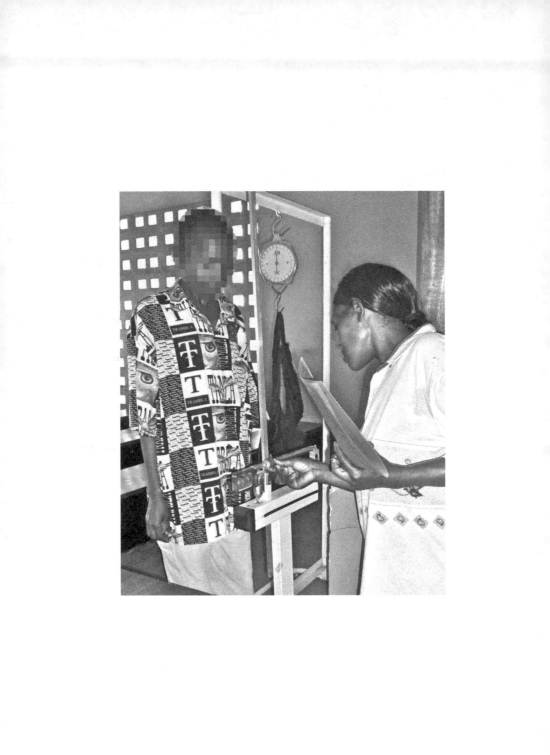

Jolly was attractive, and she knew it. During Jenipher's first meeting with her, Jolly recalled how she turned men's heads. "I used to look nice, and men really disturbed me," she said. But at thirty-four, looking back, she seemed to distance herself from the smart, pretty girl she had been. "You know, those years we were growing up and enjoying life and money," she said. "When you are young and beautiful, everybody saying you are beautiful, you are just vulnerable to men. I was full of myself; I had *kyejjo* [impertinence, stubbornness, insolence, conceit]. I was feeling great, but now . . ." She touched her cheek wistfully. She was still good-looking and took care with her appearance, but Jolly now felt that life was passing her by. Although she had had so many admirers, she was not married and, most important, had not yet borne a child.

The first time they met, Jolly and Jenipher talked for hours; by the end of the meeting, Jenipher felt as if they were already close friends. Half way through the meeting, Jolly suddenly paused and said, "But Madam, am I telling you what you want to hear, or am I going too far? What do you want to do with this information?" Jenipher explained the purpose of the project once more, and Jolly continued, "You seem to be a trustworthy person, and I will not hide anything from you. But don't laugh at me. I was naive and vulnerable."

Jolly grew up in Kampala, the second of eight children, in a family of comfortable means, a working class family with jobs and regular salaries. Her parents were employed abroad by the time Jenipher got to know Jolly, and her brothers and sisters were well educated and had good jobs. While Jolly managed to complete secondary school, she said that she had never been serious about books. She worked for three years as a tea girl and cleaner at a European embassy, then for seven years at an up-market restaurant in Kampala.

In her early affairs, Jolly said, she had always been careful, using condoms without fail. When she met a man who was very strict and insisted they go for HIV testing, she was not even worried about the results. She tested negative, and they continued to use condoms. Then she met a stout young man, Boxer. Her family did not approve of him, but she was fascinated, even though he had a child and despite evidence that he was seeing other women. ("His behavior was bad, but his looks were good," Jolly said.) For two years, Jolly and Boxer used condoms, until he persuaded her that they did not need to continue because they loved each other and planned to marry. Jolly allowed herself to be convinced and accepted "live" sex.

Boxer told Jolly that the mother of his child had given birth to a second child. This annoyed Jolly, but he assured her that he did not love the other woman and did not know how it had happened. After four months, the child died. Jolly asked what had caused the death, and Boxer decided to be tested for HIV. He found that he was HIV-positive. "He called me home and told me about the results," Jolly said. "I felt very cold. I felt *ensisi* [shock, dread]. I quarreled with him and asked him how he could tell me such news after stopping me from using condoms. It was June 1999." She repeated many times that she felt cold when she received the bad news. "I saw a death trap and felt that even if I prayed to God, this was the end of the world," she said. "I blamed myself. I got scared and decided to stay with Boxer for fear of staying alone, and I felt that he was the only one who knew about my problem. I feared to go and test again." She kept reflecting on her "vulnerability and naïveté" throughout the discussion.

Boxer developed *kisippi*, the belt of herpes zoster, then meningitis and repeated bouts of fever. Jolly feared asking about symptoms of HIV because she did not want to learn about them; she was too frightened. She was also afraid to leave Boxer because he was tough and slept with a gun under his pillow. They did separate once, but she returned to him. She conceived but had a miscarriage. Finally, they split up for good. Then life became boring and frustrating; Jolly had no one with whom to share her problem, and she kept checking her body for changes.

Soon she met and fell in love with a new man, Ali. He was different from Boxer—well-mannered, educated, and from a good family. Unlike Boxer, who threatened to beat her if she insisted on using condoms, Ali always had many condoms at home. Moreover, Jolly found bras and panties in his bedroom. On several occasions, women knocked on his door late at night when Jolly was with him. "But anyway, he was handsome," Jolly remarked as an explanation of Ali's active sex life. He had a child who was staying with his grandmother, and Jolly thought that Ali might not be sick because his child was still living at four years old. She later took over responsibility for this child, taking it to stay with one of her relatives and paying school fees.

Jolly and Ali were together for four years, then Jolly obtained a visa to go to Europe, where she got a job as a maid. With distance, she realized that Ali had used her for sex, enjoying relations with other women while they were together. Yet she still sent him money and continued to support his child, hoping to keep him. At the same time, she dated several new men, explaining that dating meant having protected sex.

To avoid being a "paperless" immigrant, Jolly was advised to acquire a

United Nations card showing registration as a refugee; this card eventually saved her life. Within a year of going to Europe, she said, she started to feel so weak that she did not even want to attend parties. She developed a painful swelling in her armpit and a terrible fever, for which she sought help at the United Nations clinic, where her card entitled her to free treatment. "You know, those people do not know some diseases," she said. "They learn about them in books but have never experienced them. Doctors liked me so much because they used to bring students to learn from me about my swelling in the armpit. In Africa, we rarely test for things like diabetes. But in Europe, they tested for each and every thing on my body, including HIV. One of the doctors used force to draw blood out of me, and I did not like it." After about three hours, the doctor returned and sent Jolly in an ambulance directly to the hospital. She was put on an intravenous (IV) drip and told to call a relative because she was badly off. She cried and asked what the problem was, but she was not told. Deep inside, she suspected that she was HIV-positive, but she did not want to hear the truth. It was not until she saw the word "AIDS" written on her IV drip bottle that her suspicions were confirmed. "I tell you, I will never forget that day," she said.

Jolly kept quiet for about three weeks until she gained courage to ask about her CD4 count. The doctor told her that it had been only 2 when she was rushed to the hospital, but it had risen to 64 and was improving. She remained in the hospital for several months. "My dear, I had many diseases," she said. "I had tuberculosis and a fungal infection. I recovered from those, but I was very weak. You know, 'slim' is a psychological disease. But I became strong and started eating and drinking well so I could gain energy and start working. I was later given Kaletra and Combivir for HIV, and my CD4 improved to 200. But they used to measure the viral load all the time, though they did not say anything to me until I asked. The swelling in the armpit was operated on and removed."

When Jolly regained her strength, her parents and aunts urged her to return to Uganda. She had told her sisters about her illness, and she asked them to come alone to pick her up from the airport because she was very weak. Above all, she begged them not to tell her boyfriend. "When I arrived, my sisters were there to welcome me, and they all started crying when they saw me," she said. "I was very thin. But I encouraged them that I was going to be fine. They suggested that I go straight to TASO [The AIDS Support Organization]. I reached home and found two of my brothers who had stayed to prepare something for me to eat. People at home really cared about me so much. I don't know how I can even thank them. I weighed 38 kilograms

[85 pounds]. They bought me repellants and a mosquito net so I wouldn't suffer from malaria, and they got me local herbal medicine in small jerricans (*budomola*), which I kept taking with the medicine I had brought from Europe." Jolly started eating garlic and *nkejje* (small fish), which her aunt bought for her.

One of her aunts had a friend who suggested that Jolly should be tested by the Infectious Diseases Institute (IDI) at Mulago National Referral Hospital, which provided free treatment. That is where she became a client. "I don't know how I can thank this government and God," she said. "Otherwise, for us, we would be dead by now." She was advised to eat well, and she started spending about 70,000 shillings [about $38] per week on fruit, sweet potatoes, pumpkin, powdered milk, porridge, and eggs. She received money from her parents every Friday. From the bank, she would go straight to Nakasero market to buy food.

Jolly slowly adjusted to her new life. "Our neighbors are primitive, because one time they saw me and started rumor-mongering, saying I was sick and looking like an old woman," she said. "I kept quiet because it is [just] a question of time for [misfortune to strike] everybody—[even] your son or daughter. You don't have to laugh at [ridicule] anybody as long as you live. Another side effect of this medicine is that I get annoyed or stressed or anxious very fast, but after some time, I settle [down]. My relatives are now used to me, and LTV [a Christian television channel] has helped me so much because they broadcast encouraging programs. You feel that there is life after death."

About four months after she returned to Kampala, Jolly finally got in touch with Ali. She said,

I was feeling better, though still weak and not looking very good. I was scared and worried about what he was going to say when he saw me. My brothers advised me not to go out with him because I might be tempted to drink alcohol when I am not supposed to. They told me to invite [Ali] home. He came the next day and greeted me with great surprise, wondering what had happened to me, and we all started crying. One of my brothers was there and tried to give us courage. We sat, and I told the whole story. He said to me, "Jolly, I loved you, and I will continue loving you. I will not hate you." I could not believe what I was hearing.

Ali kept visiting Jolly and said he was sure they were both sick and needed to support each other. Jolly suggested that they go together for HIV testing, but he initially refused. "I got confused," she said. "He says he still loves me, but he refused to test. I don't want to kill him." She kept pestering him until he agreed. "We went together, and I was the one talking for him," she said. "He was so worried, not talking and sweating." After thirty minutes, they were told that Ali was HIV-negative, but Jolly had the virus. In disbelief Ali stood up and asked the counselor to bring the right results, Jolly recounted. "My dear, everyone wants to be AIDS-free. I saw my boyfriend gaining energy in a second. Someone who could not talk or say anything, I saw light in his face. I was happy for him, because I knew I was the problem. I never minded but expressed joy for him."

As Jenipher ended the first visit, Jolly rounded off her account of life so far. She really wanted a child but was not sure that her boyfriend would agree. They were not having unprotected sex but were moving in that direction. She did not want to infect him and had heard about a fertility clinic in Kampala that could "put a man's sperm into a woman," as she phrased it. Her doctor had advised her not to get pregnant until her CD4 count reached at least 900. "I have a million-dollar question for Ali: will he agree to have a child with me?"

When Jenipher returned for the second visit, Jolly looked good, though she remarked that she had developed a small rash on her arms and around the neck. Always concerned about her body, she suspected her new jewelry had caused the rash. During a later visit, Jenipher accompanied Jolly to her new workplace. She had started operating a canteen at a school owned by her family. Jolly sounded happy and busy. "My dear, I am there trying hard to survive and not to think that I am sick," she said. "Don't you see I have put on weight?" However, she said that Ali was neglecting her: "I miss having a boyfriend. My friend cares, yes, but he does not give me enough time."

Jenipher asked Jolly about her health, and she said, with confidence and happiness, "I am doing well. My CD4 is 357, and they have told me to eat well so I avoid falling sick. The only problem I have is people asking me why I don't have a child, and that disturbs me a lot. I think I am growing old. I don't see anyone who can accept having a child with me, so I don't know." Jenipher asked Jolly whether she had put the "million-dollar question" to her boyfriend, and she said she feared mentioning it when she knows that she is sick and he is not. "I actually asked my doctor, who told me that she will let me know when I can have a child, and I am patient," Jolly answered. "But when people keep asking you, they take you back [remind you]."

About two months after Jenipher's first visit to Jolly's place, she came to see Jenipher in her office with some disturbing news. She had run into her old boyfriend Boxer, who had begged for forgiveness. He proposed that they live a "positive life" together and have children. Jolly knew her family disliked

Boxer and did not follow this up, but she was upset. "It is now some time since I met him, about two weeks," she said, "but I have checked my CD4, and it is 305. It has reduced! My counselor asked me what the problem is, and I feared to explain to her, but when I went to see a doctor, he mentioned that I could be having worries and most likely about relationships. He asked me whether I have a boyfriend, and I deceived him [and said] that I have one. [The doctor] told me that I should tell [the boyfriend] to give me more time."

Jenipher's next visit occurred a couple of months later, after Jolly had again been to the hospital. "My CD4 count was 330 last month, but now it is 307," she said. "They have told me I am worried about something and, I think it is this issue of the baby. I want to have a baby, I am growing old, and I was told that when one goes beyond forty, it is difficult to have a child. If my mother managed to produce eight of us, why can't I have at least one kid?" Jolly's determination on this point was evident. She had discussed it with her counselor, who advised her to bring Ali in so she could explain to both of them about the decreased danger of infection when a person has been on antiretroviral therapy (ART) for some time. Jolly had also visited a private fertility clinic to learn about assisted conception and obtained a promise from a sister working abroad to pay for the treatment.

Yet these plans did not come to fruition during the time Jenipher followed Jolly. Her boyfriend started doing business in South Africa, and she embarked on a one-year course in catering and home management. "I am OK and now weigh 68 kilograms [150 pounds], and I am going to pick up my CD4 results," she said. " I don't know what I have. I got these skin patches because I used an expired soap that almost brought me problems, but I got treatment from a private clinic and I am improving." During Jenipher's last visit, Jolly looked happy and very chic. Smiling, she announced,

I went to check my CD4 count, and I [am at] 452. I felt so happy and thought, "I could now have a baby!" I am waiting for my boyfriend, who is in South Africa, to tell him about it and see whether he will agree. He told me he will come back in November to visit me, and I will wait for his word. I no longer get worried, like you have been telling me, and it has helped me. I have come to realize that AIDS is not the only killer. You can die of anything. The only problem [with HIV] is that you live rather an uncertain life.

CHAPTER NINE

Bodies

Susan Reynolds Whyte,
Lotte Meinert, and
Hanne O. Mogensen

Jolly was preoccupied with her body—more so than most of the people whose lives we followed. Yet all of them, to some extent, shared her concerns. It seems obvious that bodies should be a central theme in life with ART. Infection with HIV is an assault on the body, and treatment brings alleviation and a return to strength. But to say this is to leave unexamined the question of what the body *is* for the first generation and how understanding and experiencing it has changed as a consequence of living with ART.

Many distinguished scholars in anthropology and sociology have underscored that bodies have multiple dimensions and can be studied from different perspectives. Mary Douglas wrote about the two bodies—the physical and the social—arguing that society shapes the way we imbue the body with significance. Margaret Lock and Nancy Scheper-Hughes proposed a threefold research agenda for what they called "the mindful body" encompassing perspectives on an individual experiencing body, a social symbolic body, and a body politic—that is, a physical body regulated by political means. John O'Neill traced perspectives on the world's body, social bodies, the body politic, consumer bodies, and medical bodies. Annemarie Mol showed how different knowledge practices in the same hospital generated multiple bodies.[1] Keeping to the concerns of the first generation and in the interest of simplicity, we will make an analytical distinction between the lived body and the measured body.

The lived body is the locus of experience, the structure through which our world comes into being as we attend to people and things through our senses, our limbs, our cognition. The lived body is also eminently social in that we are always both experiencing subjects and objects for others with whom we interact as bodies. Their gazes, their responses to our embodied selves, are part of our experience as subjects. Jolly was worried and pained by her symptoms, but she was also keenly aware of how she looked to others, such as her sisters and her boyfriend. Erving Goffman, whose term "stigma" has become so popular in discussions of AIDS, conceived stigmata first and foremost as marks on the body that in some way were discrediting in the eyes of others.[2]

What the medical treatment of HIV has introduced to this lived body is a set of seemingly objective measures and procedures for determining serostatus, and monitoring weight, CD4 counts, and viral loads. These are key indicators for medical professionals, who relate them to scientific knowledge about biology and pathology; the measured body is founded in a biomedical position and clinical practice. But the measures take on significance for those who are living the bodies under treatment. People relate test results and measures to their social situations and possibilities. The outcomes become indications of the directions their lives might take. Jolly perceived her CD4 values as hopeful or not for her life project of having a baby. Thus, measurements come to take on relevance for the lived body that goes far beyond the medical significance they have inscribed as writing in a client's file.

Symptoms

Most of the time, we take the lived body for granted. You have and are a body that is oriented beyond itself. As the philosopher Drew Leder writes, "One's own body is rarely the thematic object of experience."[3] Of course, you tend to your body and may even adorn and enjoy it, as Jolly did, but mostly you take it for granted. It is when discomfort is extreme or persistent that we become unpleasantly aware of our bodies. As Leder terms it, the body "dys-appears." That is, the body appears in a negative way to our consciousness rather than disappearing as we go about our business.[4] In the era of AIDS, the "dys-appearance" of the body through prolonged or characteristic symptoms is worrying to the extent of seeming fateful. Jolly said she did not even want to know the typical symptoms of HIV because she was so afraid she might develop them. Yet in the Ugandan context, certain symptoms—recurring diarrhea, weight loss, skin rash—are known to everyone as likely indicators of infection.

In recounting their stories, many of our interlocutors said that their bodies began to insist on attention. Some had repeated bouts of indeterminate sickness that resembled the fevers often assumed to be malaria. Alice (case V) said, "I used to get constant sicknesses, not very clear, sometimes malaria, then they said I had a problem with my salivary glands." Rosette remembered, "I started suffering on and off from malaria and also had a cough." Matayo, a health professional, recounted, "In 2004, I fell sick and could not easily identify clearly what I was suffering from. But I was presenting with chest pain, ulcers, and some swellings, as though [I had an] allergy." Some, such as Dorothy, Norah, and Julia, were first diagnosed with tuberculosis but continued to be sick despite TB treatment. Grace was found to have diabetes and thought that was the reason for her weight loss. But diabetes treatment did not resolve her problems and later she tested positive for HIV. Others remembered a single focal point of pain rather than indefinite fevers and weakness. It was the swelling in Jolly's armpit that sent her to the clinic where she finally had an HIV test, after avoiding it for so long. James got a terrible pain in his knee, and his thigh swelled so much that he could hardly walk. At the clinic, blood was taken for an HIV test.

For almost everyone, the body also became dysfunctional to some extent in that they lost strength. It was not just blemishes in appearance or pain that pushed the lived body into unpleasant awareness. As we saw in chapter 7, weakness and the inability to work had far-reaching social implications.

Once they started treatment, most people reported a diminution of symptoms. As chapter 10 shows, they often went through a period of side effects as their bodies adjusted to the powerful medicine. Some continued to have various symptoms, even after they had been on treatment for months, and it was hard to know whether they were due to HIV infection, the ARVs, other conditions such as diabetes or high blood pressure, or merely the common illnesses that affect everyone. Ivan had been in treatment for more than two years and was much better, but he still found that his body made itself unpleasantly noticeable from time to time. "You know, AIDS is funny," he said. "It comes in many ways. Today you may develop a running stomach; the next day, body itching; another time, vomiting; and another day, you are OK. Or the whole day you are OK, and in the evening you start shaking. Like now, I have pain in the legs and I don't know why. And my wife feels very cold at night and during the day, she is OK. It is a funny situation, but I am OK, and I appreciate ARVs." For Ivan, as for many others, bodily discomfort—the "dysappearance" of the body—was a reminder of being HIV-positive. Aside from the dis-ease of symptoms, they indicated a life situation that could be ameliorated but not fundamentally changed.

Appearances

Much as people reported their own experiences of discomfort and pain and alleviation, they were equally preoccupied with how changing bodies presented to others. "Dysappearance" was not only about how people became distressingly aware of their own bodies, but also about how their bodies appeared negatively to others and how they read the sick signs on the bodies of their partners and children. As they improved with medication, they were keen to note how their looks impressed others. Bodies revealed sickness and health, without any words being said. The eloquence of bodily "dysappearance" renders the simple question of intentional disclosure superfluous in many cases.[5]

Many health workers to whom we spoke said that the figures of current patients were generally less grim looking than had been the case before ART became widely available. Because people tested earlier and started in treatment, it was less common to see the emaciated skeletons of feeble people in advanced stages of AIDS. Among our informants were people who had started treatment in time, and their appearance did not suggest their serostatus. Yet there were still those, such as Jolly, whose bodies had wasted drastically before the ARVs took effect. Their appearances spoke to others without any words being said.

Robinah (case I) hardly had to tell people about her illness. By the time she decided to take the HIV test, they were already pointing fingers at her. Whenever she went to funerals, church, and other gatherings, people stared in dismay. This helped her in that she was already used to being seen as HIV-positive, so disclosing was not a major problem. "Before I started ARVs, I did not look human," she said. "My hair had mostly gone, and the little that was left had become brown; my body, too, was untouchable and looked terrible. Only a few daring people would come near me and associate with me. But all this has now changed. People seem to say, 'So this is a real person, a person like us.' Now many people know about my status, including my children, and they appreciate me like that." Even those who previously would not touch Robinah have dropped their negative attitude.

We found ourselves noticing the marks of sickness on people's bodies and taking pleasure with them when signs of recovery appeared. In notes from her first meeting with Juma, Phoebe wrote:

> Juma is a tall Kenyan, aged 37 years, but the sickness has made him look older. He looked so frail and very weak, had spots all over the body, and had lost almost all his hair. The remaining hair was very scanty and grey in color like that of an old man. He really looked as if he was just recovering from some serious sickness that has made him walk with difficulty.

The entry written three months later read:

> Juma looked totally different, very strong, had really put on weight and I am sure we would have missed him if we had met him on the way. The rash scars on his body were disappearing except he looked much darker than the first time we saw him and his hair had started growing and it is curly and some of it is gray. Juma was happy to see us; he greeted us, shook our hands, and said proudly that he had come to make sure that we saw how healthy he looked!

The heft and robustness of the body were perhaps the most revealing aspects of appearance.

As time goes on, the shape of the body is also being read in another way. Those who have been on ART for years experience a redistribution of body fat, known to medical professionals as "lipodystrophy." Anna, who had been on ARVs for a decade, noticed the changes in her body. She explained to Lotte that she easily recognized others who had been on the medicine for a long time by their sunken cheeks, skinny limbs, and potbellies. Presumably, this will come to mark the appearance of more and more people and will be read by the first generation, just as "slimming" reveals untreated HIV.

Skin, the visible surface of the body that we present to our fellows, was a concern for many. Marks on the skin took the form of rashes. Some appeared with the onset of HIV, and others were apparently reactions to medicine. Sores on the lips and in the nostrils were also obvious blemishes on the body surface. The most distinctive marks were the painful stripes of raised blisters called kisippi, meaning "belt" in Luganda. Kisippi was so well known as an indication of HIV that it could be considered a stigma in the original sense of the term: a bodily sign cut or burned into the flesh that exposes something unusual and bad about the moral status of the bearer.[6] Jessica remembered how her husband's illness first manifested itself and how he tried to deny the evidence. "He started showing the signs, like herpes," she said, pointing to three parts of the body where he had rashes. "During those days, he would be deceiving us that it was spiders—the kind of spiders that burn your skin and make it peel off."

All kinds of rashes could be socially painful. Jessica stopped selling food items when she was very sick because, her health worker said, she felt uncomfortable selling groceries with skin rashes all over her body; she used to scratch herself a lot. MamaGirl (case IV) recalled that her biggest problem was skin rashes. For two years before and one year after she started ART, she had "too many rashes," she said. She showed Godfrey dark scars on her arms and legs, which were still visible five years later. Goretti raised her dress to show black spots that remained from a severe skin rash and sores she had suffered. Antiretroviral therapy helped enormously, but she sometimes still got a funny rash on her face and chest and had to buy cream for it.

Women more than men seemed to be bothered by the skin blemishes (although Juma showed Phoebe a small bottle of medicine he had bought to remove the marks left by his rashes). Hanifa was explicit about how much she disliked rashes:

I had herpes zoster three times before I started ARVs. In 1996, I got a rash, and I went to check for syphilis. It tested positive, and I got treatment. The syphilis went, but the rash stayed. So I went to Swissgarde [a South African firm that sells nutritional supplements] and bought some medicine from there at 18,000 [shillings]. They are vitamins but good. When you take them, you feel improvement in your life/health (obulamu). I was starting to develop herpes in 2000 on the right leg, but one of my friends told me about medicine, which I used before it got severe. It came back in 2001, and it was starting on my face. I used the same medicine, and it went away, leaving only a small scar on my lower lip. Usually when I get a problem, I write down the medicine I have used to treat it with, so when it comes next time, I just go and buy it. But before the third time with herpes, I had developed TB, and I was put on an eight-month treatment. Just as I was finishing the dose in 2003, the kisippi also came. I was in Rwanda, and it came again, around the chest. This time I thought, 'Let me leave this disease to come out [lufulume].' Maybe previously I had been suppressing it and not letting it out; maybe that is why it kept coming back. This time I didn't apply anything except painkillers. I let it come, and see here. [She opened her blouse to show scars on the left side of her chest.]

Recently I wanted to use [a] Swissgarde product, because my hair was not looking good, and found it cost 28,000 shillings. I didn't buy it because I did not have the money. I don't want to have any health problem. At home I was nicknamed "Kakelenda" [Tablet]—any slightest ailment, I seek treatment. What I hate most is a skin rash; the rest, like those inside the body, I can tolerate, but not a skin rash. Even if it is a small rash, I would rather go hungry and buy a tube of ointment to remove it.

Once when David called Hanifa, she did not want to meet him. She had a headache on one side and sounded frustrated. She had developed a pimple in one of her nostrils, which made one side of her face swollen. "I hate myself now," she said. "Here I am looking like a funny insect—you just can't recognize I am the usual Hanifa." From previous interactions with her, David knew she was sensitive about her skin. Hanifa, like others, used concealment tactics when her body stubbornly showed the stigmata of HIV and the side effects of treatment. Keeping out of sight, wearing clothing that covered arms and legs, or using creams were common.[7] Such tactics of information control and presentation of self were part of Goffman's framework for understanding stigma.

But it is important to remember another of Goffman's central points about stigma: it must be seen in terms of social relations. An attribute is not discrediting in itself, always and for everyone. In some relationships, it does not detract from the moral value of the person and does not require hiding or denial. On the contrary, it may evoke concern and sympathy. Benjamin described how he had been weakening and losing weight. "When my wife and sister came from Busia to visit, they found that I was not doing well and were shocked at how I looked," he said. "My wife said I didn't look the same anymore." When he shared his suspicions about the illness with his wife, she insisted that he go for an HIV test and get treatment if he needed it. When Joyce came to see Robinah and found she had lost weight, had skin rashes and long nails, and was eating alone, she immediately started caring for her by giving her a bath, cutting her nails, and eating with her. What were discrediting signs to some family members were reasons for Joyce to care for her sister.

The Measured Body

While experienced symptoms and concerns about appearance have long been part of living with grave illness, the members of the first generation have appropriated new ways of understanding bodies. Biomedical technology for testing and monitoring treatment has added new dimensions to bodily experience for everyone, although in different ways, depending on treatment programs and levels of education. Everyone had to take an HIV test, and all were regularly weighed. At the time of our study, CD4 counts to measure the strength of the immune system were standard in many programs, but not, for example, in the Ministry of Health rollout at Busolwe Hospital. Tests of viral loads, which measure the amount of HIV in the bloodstream, were expensive and much rarer; most patients were not familiar with viral load measures.

The HIV test itself, a simple procedure that gives a digital answer—yes or no—was mentioned by all as decisive in how they interpreted their symptoms. In other areas of health care, diagnostic tests are also known: people have their blood tested for malaria parasites or hemoglobin levels, their sputum tested for tuberculosis, and their feces tested for microbes. But only the HIV test is strictly required and ceremonious. The way people are asked whether they are ready for it, the obligatory counseling, the portentous announcement of results: all of these aspects make it exceptional and lend it an authority that no other test has. They also contribute to the sense that the test unveils the hidden truth about the body. It was evident that for most of our interlocutors, receiving the finding that they were HIV-positive was taken as a fateful revelation. Even those who already had strong suspicions credited the test with the authority to confirm the reality of their fears. The body measured by the lab test became a dimension of the lived body. When people told others what the test had shown, the result entered into the intersubjective relations they had with those others. And, of course, the laboratory truth has other social consequences in that a positive HIV test is the necessary ticket for admission to programs for treatment and other benefits, and thereby for changing social relations as well as the body. With so much riding on the outcome, it is not surprising that the majority of our interlocutors confirmed their positive test by testing again somewhere else, often at their own initiative, but sometimes at the behest of a treatment program that retested new clients as a matter of course.

Nearly everyone mentioned their weight when talking about changes in their bodies. Very few people in Uganda have scales at home, so following changes in one's weight is not routine. People might weigh themselves at health units; urbanites can pay a bit to stand on scales placed on sidewalks by small-time entrepreneurs; country people weigh themselves on the hanging scale at the mill where they take their grain to be ground.[8] But members of the first generation were weighed regularly when they attended the HIV clinic, and they adopted those numbers as a way to talk about the directions their bodies and lives were taking. This was facilitated by the fact that for some programs, at least, body weight was noted in the papers that clients kept.

The very first time Phoebe met Jessica, she showed the weight recordings in her TASO notebook: 52 kilograms (115 pounds) on 11 May; 48 kilos

(105 pounds) on 13 July. During Phoebe's final visit, Jessica declared that she would have died by now without treatment. "I started ARVs on 19 August 2005," she said, "and that time when I weighed myself, I was only 23 kilograms [50 pounds]! Now look at me. When I tell others that I am positive, they can't believe and they say I am deceiving them." Suzan (case III) said, "Even the weight—it had been 54 kilos [120 pounds] at the test in Mengo and reduced to 48 kilos [105 pounds], but after that treatment, it went to 50, then 54. Now I weigh 63 kilos [138 pounds]. It makes me love this treatment. I have seen the improvement, and I can't miss even a day."

Many people had experienced dramatic weight loss before or just after starting treatment. Saddam (case II) thought he was bewitched when his weight went from 105 to 88 pounds. Rosette went from 190 to 100 pounds; William, from 158 to 123 pounds. Like Jessica and Suzan, most put on weight under ART. Joseph reported that when he started treatment, he had weighed 80 pounds; two years later, he weighed 120 pounds. But once they were focused on body weight as a measure of improvement, people worried when the scales showed loss. They related diminishing weight to episodes of sickness and concomitant loss of appetite, to overwork, or to worries. William had been gaining on treatment but lost a few pounds when he fell sick with malaria. "When you get any disease, you deteriorate back to the level where you were before starting on ARVs," he said. For William, as for many, changes in weight indicated possible changes in the direction of health.

Although the numbers provided a concrete and systematic way to register differences, a scale was not really necessary to recognize changes in body size. The relationship between pounds and appearance was evident. This was not true of the relation between bodily appearance and CD4 counts, the other common method of monitoring the progress of HIV. A few people reported that they had no visible signs of HIV infection yet were found to have very low CD4 counts. When Rachel's husband (see case X) finally had his CD4 checked, it was 50. The doctors could not believe it, he said, and thought they had made a mistake. "I had never been sick," he said. "I was not weak. I had been working." Thus, CD4 counts were not directly related to apparent symptoms. Looking ill did not necessarily indicate that things were going badly, either. Remember that when Saddam seemed poorly during one visit, he challenged Phoebe to check the CD4 count in his file. He was convinced he was improving.

Even though most Ugandans did not monitor their weight, it was a known measure of health, whereas CD4 counts represented a new value that came into public awareness together with the rollout of ART. Health workers explain CD4 as a count of the *askaris*, or guards, in the blood that protect against sickness. The more askaris one has, the safer and stronger the body. Many learned that ART was started when the CD4 count fell to 200 (or, in some programs, 250). Nearly everyone remembered what his or her CD4 was the first time it was checked, and everyone noted changes with keen interest. The numerical trend was taken as an indication of the development of their disease. Though abstract, CD4 counts tended to have an authoritative status that surpassed even people's own lived bodily experiences. It was as if CD4 monitored the true state of the body. It confirmed that the treatment really was working, even though the medicine had side effects and various symptoms emerged from time to time.

Although doctors explained CD4 counts in terms of the body's defenses, our informants related it to their social and existential situations.[9] The rise in values as they undertook treatment gave them hope, which they shared with others. Husbands and wives often knew each other's CD4 counts. Once when Jenipher arrived at Herbert's place, his wife said he had been wanting to see her to share the good news about his recent CD4 test. "I had never been happy like I was when I got my results," he told Jenipher. "My CD4 count is 525. I am now OK and doing well." Juma remembered that when he first tested, his CD4 count was 1. "Even the technicians could not believe that I was still alive," he said. He immediately noted that his wife was tested at the same time and had a CD4 of 314. After six months on ART, his count rose to 100. But as Phoebe followed him, his wife's count fell steadily, and she confided her worries about losing weight although she was not sick. When her count reached 198, she was advised to start ART.

People compared their current numbers with their earlier ones and with those of others they knew, and took the measure of their social well-being. They appropriated the numbers, including the authority of biomedicine, which was linked to these objectifying and quantifying devices. In this numbering process, people were able to contribute added significance to the worries and hopes they were living. As "symbolic forms," numbers became a way of apprehending the body. At first glance, they seemed to formulate sickness from a materialist and individualizing perspective.[10] But the way people used quantification was never so simple. Turning numerical information into relevant knowledge about oneself was fundamentally a relational act.[11] It was as relational agents in a life-world that people used the numbers.

Like Jolly, whose hopes for a baby were linked to her CD4 count, people looked forward to the social possibilities opened by a positive trend in their CD4 numbers. But they also linked the numbers and their social lives in another way, when they explained numerical changes in terms of their relations to others. Counselors and health workers seemed to encourage this kind of interpretation, as when Jolly's doctor asked her about her boyfriend when her CD4 value fell. Robinah and her sister Joyce were very keen on trends in CD4 tests. Joyce explained how she started on ART some years after testing positive: "My CD4 had fallen to 163 down from 360 and I was very upset. I had high CD4 and did not expect it to fall so rapidly. Maybe because of too much work—I have been too busy and was psychologically unsettled. I had a problem because my daughter [Robinah's daughter] conceived yet she was still in school. I think this is why my CD4 started falling so fast." Worries and problems were blamed for declines in CD4 counts, both before and after starting on ART.

The notion of the measured body raises a very particular set of issues in relation to HIV. While most symptoms of the lived body are very evident to the self and to others, certain measured qualities are not. First and foremost, the presence of the virus in the body is not manifest in the early phases of the disease. We remember a poster from the 1990s showing pictures of many different kinds of people, young and old, male and female, prosperous and poor. The caption read: "can you tell which one is HIV positive?" It was an effective reminder that you just do not know by looking. In those days, it did become evident as people's health declined. Nowadays with ART the question of whether you can tell takes on new relevance. Many of our interlocutors rejoiced that they now looked so good that no one would guess. As Alice remarked proudly: "I look better even than those who are not sick!" Those who had been reduced to bones and rashes recounted with satisfaction the reactions of their families and friends to their re-won appearance of health and vitality. "Are you really the same one who was so sick?" Only the results from the HIV test and the CD4 measures told a different truth. The stigmata were no longer apparent and it was thus possible to "pass" as a perfectly healthy normal person. People regained latitude in respect of whether to reveal their positive status or not, because their bodies no longer spoke about it. They could choose to disregard the "confessional imperative" in some situations and tell or imply details about their health to selected people.[12]

Embodied Sociality

Of all the topics of concern to the first generation, bodies might be the most individual. Waves of nausea, cramps of diarrhea, and incessant itching of the skin are all sensations of the individual body. Pain and exhaustion are felt by individuals. The relief of being able to sleep, the pleasure of a returning appetite, and the growing strength of a body on the mend are likewise individual experiences. Biomedicine reinforces the individual delimitation of bodies almost by definition. Testing blood, examining signs, giving medication, and monitoring outcome are focused on single bodies. But people were not preoccupied with the experience of their own bodies. In important ways, they embodied sociality.

People did recount their symptoms, but they did not dwell on them. They described changes in their bodies, for the better or the worse, but very often these were told in terms of what they meant for the ability to act and interact. In chapter 7 on Work, we have seen how strength and weakness of the body were important because they affected the extent to which people could be "useful" in sustaining themselves and caring for others. Even the pleasure of enjoying re-found energy took on a social dimension, as Phoebe noted when she talked to Hassan (case VIII) on the sidewalk, where a group of boys were passing the time. With a happy smile, Hassan reported that he was in very good health: "I even go to the football [soccer] pitch, where I play football and run races." The boys found his delight highly amusing; he seemed to them to be bragging. Hassan's returning strength allowed him to play football with others, and even the way he spoke about it evoked a response from his companions.

The sociality of bodies extends to bodily care. The "technologies of the self" about which Michel Foucault wrote are often taken to be matters of individual self-discipline.[13] People did develop disciplines of taking their medicine, trying to eat well, getting enough rest, and treating symptoms as they developed. Yet most took care of their bodies with the help of others. As we saw in chapter 8 and as chapter 10 shows, people often emphasized that others helped them to eat well and remember to take their tablets. Even in relation to the problems that are thought to cause CD4 counts to drop, several informants said that they had been advised not to worry—as if the friendly counsel of a health worker or relative could really help deflect gloomy thoughts and persistent anxiety.

The state of the body reflects intersubjective experience and our involvement with others. Herbert Muyinda, who worked with disabled people in Uganda, used the term "embodied sociality" to capture the way that the disabled body incarnates social relations. Those who were cared for and who had been able to establish relations with relevant nongovernmental organizations extended their bodily competences through assistive devices.[14] In the same way, people on ART who receive affection, good food, attention to health problems, and medical treatment embody the relations they have with others. Embodied sociality means that the fate of the physical body reflects the social relations in which it is embedded.

Measurement and Health Consciousness

In many Ugandan languages, the same word denotes health and life. People infer from others' bodily appearance information about their general well-being, as well as about their biological health status. Corpulence suggests prosperity; cleanliness and neat hair reveal discipline; smooth, glossy skin indicates care (and the ability to buy skin-lubricating products). In the time of AIDS, people learned to read bodies for disease. Slimness was no longer necessarily an indication of poverty. Moreover, they learned that appearance did not always reveal health.

The widespread use of measuring techniques, from HIV tests to regular monitoring of weight and CD4 counts, seemed to contribute to a separation of health from life and well-being. Health increasingly became something to be objectified and quantified. The new techniques differed from the well-known tests for malaria, anemia, and venereal infections not only in that HIV testing was so momentous, but also in that a positive test led on to a whole regime of systematic measuring. The first generation developed a new consciousness of health as something to be made visible by continuous revelations of hidden technical information and meticulous quantification of the body's weight. In this respect, the response to the AIDS epidemic may be preparing the way for interventions against other, increasingly common chronic conditions, such as hypertension and diabetes. Like HIV, those conditions are initially treated only after a positive test—not symptomatically, as is often the case with malaria and respiratory infection. Ideally, they should also be monitored by lifelong regular measurement of blood pressure, glucose level, and weight.

Health is being quantified in clinical practice, and numbers are recorded in journals kept at treatment facilities. But the separation of health from general well-being is not maintained in everyday life. The "values" that are measured in blood are always contextualized in terms of the values of social life. As the next epidemic of chronic "lifestyle" diseases unfolds, this is not likely to change.

Notes

1. Douglas, *Natural Symbols*; Lock and Scheper-Hughes, "The Mindful Body"; O'Neill, *Five Bodies*; Mol, *The Body Multiple*.

2. Goffman, *Stigma*.

3. Leder, *The Absent Body*, 1.

4. Leder, *The Absent Body*, 84.

5. Hardon and Posel, "Secrecy as Embodied Practice."

6. Goffman, *Stigma*, 1.

7. Kyakuwa and Hardon, "Concealment Tactics among HIV-Positive Nurses in Uganda."

8. S. Whyte, "The Publics of the New Public Health."

9. Meinert et al., "Tests for Life Chances."

10. Good, "The Narrative Representation of Illness," 83, 87.

11. Konrad, *Narrating the New Predictive Genetics*, 85–86.

12. Hardon and Posel, "Secrecy as Embodied Practice."

13. Foucault, "Technologies of the Self."

14. Muyinda, "Limbs and Lives."

CASE X

Rachel

BUCKETS OF
MEDICINE

Susan Reynolds Whyte
and David Kyaddondo

MEDICINE

(overleaf)

Antiretroviral tablets
hung up at home,
out of children's reach.

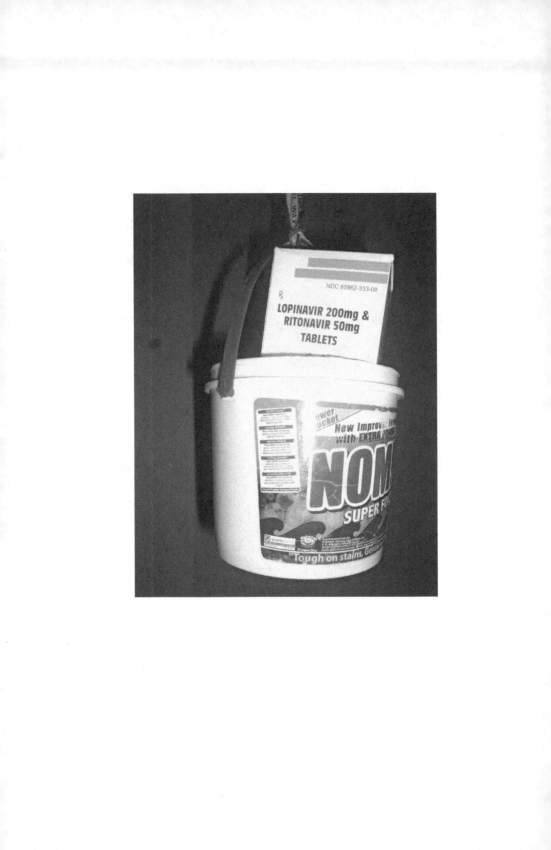

On a narrow alley in Kampala, in a rather new one-story building, Rachel and her husband, Steven, rented two rooms. The sitting room was bare except for wooden benches and stools; there was also a television monitor and a music system. Chalked on the wall were the words: "To avoid corruption please pay cash with your order." As David and Susan sat conversing with Rachel and Steven in the late afternoon, customers came by for small jerricans of waragi, the popular home-distilled alcoholic spirits, also known as *enguli* or *kasese*. Steven gestured toward the neighboring buildings and laughed: "the whole place is a bar." Men sat on the foundation shelf of an unfinished building across the way, chatting and enjoying their drinks with pieces of pork fried by an enterprising woman in the next house. A few doors away, people were gathered around a pot on the verandah sucking warm millet beer through long straws.

Rachel and Steven were from eastern Uganda and had many people from their home area in this part of Kampala. Steven's brother lived nearby; he was receiving antiretroviral therapy (ART) from the nongovernmental organization (NGO) Reach Out Mbuya, and when Rachel fell sick with an illness that refused to respond to treatment, he took her to Mbuya Catholic church for testing. A few months later, he found these rooms so they could move into the Mbuya catchment area, where Rachel would be eligible for treatment. Two of Steven's adult brothers came to stay with them. His sister, who worked in a blanket factory, lived close enough to stop by every evening after work.

Rachel was twenty-six years old and had completed four years of secondary school, followed by a two-year secretarial course, although she had never had a paid job. Steven was an electrician and had worked for several construction companies. They had a son, who was five. Rachel was not as talkative as others, but she was open and self-confident, expressing no grief or bitterness about their situation. She recounted what had happened after she tested positive in May 2005.

She was started on Septrin. When a blood test revealed that her CD4 count was 84, she was advised to begin taking antiretroviral medicine (ARVs). First she went to "study ARVs" at the Mbuya church—that is, she attended three counseling sessions with a doctor about how to take the medicine. "I signed, and they started giving ARVs," Rachel said. "There is a form they give clients to sign. You go with someone who will help you to take the medicine properly. I went with my husband's sister. She comes to check every day—

sometimes she watches me take the medicine, sometimes she just asks. The CATTS [Community AIDS and TB Treatment Supporter] comes every Sunday and counts the tablets remaining."

When David and Susan first met Rachel in December 2005, she had been taking Triomune for three months. "When I started the medicine, the skin rashes increased," she said. "I had headache and felt like vomiting. But I was getting improvement. The diarrhea went away. Even the weight—I used to weigh 60 kilograms [132 pounds] before I fell sick. I went down to 54 [120 pounds], now I'm up to 59 [130 pounds]. I started eating well. Sometimes I have a headache, but if I take Panadol, it goes away. Now only the skin rash is disturbing me, but not as before."

Asked how she keeps her medicine, Rachel said that she stores it in a small bucket hung high up in the bedroom so their child cannot reach it. We wondered whether the child understood that his mother was sick, and Rachel explained about a second bucket: "he sees me taking medicine, but he doesn't know the sickness. But he takes medicine, too. He has been sickly since he was born. He was tested at Mulago in September. He doesn't know which sickness he has, but he knows he has to take medicine because he falls sick. His medicine is separate. For his there is another bucket." Steven interjected, "You can't get the medicine mixed up. If the child gets the medicine for an adult, it's bad."

Then Rachel revealed that Steven also had tested HIV-positive. That was the reason the Reach Out staff had advised them to take their child for testing. Steven took up the story. His chest X-ray was OK, but a blood test in September showed a CD4 count of 50. "The doctors couldn't believe it," he said. "They thought it was a mistake, because I have never been sick. I'm not weak. I've been working." We asked why he had not yet started on medication and he explained that he sometimes gets called for work away from Kampala. "But I'm supposed to start," he said. "Yesterday I went to study ARVs, but they weren't there. I'm supposed to go on Monday. Soon we will have a third bucket."

When David called again six months later, he learned from Rachel that Steven's health had failed soon after the first visit. Despite the support from Reach Out Mbuya, the financial burden had been heavy. At first his illness seemed like malaria, with joint pains and vomiting. A nearby private clinic put Steven on a drip at home, and the couple bought medicine. The total bill was 35,000 shillings [about $19]. The Reach Out staff suspected tuberculosis, and Steven started on TB drugs but stopped again after further tests ruled that out. Then he got swellings on his neck (Rachel later speculated that they might have been side effects of the ARVs). Reach Out referred him to a private clinic in another part of Kampala and covered the cost of transportation and surgery. A sample sent to Mulago showed that the swelling was not cancer. But then swelling on the other side of his neck needed to be opened, and this time Reach Out said the couple had to pay themselves. They chose a less expensive clinic nearby, where they were charged 30,000 shillings. Steven had not been able to work, and Rachel raised the money by borrowing and using the capital from her waragi business. But at least Steven was improving and the swellings had disappeared.

Three buckets for medicine now hung in the bedroom. Rachel took her ARVs at 9 AM and 9 PM. Steven and their son took their medicine at 7 AM and 7 PM, because the child had to go to school and Steven left early for work. "It's me who usually reminds them," Rachel said. "For me, I can't forget, although when I am busy I may delay by maybe thirty minutes. And the child is now getting used to it. When evening comes he reminds me about the drugs." Because she and Steven had both been on the ARVs for more than six months, the CATTS were no longer monitoring them.

Subsequent visits in September and October 2006 revealed that the family drug regimen had become complicated. The child received medicine from a different program from his parents, which always presented challenges. When he was first tested, Reach Out Mbuya did not treat children younger than twelve, although that had changed by the second half of 2006. He was enrolled in a three-year research project at the Mulago National Referral Hospital's Pediatric Infectious Diseases Clinic. He was given medicine for three weeks at a time, but if he fell sick between visits, his mother took him there for treatment. The clinic gave soybean flour and refunded transportation costs at 3,000 shillings [about $1.50] per visit, an important consideration. When Rachel applied to the Reach Out program for help with her son's school fees, she was turned down because he was not receiving medicine from that program. By that time she could have switched him. She regarded the medications for children available at Reach Out and Mulago as equally good but felt that her son should remain in the Mulago program because he had only completed one of the three years on the research project. So she continued to spend a day every three weeks traveling across town to the hospital and waiting for her son's turn to be examined and given the next supply of drugs.

Keeping Steven provided with ARVs proved to be a much greater challenge once he grew strong enough to go back to work. His employer obtained a contract in Juba, southern Sudan, to work on a large public building. Like many Ugandans at the time, Steven was attracted by the opportunities and the high wages, even though the journey was long and there was always fear that conflict might erupt again. The problem was that Reach Out supplied medicine for one month at a time, which was the amount Rachel received. In special cases, it would provide two months' worth, but as a staff member told David, the program did not want to give larger amounts because it wanted clients to come in for health checkups and to ensure that people were taking their medicine properly. Steven explained, "They want to see me; they want to know if I am healthy. I look healthy, but they want to see me. The doctor checks and asks you, 'Are you OK? Do you have any complaints?' If you say how you feel, they may ask you to go and check the CD4. But coming here from Juba costs 100,000 shillings [about $55], which is very expensive. And the company can only give you transportation after three or four months."

The journey between Juba and Kampala was not only expensive; it was also dangerous. Steven talked about a time he had been in a bus that went out of control and overturned three times. People died, and Steven suffered a severe wound to his right arm. "I thought the bus had been ambushed and ran to the bush," he said. "When soldiers ran after me, I thought they were chasing me. They caught me and started tying my wounded arm, and I boxed them, saying I would also fight. Later I realized that the whole bus was full of blood. Then I surrendered my hand to be tied. They took me to the International Air Ambulance (IAA) hospital—it has a branch there. The medical fee was 900,000 shillings [about $493], and the company paid." If Steven had been traveling on his own—for instance, to pick up medicine in Kampala—he would have had to pay his own expenses for treatment after the accident.

Steven said that he calls Reach Out Mbuya when he cannot come home from Juba to fetch his ARVs and asks the program to give Rachel the supply so she can send it to him. The NGO's staff is not happy about it but has allowed her to send him a further one-month supply as he finishes the two-month supply he took with him. Rachel explained that she packs the tablets carefully in an envelope and gives them to Steven's boss. The boss, who flies to Juba, then calls Steven into his office and hands the envelope directly to him. The Sudanese authorities are strict about bringing medicine into the country, Steven explained. "There is even a time when they were arresting people with drugs because there were people who were bringing expired drugs. Mine can be brought because they come by plane. Even me, I have my briefcase where I carry them with the documents. If they ask, I can explain." Asked whether he had ever run short of ARVs, Steven asserted, "Never, because I always call these people in advance when remaining with drugs for two weeks—unless the disappointment will come from their end and they refuse to send to me."

By September 2006, just a year after she started on ARVs, Rachel had become a "professional" in ART in that she had obtained a job working for Reach

Out Mbuya program. She was assigned to monitor adolescents and children, who by this time were also eligible to receive ARVs. "I monitor them, count their drugs, and remind them to go to the clinics," she said. "Most of the children are orphans with no parents. Many of those who care for them are not on drugs, so they easily forget. I keep visiting them and remind them." Rachel had to make twenty-one home visits each week, about which she submitted a written report, in addition to helping in the clinic three days a week.

Rachel was knowledgeable about the drugs in her buckets:

They changed me to Combivirpack; it combines Nevirapine and Combivir. They told me that Triomune was out of stock. That time, they changed many people. Even sometimes it used to make me feel that I was not breathing well. But now I don't have any problem with it. This one [nodding at Steven] takes Combivir and Efavirenz. He takes one in the morning and two in the evening. Even the boy takes Combivir and Efavirenz, but now he was changed from red to white, because of increase in age. They give him for three weeks—he gets twenty-eight each visit.

The effects of the medications were evident—physically, socially, and economically. Rachel's CD4 count had risen from 84 in September 2005 to 282 by April 2006. By June, her skin rash had disappeared, and when David last saw her, in October 2006, she looked well and had gained weight. From a new resident of Mbuya Parish and a novice consumer of ARVs she had become an "expert," a pillar of the program, who guided new clients at the clinic and monitored how they medicated children in their care. Antiretroviral therapy had become a source of income for her, supplementing her bar business, which now had limited opening times in the evening because of her work obligations in the program.

As for Steven, he might have died in early 2006 had he not started on ARVs. His health, which had been amazingly good, collapsed in late December. He could not work, and medical expenses made a dent in the family budget. Fortunately, he and the family benefited from rations of yellow maize meal, beans, soy and cooking oil that they received through the treatment program. With ARVs and good feeding, Steven improved so much that his CD4 count rose to more than 200. In August, he was able to return to work, earning good wages in Juba. In September, while he was back in Kampala for a visit, he confided to David that he had finished building a house in the village and was looking for a plot of land in Kampala. He was going to take the family's city furniture to the new house in the village and buy new furnishings for their town home. There were plenty of contracts in Juba.

Not everyone was aware that the family was taking ARVs. Rachel said that most of their immediate neighbors knew. After all, her brother-in-law and neighbor had brought them to the area so she could get the ARVs. Many knew the Reach Out Mbuya program; the man in the next room worked there. The weekly visits of the CATTS could not be kept secret—and, as people say, there are no secrets in this type of dense urban housing. But Rachel and Steven had not told the teachers at their son's school; indeed, they had not even told their son. Steven's immediate boss knew, of course, since he carried the medicine to Juba. But, Steven said, he had not told the "big people. When you tell them, you may lose your job."

When we first met Rachel and Steven, they had not told their own parents in eastern Uganda. Steven had already lost a brother and a sister to AIDS, and another brother (the one who had introduced them to the Reach Out Mbuya program) had almost died. He thought the shock of hearing that he was also infected would be too great for them. Rachel said she would tell her parents when she went home for Christmas, but in the end, she did not go because Steven fell so gravely ill. The last time David visited Rachel and Steven, in October 2006, they were looking forward to seeing their parents at the coming Christmas. In the interim, Steven's parents had learned that the couple were infected; Rachel suspected his sister (the one who had been her treatment supporter) told them. She also speculated that her own parents might know, although she had not mentioned her sickness to anyone in her family. In any case, she said, "I think now I can tell them about my situation."

CHAPTER TEN

Medicine

Susan Reynolds Whyte
and Godfrey Etyang Siu

High up in Rachel's bedroom hung three small buckets, each containing the
ARVs for a family member: one for herself, one for her husband, and one for
their young son. Rachel claimed that she had thought up this storage system,
and we never saw anyone else keep their medicine in this particular way. But
the handling of ARVs as something special was nearly universal. Acquired
immunodeficiency syndrome has been made an "exceptional" disease, set
apart from others in the way it is diagnosed and treated and surrounded with
special guidelines on confidentiality and counseling. It has its own programs
and, to a large extent, its own funding sources that are separate from those
available to deal with malaria, respiratory infections, and the other illnesses
that plague people in low-income African societies. There are debates about
whether AIDS should continue to be treated as exceptional and whether the
exceptional response has meant the neglect of other health problems.[1] But
there is no doubt that HIV and AIDS have been made unique among diseases
in Uganda, and so has the medicine to treat them. Perhaps it is equally useful
to speak about "ARV exceptionalism." The uniqueness of ARVs is partly a
creation of the programs that surround them with such strict rules and procedures and partly an attribution of the clients who experience their powerful
sickening and healing effects. To understand their singularity, we must see
them against the background of other types of medicine, and we must recall

the medicinal context that the first generation experienced before free ARVs became widely available.

Antiretrovirals are medicines for life in the double sense that they are life-saving and lifelong. Although other medicine has these two qualities, as well, ARVs have come to embody them more explicitly. When AIDS first became known to the Ugandan public in the 1980s, it was as a deadly disease. "AIDS Kills!" was the warning in many of the first educational campaigns. Malaria kills, too, but not inevitably, as AIDS was seen to do. In the history of the disease, and in the experience of the first generation, ARVs came onto the scene as a savior in the face of death. With the rollout of ART in 2004–2006, the warnings that AIDS was a killer were replaced by messages on signs and in the radio that HIV was treatable at your nearby health center. Antiretroviral medicine was a new blessing, not something taken for granted—at least for the first generation. The great accomplishment of the programs that delivered ARVs was that they established frameworks for consistent and enduring treatment. This was revolutionary in the Ugandan context, in which treatment for chronic diseases is often sporadic. People in treatment for epilepsy, diabetes, severe mental illness, and cardiovascular disease also need to take medicine daily for life. But few manage to do so with the commitment and regularity that characterized the ART clients in our study.

In Uganda, ARVs entered a setting in which presumptive treatment and self-medication were common. At public health facilities, fevers were commonly treated with both antimalarials and antibiotics, since accurate diagnosis was often impossible. Drugshops and small private clinics sold a wide range of medications, including prescription-only drugs, on demand or according to the judgment of the drugshop attendant. The private sector supplemented the public one, which was marked by understaffing, short opening hours, and medicine going out of stock. In this situation, it was not surprising that antibiotics and antimalarials were not prescribed, dispensed, or taken according to biomedical guidelines. Full courses of medicine were often not completed, and sometimes they were not even purchased or provided. Pharmaceuticals had a lively social life as they took on values beyond the biomedical knowledge that was supposed to guide their use and were transacted with little regulation by authorities.[2] These were exactly the circumstances that made early observers fear antiretroviral anarchy once AIDS drugs were introduced in sub-Saharan Africa.[3] Yet the experience of the first generation was that ARVs were kept apart from the conditions that prevailed for other kinds of medicine.

Rules and Procedures

"These drugs have their rules," stated several of our interlocutors. The acknowledgment of rules was one of the most striking features of life on ART.[4] The medicine had to be taken every day, without fail, at a fixed time, preferably after eating something. It could not be shared with others, and it could be obtained only with a health worker's prescription. People learned the rules from their treatment providers, as Rachel and Steven did when they "studied ARVs" for three sessions before starting on the medicine. Other programs offered "pre-treatment counseling" to impart the rules to prospective clients. But the stringency that is part of exceptionalism starts even earlier. No one can start ART without testing positive for HIV. Those who tested positive and joined the programs we have described were put on a daily dose of Septrin (co-trimoxazole) even before they started ARVs. They were given appointments to come in for a checkup and to pick up more Septrin. Their compliance in keeping the appointments and their adherence to Septrin were taken as an indication of their suitability for the strict regime of ART.

Our interlocutors were aware that starting ART meant crossing a threshold that was controlled by gatekeepers. The Joint Clinical Research Centre (JCRC), Infectious Diseases Institute (IDI), Reach Out Mbuya, and Home-Based AIDS Care (HBAC) insisted that their clients' CD4 counts be tested before they started. The general rule was that ARVs were initiated when the CD4 count fell below 200; our "numbers-literate" interlocutors explained their start, or the fact that their HIV-positive partners had not yet started, in terms of CD4 levels. But the government rollout program at Busolwe Hospital made the decision to start people on ARVs on the basis of clinical stage. It did not require patients to make the journey to the nearest large town and pay for a CD4 test. Consequently, its clients spoke of starting in terms of their general state of health. Dominic (case XI) explained that when he first tested HIV-positive, he begged the health worker to give him "RVs" because he did not feel well and even offered 30,000 shillings (about $16) to buy them, but he was told that he was still OK and was not yet ready to start.

People who started on free ARVs were monitored by their programs to ensure that they took the tablets without fail. This was done in three different ways, depending on the treatment program. All who initiated treatment were asked to identify a "treatment companion" (or "buddy" or "partner") who would remind them to take their drugs. (They did not, however, necessarily directly observe them swallowing the drugs, as in the Directly Observed

Treatment System approach to TB medicine.) This was a formal requirement; the name had to be entered in the client's papers. Thus, Rachel brought her husband's sister when she signed up to start treatment. A second way to monitor observance of ART procedures was the requirement that the client bring the remaining medicine when he or she fetched the next supply of ARVs. By counting the pills, the dispenser could check whether the client had taken the medicine every day. Some programs had a third method of monitoring medication: the two geographically delimited, comprehensive treatment programs arranged to have fieldworkers visit their clients at home once a week to ensure that they were taking their medicine and to see how they were. As we saw in Rachel's case, CATTS checked on their clients weekly for the first six months. After that, it was assumed that such close supervision was no longer necessary because clients were habituated to taking their medicine regularly. The HBAC project delivered medicine to clients' homes each week, providing an opportunity to see whether all medicine for the previous week had been taken. Moreover, counselors talked to clients at home about their adherence to the ARVs.

In addition to monitoring medication, treatment programs required that the clients' health be checked regularly, usually when they came in for the next supply of medicine. The consultation with a health worker was augmented in some programs with regular CD4 tests, and even, in the case of the HBAC research project, tests for viral loads. This health surveillance imperative, together with concern about whether ARVs were being taken punctually, meant that clients had to come at fixed intervals to get refills and talk to health workers. Rachel's young son was checked and given a supply of medicine every three weeks; Rachel herself went in every month, and her husband, Steven, as we saw, was given two-month supplies. This binding of clients to a place and a tight time schedule was most pronounced in the first months of treatment, when programs followed their clients closely. Later, the stringency was relaxed somewhat in that relatives or friends were allowed to fetch the refill, as Rachel did for Steven. Yet the conscientious manner in which clients adhered to their schedule of appointments at the clinics suggested that they were fulfilling their part of a contract.

Agreements between clients and programs were written. As we saw in chapter 2, paperwork was an essential part of clientship. All clients had cards or papers on which their schedule of appointments was recorded, and these were kept carefully, as the medicine itself. Once, David and Susan overheard a health worker giving an educational talk to clients waiting at the IDI. He held up an appointment card and asserted: "This paper is your life. Keep it well!" William kept his medical forms at home in Luwero. Once, he left them there when he had an appointment at the IDI. He called his wife, who sealed them in an envelope and sent them by taxi to Kampala, an hour away, where William waited for them in the taxi park. Some clients, such as Tom, claimed that they carried their papers with them at all times. But no matter where they kept them, the papers served as an important record, indexing their clientship and documenting the schedule of medicine refills.

The rules were a fundamental aspect of ARV exceptionalism. Few, if any, other types of medicine were surrounded by such formality: the need for accurate diagnosis through testing, initiation through "study" or counseling, adherence monitoring, scheduling of refills, and health checkups were all requirements of programs that set ARVs in a medicinal class unto themselves. One might ask whether these rules represented control or care—an attempt to impose discipline or to offer high-quality health services. Clients did discipline themselves; they learned to be virtuous, responsible medicine consumers. But they did so because the provision of medicine was relatively dependable, and the providers seemed attentive and concerned in a setting where these qualities could not be taken for granted. Care and control were combined in the medicine and its rules.

Medicinal Variety

Our interlocutors benefited from the advent of the relatively inexpensive generic antiretroviral Triomune, produced by the Indian firm Cipla. Triomune, the first generation of widely used ARVs, was a fixed combination formulated as a single tablet, making it easy to take as well as cheap to supply. Of the forty-eight people we first interviewed, at least twenty-eight were taking Triomune. Eight were not sure about the names of their ARVs and we were not able to confirm, but some of them may also have been taking Triomune. Twelve were taking other combinations. The type of ARV taken depended partly on the program to which a client belonged. The national rollout at Busolwe Hospital and elsewhere provided only Triomune. At the time, the HBAC program used only brand-name medicine (in several tablets), while other programs offered both generic and branded medications.

Most people knew the name of their ARV. Triomune was easy to remember, and it was a single tablet. The HBAC clients, who received three different tablets, remarked that the names were difficult and they could not remember. The medications were delivered to their homes pre-packed in daily doses, so they did not handle the original packages with the brand names. MamaGirl (case IV), an HBAC client, said that her medications were just called "ARVs," but she also showed us a paper with the names 3TC/Lamivudine, D4T/Stavudine, and Nevirapine.

About half of our interlocutors had experienced switching ARVs or formulations, either because they had moved from one program to another or because their health worker had changed the prescription. At the time of our study, people were being moved between Triomune 30 and Triomune 40. Some thought that the 40 milligram (mg) formulation was for people who weighed 130 pounds or more, and they were switched according to weight gain or loss. Others were unsure of why they were switched, and many associated switches with side effects.

Hanifa started out buying ARVs at the JCRC; she was later referred to The AIDS Support Organization (TASO) for free ARVs, then joined the IDI program. She recounted the implications of these moves for her medication. "I have been using Triomune 30 since I started," she said. "I have never changed. I even asked the doctor at Joint [the JCRC], 'I see other people changing, so will I also be changed from Triomune?' He told me that they give drugs according to one's health status and that Triomune is OK for me. But when I went to TASO, I was worried, because at TASO they have three tablets, not one. Their Triomune is in three tablets, which you have to take. But now at the IDI, I take Triomune and Septrin. At Joint [the JCRC], I was not taking Septrin." Later in the discussion, she added, "What I am worried of most is changing regimens."

Those who were paying for their drugs worried about being switched to medicine that was more expensive. Jackson was being treated at a private clinic and was buying his ARVs. His doctor had excellent connections at the IDI, and Jackson was referred there when he failed to improve on Triomune 40. Three new drugs were prescribed, of which two were expensive and one was impossible to obtain from the private clinic and from the IDI. "What about second-line drugs?" Jackson said. "When I fail to get them with the connections I have, then how will others manage?"

Antiretrovirals are the focus of public consciousness; they are the revolutionary breakthrough that became widely available for the first generation. But it is important to bear in mind that people have been, and still are, taking other medicine, too. Before they were diagnosed as HIV-positive, many went through periods of illness for which they were trying a variety of medications. As Loyce noted, "I suffered from every illness you can imagine, including fever, flu, cough and anemia. I used every type of medicine. I never thought about it at all that it was AIDS." Other people mentioned severe bouts of malaria, for which they had been taking antimalarials, and diarrhea that they were treating with Flagyl.

When their health continued to deteriorate, some tried alternatives to biomedicine. Hope recounted that she did not want to go to TASO to start ARVs because people would know she had AIDS. So she got friends to discreetly bring her herbal medicine commercially marketed and sold in small jerricans called budomola. She, like others, also tried commercial vitamins, tonics, nutritional supplements, and over-the-counter preparations for a variety of ailments that were being promoted in Kampala, such as those sold by the South African companies Golden Products, Swissgarde, Zinunula, and House of Health. They were expensive; Hope was spending 100,000 shillings [$58] per month for them. MamaGirl spent the greatest part of her deceased husband's money on Swissgarde products.

Once they were diagnosed as HIV-positive, nearly everyone had started taking Septrin, which they continued to take daily alongside their ARVs. Many were diagnosed with tuberculosis and took several tablets a day for up to eight months to treat that condition. In addition, people used medicine to treat opportunistic infections such as oral thrush and pneumonia, the side effects of ARVs, diabetes, and all of the other "ordinary" ailments that HIV-positive and HIV-negative people suffer from time to time. Some of the supplemental treatments people mentioned were uncommon—for example, William took honey as medicine; Cathy took vitamin B to increase her strength and appetite; Tom said he could not sleep without Valium; and Hanifa, who had been nicknamed "Kakelenda" (Little Tablet) because of her keen interest in self-medication, bought a product from the Chinese company Tianshi. Moses took Triomune for HIV but used herbal medicine for his diabetes.

No one was able to get all of the different kinds of medicine he or she felt was needed from the same source all of the time, even though most programs offered some medicine for common ailments in addition to ARVs. The programs that offered the most comprehensive health care—HBAC and Reach Out Mbuya—provided treatment for all kinds of complaints, but they were not open on weekends. Sometimes people bought other medicine from nearby drugshops, because that was easier or because they wanted medication that was not available where they got their ARVs. Cathy explained that she bought Flufed (for colds) in local shops instead of taking advantage of the free medicine at Reach Out Mbuya because "one goes through a lot of bureaucracy and spends the whole day there, and at the end you go out with only vitamin C tablets." In contrast, James held off on getting treatment for a severe cough until his next appointment at the IDI; he did not want to self-medicate when he had a clinical appointment in a few days and could ask a doctor to pre-scribe medicine that he could get along with his ARVs.

Viewing ARVs in relation to all of the other types of medicine people take underlines their exceptionalism, but it also reminds us that no one is totally a client of one program in the sense of getting *all* of his or her medicine from one place. And certainly, no household is dependent on a single ART program for all of its medicinal needs.

Fee and Free

The first generation includes those people who started buying ARVs when the price began to fall. Twenty-seven of the forty-eight people whose life stories we heard in late 2005 and early 2006 had paid for their ARVs when they be-gan treatment. But by the time we met them, ten had already moved from fee to free arrangements; almost all of these were clients of the IDI or the JCRC programs. Of the twenty-three people we followed over the ensuing year, six received their medicine on a fee basis at the outset, and three moved over to free provision during the course of our study. The movement from fee to free was a historical shift, as was the access of tens of thousands of new clients who would never have gotten treatment if they had had to pay.

Clearly those who were in fee-based treatment had some resources. They were people who had jobs or had relatives who could afford the cost. Even so, we heard many accounts from people who had to break off treatment because paying for medicine became too great a burden. Ivan tested HIV-positive in early 2003 and started on ARVs after learning that his CD4 count had fallen to only 4:

> In Mbale, I was buying drugs, but it was a gambling situation because they gave only whatever I could afford to buy, not according to the dose I was supposed to get. They could give me drugs equivalent to the money I had at a particular time and the type of complication I had. I would spend 30,000 shillings or 40,000 shillings [$17–$23] per week. Sometimes I would not go because of lack of money, but whenever I would go for treatment, they would just give me drugs for the money I had, not even asking me where I had stopped and why I had not come back. I realized I was playing with my life. One time I was coming from Mbale and felt hungry and wanted to buy fruit. As I took the money from my pocket, the small envelope with my tablets fell out, and I did not realize that I had lost my drugs. I ate the fruit and went home. At the time of swallowing the drugs, I checked in my

pocket. There was nothing! I lost hope and just gave up, and I said, "Let me just ignore [this] and pack [die]!"

Even though the price of ARVs fell from $900 to $350 a month when generics came on the market in 2001, buying the medicine was a dreadful strain. Some said that they could afford to buy medicine for only a week at a time, and sometimes they had to borrow money or sell property to get funds for the next week. Julia, a health worker at an up-country hospital, started ART in 2001, traveling to the JCRC in Kampala. "It was a big problem paying this amount of money every month, and it was very inconvenient going to Kampala from Pallisa," she said. "I could pick almost the entire salary and take it to pay for the drugs, yet at that time, the salary was also low." She was later transferred to the Mbale branch of the JCRC, which was closer to her home, but still found the costs onerous. In 2004, when her son was registering for the fourth year of secondary school, Julia dropped out of treatment for two months to pay his fees. Two other people reported that they also had not been able to afford their diabetes medicine for some months while they were paying for ARVs.

Being switched to more expensive medicine could be disastrous. When Benjamin went to the JCRC for his third month's supply in mid-February 2006, the doctor said he had to change the medicine; the new one cost more than twice as much and was supposed to be stored in a refrigerator, which Benjamin did not own. He also had to pay for Septrin for himself and his wife, for a CD4 test, and for medicine to counteract the anemia he had developed when he started taking ARVs. He was dismayed when Godfrey met him on that occasion, wondering how he would manage if he had to stay on the more expensive medicine. He left the center with ARVs for only two weeks yet had paid 184,000 shillings [around $101], not including the cost of transportation.

Medicinal Practices

People who started taking lifelong medication developed habits of incorporating medicine into their everyday lives. Partly, these habits had to do with following rules: remembering and taking tablets at appointed times. Partly, they had to do with the social implications of taking ARVs and what keeping and swallowing pills communicated to others. Where people were open about being on ART, others became involved in helping them to follow the rules. Those who maintained degrees of discretion had to store and take their drugs with care—at least, in relation to those who were not privy to the knowledge.

Rachel maintained that she developed her system of storing the medicine in small buckets for safety: she needed to keep the ARVs for herself, her husband, and her child separate and out of her child's reach. Like Rachel, most people stored their medicine in their sleeping area—the most private place in living spaces that were often small and crowded—in locked boxes, cupboards or wardrobes, or, sometimes, under beds. Many people said that they had to keep their ARVs where children could not find them. Hassan (case VIII) said he kept medicine on top of a house wall where even rats could not reach them. But storing ARVs out of the way met needs for discretion, as well as safety, especially in homes in which people had not told their children that they were being treated for HIV infection.

Many people mentioned that it was important to be able to take ARVs openly, at the proper time, no matter who was watching. Of course, this was not a problem for those who had disclosed their serostatus. But some people remained secretive and took the pills without revealing their purpose. Although Matayo talked about the importance of taking medicine openly and publicly, for example, Godfrey noticed that he carried his ARVs in a plain envelope so no one would see what he was taking. And Paul recounted that his daughter had asked him why he was taking medicine when he was not sick. "So she knows that I am taking drugs, but not why," he said. "I only try to convince her that I am trying to keep healthy by taking these drugs. Sometimes I take them in my bedroom, where the children do not see." Several people had not revealed to their partners that they were HIV-positive and in treatment. One had diabetes, so her husband was used to seeing her taking medicine for that; she, like Alice (case V), was convinced that her husband never looked in her personal possessions and thus had not seen the medicine. The most extreme example of secrecy was a man who not only had not told his wife but connived with a doctor to start her on ARVs under the pretext that she was being treated for TB.

People were told to take their ARVs twice a day, at twelve-hour intervals, and never to ever forget. Like Rachel, they chose their own, most convenient times—one university student taking night classes, for instance, took ARVs at noon and midnight. At first, the schedule was hard to remember, some people explained. They might miss a dose or remember a little late. However, over time, they claimed, they became so habituated that they never forgot. Juma had set his mobile phone to remind him. But for most people, the important reminders in the initial period were those offered by other people—some of them designated "treatment companions," and others supportive household members or neighbors. What was striking was the way in which the rules that made ARVs exceptional were acknowledged and encouraged by others as a way to show concern.

William's eldest brother was his registered treatment companion, but another brother and sister-in-law with whom he stayed during the week reminded him. "I can't forget," he said, "because the people I live with here seem to care even more than I do. Even madam at home [his wife, whom he stayed with on weekends], she always asks, 'Where are the drugs?' Even here, he [nodding at his brother] looks at the watch, and then I have to remember. But there was one day I was in the taxi, and it was delaying, I felt so tensed up. I was late by about one hour." Jessica's adult daughter was her treatment companion, but others also supported her—even her landlady. "I told everybody. Friends, neighbors—everybody. Even the owner of this house," Jessica said. "She was very happy. 'Thank you so much for enrolling in TASO,' she said. 'Please never forget to take the ARVs.' She is an old woman. In the morning she always passes, knocks, and says, 'Did you take your medicine today?'" Even children who are informed play a role. Hope explained, "My children keep reminding me to swallow drugs. For example, when we are going to the village, they ask me whether I have packed my medicine. They say they don't want me to die." Joyce (case I) provided a striking example of the social relations of adherence when she mentioned that her sister, as well as the headmaster and pupils at the school where she taught, conveyed her ARVs to her when she forgot.

Like Hope's children, most people were conscious of the need to carry their medicine when they traveled and even when they thought they might be delayed somewhere beyond the appointed time. Philip proudly showed us a black computer bag he had obtained. "I go with this bag when I travel," he said. "This is where I keep all the medicine. I always go with this bag. It is now part of my life. Like last week, where I went to a funeral, I went with it." William said that he always makes sure he has enough medicine with him: "I carry a tablet when going to work," he said. "I keep it in the money purse, sometimes more than one tablet. Usually I take my ARVs at about 8 PM [when he expects to be at home], but I may take long before returning to where the drugs are kept. When I am traveling, it is the first thing I pack. If I intend to stay for two days, I pack medicine for three days just in case I stay longer."

The ability to take ARVs on a regular schedule requires obtaining them in a timely manner so the supply never runs out. As we have seen, the programs had policies in place governing the size of the supply they would provide at a time. They also differed in terms of whether they would give the medicine to someone other than the client. The HBAC field officers were strict about placing the following week's supply into the hands of the client. Other programs seemed willing to be more flexible. But sending others to fetch one's ARVs is possible only if those others are part of the "treatment alliance" in the sense that they know one is in treatment, accept the importance of following the rules, and can manage the interaction at the clinic.

Drug Power

It was widely recognized that ARVs had great power to heal, but their strength was also evident in the many grim side effects they caused. In fact, several of our interlocutors said that they had been afraid to start on ARVs for that reason. As Mary explained, "I feared to start on the medicine because my CD4 was so low. I thought the drugs are strong and needed a strong body."

Almost everyone reported difficulties when they started ART. "It was as if my body was in a fight with the drugs," Goretti said. The most common side effect was severe pain and swelling in the legs and feet, which sometimes affected one's ability to wear shoes or walk. Many people had their dosage of Triomune reduced from 40 mg to 30 mg, or they were given a different medication altogether, because of this complaint.[5] People mentioned nausea, diarrhea, sleeplessness, nightmares, headache, and thirst. Some said that their appearance changed. "When I started, my face got so swollen, it got blown up like a balloon, the eyes became red, I got a skin rash all over the body," Harriet said. "Before taking the drugs, I was light-skinned, but when I started taking the drugs, I became pale like cement. People could only recognize me after I told them, 'I am Harriet.'" When Rosette was switched from Triomune to a combination of three other drugs, her toenails fell out. "They have just grown back," she said, leaning down to feel them. "My feet pained so much I could not touch them."

Some people were given medicine to counter the side effects of ARVs; others thought they could be mitigated by right living. "Some people threaten to throw away the drugs, especially when they see those with side effects like black patches that make them look as if they were burned by the drugs," said Loyce, recounting conversations she had had with fellow clients of the IDI. "We encourage such people to eat greens, fruit, and other food that strengthens the body, like sweet potatoes, posho, and cassava, so that they don't get such side effects." Cathy was happy that she had escaped severe side effects and made a quick recovery and credited her healthy habits. "Some clients don't respond; their drug adherence is not OK, maybe because they don't go to bed very early," she said. "I know one person whose skin is bad because she drinks waragi. Me, I don't drink waragi. I don't smoke. When I get money, I buy milk." Still others thought that they were able to evade side effects because their bodies "matched with the drugs."

For most people, side effects diminished within a few months. Those who had more experience encouraged ART novices to hold out. Like Rachel, several mentioned that they were heartened because they felt they were growing stronger, despite the side effects. Indeed, all of the people we talked with were grateful for the power of the medicine.

Exceptional Medicine

Drug regimens have continued to change since we ended our visits to Rachel and our other interlocutors. New medications have become available; policies and prices have shifted. Soon it may be hard to remember just what it was like in the years before widespread access to ARVs and how exceptional they were when they became part of Ugandan life in 2004–2006. Lest we forget, Peter Mugyenyi, who has been the director of the JCRC since 1992, describes the desperate search for effective medicine in A Cure Too Far.[6] When the AIDS epidemic was at its peak in Uganda in the 1990s, all kinds of remedies circulated. Exaggerated claims about herbal preparations were common. The JCRC ran trials in the hope that one might prove effective—or, failing that, in the conviction that evidence of their uselessness would prevent dying people from spending the few resources they might leave to their families. In addition to Ugandan herbalists, medicinal entrepreneurs from all over the world approached the JCRC to get scientific approval for their AIDS medicine. Candidate medicine came from China, Israel, France, Britain, the United States, and Norway. Mugyenyi was disillusioned with many that seemed to be dubious attempts to spin money out of families' despair. A few were better founded scientifically but failed to show convincing effects. Rumors circulated that a cure had been found but that it was being kept secret.

In 1996, highly active antiretroviral therapy—not a cure but a means of control—became the standard treatment in Europe and North America. It was soon available in Uganda, as well, but at a price that was prohibitive for all but the wealthiest people. This was bitter knowledge for the Ugandans who were aware of it, and Mugyenyi devoted another book to the years in which the healing power of ART was kept inaccessible to millions of Africans who suffered largely preventable deaths. "Carnage" is a word that he uses frequently, and "genocide" figures in the title.[7]

Antiretrovirals were exceptional not only because they had singular rules and were powerful. The early years of the epidemic were years when public health facilities had been enfeebled by misrule and economic collapse. Overwhelmed by AIDS patients, they had few drugs to offer. Families struggled to buy all kinds of pharmaceuticals from privately owned drugshops. Most also tried herbal medicine, some of which was promoted as curing AIDS and priced exorbitantly. The advent of drugs that were free, effective, and in reliable supply was truly extraordinary.

Antiretroviral medicine instilled a new confidence in biomedical health care. Against years of experience with stock-outs in government facilities and shopping from one source of pharmaceuticals to another, the rollout gave a revolutionary model of how medicine could be supplied, dispensed, and monitored. Of course, it was not perfect, and grave problems arose in the years after our study ended. But it was immensely impressive in relation to what had gone before.

Notes

1. Smith and Whiteside, "The History of AIDS Exceptionalism," 10.
2. S. Whyte, "Pharmaceuticals as Folk Medicine"; Van der Geest et al., "The Anthropology of Pharmaceuticals"; S. Whyte and Birungi, "The Business of Medicines and the Politics of Knowledge in Uganda."
3. Harries et al., "Preventing Antiretroviral Anarchy in Sub-Saharan Africa."
4. In her doctoral thesis, Louise Mubanda Rasmussen describes how the rules are imparted and understood: see Rasmussen, "From Dying with Dignity to Living with Rules," 139–46.
5. After our study ended, Triomune was discontinued in Ugandan ART programs because of its side effects.
6. Mugyenyi, *A Cure Too Far*.
7. Mugyenyi, *Genocide by Denial*.

CASE XI

Dominic

A MULTITUDE OF
ADVERSITIES

Jenipher Twebaze and
Susan Reynolds Whyte

LIFE

(overleaf)

Everyday matters such
as laundry continue.

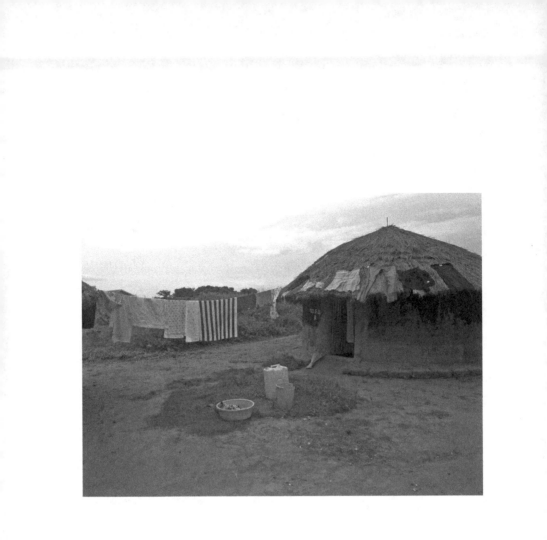

"I wanted to marry, and as you know, here we buy women. We buy women with five cows. When I told my father, he said, 'My son, we are poor, and you know you don't have five cows. What plans do you have?' I told him that I was relying on him. We had grown rice, and we had many acres." When he first met Jenipher in December 2005 in the waiting area at the hospital, Dominic was friendly and forthcoming. He launched into a long and complicated story about marriages, work, and money but also about adversity and being cheated and misused by others. Despite his Christian name, Dominic was from a large and well-established Muslim family in eastern Uganda. "My father is a farmer and a Hajji [one who has made the pilgrimage to Mecca]. He has four wives and about twenty-six children, though I don't know them all, and there may even be others, too. I went to Kiwarabu [Arabic-language Koran] school in Mbale for seven years at the home of my father's brother, who was teaching young boys Islam."

When Dominic returned home after seven years, he wanted to attend a government school, where other subjects were taught, but there was no money and, besides, no one else in the family had gone to school. So Dominic started to work looking after people's cows. His payment was a small jerrican of milk every day, which he sold. He was fourteen years old when he decided that he should marry. Jenipher asked him whether his father thought that was young for marriage, and Dominic replied, "How? All he wanted was to see me grow, and here for someone to become a man, he must have a wife." Dominic's father called his friend, a sheikh, to take twenty bags of rice to sell for them in town so they could buy cows for bridewealth. Three days later, the sheikh returned to report that the rice had been stolen. "My father just kept quiet," Dominic said. "Because the person talking was a sheikh, my father could not doubt his words. He just said this is OK because that is what Allah decided." So Dominic herded cows for four more years.

Then one day, the sheikh offered to make up for the loss of the rice by providing one of his daughters as a wife for Dominic. Dominic and his new wife went to stay with her mother, who was farming and trading matooke (cooking plantains) in Masaka and Mbarara. They spent a year working in her gardens until Dominic returned home because he felt that others were laughing at him for serving his mother-in-law with no prospects of establishing himself independently. His young wife refused to go with him, and within a few months he had received a message that their new baby had died. He had no money to transport the corpse from Masaka and had given up on burying his child at home, as is proper, when his mother-in-law arrived, carrying her bag. "She boarded a taxi with a body in her bag, and you could not tell that there was a human being [in her luggage]," he said. After the child's death, Dominic tried again in early 1995 to persuade his wife to return. But she refused, having become involved in trading, and she only returned briefly in 2004 wanting to resume the marriage. Then it was his turn to refuse, because he had remarried in 2003.

Dominic struggled to raise the bridewealth for his second marriage, growing rice and exchanging it for cows from the man for whom he worked as a herdsman. He also began working as a butcher, putting aside a little money every day in a small bag. Dominic's new wife moved in with him before he had amassed the amount agreed for the bridewealth. Her parents had said that the balance of 180,000 shillings [about $70] could be paid later. But when she failed to conceive, Dominic was convinced that her parents were preventing her from having children. "I worked hard and raised 100,000 shillings, leaving a balance of 80,000," he said "I asked the parents to allow my wife to have children and said I would complete the rest with time. They accepted, and my wife became pregnant." (That senior relatives can curse the bride to barrenness if the bridewealth is not paid is a common belief in the part of Uganda where Dominic lived.) When Jenipher pushed Dominic about whether he had had other relationships between his first and his second marriages, he explained that he had in fact had six children during that period with six different women. Three of the children were staying with him and his second wife, while the other three lived next door with his mother.

He continued,

It was at that time when I had a [bridewealth] debt of 80,000 shillings that I started falling sick on and off. I was not spending a week without suffering from malaria. I could be admitted here at the hospital. One time they put twelve bottles of water in me, and I said this time I am dying. That was May 2005. Also, my mother ran mad in early 2005. She was bewitched by her co-wives. But one of my in-laws, my sister's husband, took her to *abagangi* (healers or so-called witch doctors) and she recovered. She is now OK. My father landed on this doctor here [referring to a clinical officer who has worked at the hospital for many years and is now in charge of the HIV clinic]. He told him, "My son is falling sick all the time. What can I do with him, because now I am struggling with his mother?" Then this doctor advised that I should be brought to the hospital for treatment.

Dominic was tested for HIV at his local hospital on 3 May 2005 (he remembered the exact date) and was told that he had the virus. "I felt bad, but I almost suspected it since I was understanding what the problem was," he said. "They asked me how many sexual partners I had had, and I told them eight. They asked me whether I had lost any of them, and I said all were alive except the Masaka woman who had just died. I told the doctor, 'I hear you have drugs here. Why don't you give them to me?' He said that I am still OK and not yet ready to start on them."

When Dominic learned that he had HIV, he did not tell anyone, but when he started on antiretroviral medicine—or "RVs," as he called them—on 12 June 2005 (again he remembered the exact date), he was instructed that he had to tell at least one person at home who could help him remember to take his tablets. "So I told my wife, and she quarreled and packed her things and left me," he said. "She went to her [parents'] home crying and quarreling. But she stayed only for four days because her people kept asking her how she could leave me alone in the house sick. She came back after she had cooled down. She even reminds me now when I forget to swallow tablets. Sometimes she gets annoyed with me, but such things happen in marriage. Otherwise, we are OK." Later, his wife was tested for HIV, but she had not gone back to learn her results, and the couple had not had their child tested.

After starting on ARVs, Dominic recounted,

I was given a TASO [The AIDS Support Organization] card that has my name and number. One of my stepmothers came and took the card away from me, saying that she was going to collect food for me. That was in August, and I have never seen the food. I came and told my health worker, and he said that I had better get my card from her. When I asked her to bring back the card, she said I should give her 5,000 shillings so she can start getting food for me. I sold my chicken and sent 5,000 shillings, but still she never brought anything. When I came back to hospital, I told my health worker. He said he would talk to her. One time, he found my stepmother at my butchery and asked her why she had taken my card and asked her to bring it back. She promised to bring it. I think she used the card to get food from somewhere, but I don't know where, because in the evening, she sent one kilogram of sugar, one kilogram of posho [maize meal], and one kilogram of beans, but she kept the card. I think she was bribing me not to tell that she has not brought the card. I am supposed to come back [to the clinic] on 22 December, and that is when I will tell my health worker that I have not received it up to now.

Jenipher's first long conversation with Dominic ended on a positive note. After all the struggles to start his own family, he concluded, "We are OK. My child is doing well because he weighs 12 kilograms [about 25 pounds]. For my wife, she is like you: fat and good-looking. If you see her, you can't think she is my wife. She looks so healthy, and you cannot tell that she has a problem."

The next time Jenipher went to visit Dominic, she looked for him at the trading center, where he had told her he used to work. She located people who knew him but learned that he was in jail for stealing a sheep. At Dominic's butchery, she talked to his younger brother, who was minding the business. At the butchery, people were stopping by to hear about the case. Everybody was saying, "But Dominic has never stolen anything. How could he steal a sheep?" After some hours of waiting, Dominic's mother came and took Jenipher to the jail cell at the police station. Jenipher was uncertain about how to introduce herself and how to explain to the police officer that she needed to see Dominic. Dominic's mother introduced her as a visitor from Kampala who had to return to the city soon, and the policeman on duty agreed to bring Dominic from the cell for a visit. As they sat on a small bench under supervision by the guard, she heard what had happened.

The owner of the cows that Dominic used to graze had sold them, giving him two. One he slaughtered and used to reinvigorate his business as a butcher. He had been doing well enough to buy a "tipper," or dump truck, with which he and a half-brother were getting contracts for construction work in a town about 40 kilometers away. For the butchery, he bought sheep and goats in the local market; the day before, he had bought a sheep from his stepmother, who needed cash to repair her house. He sold the skin, which was put out for sale in another trading center down the road. A passing man saw the skin and identified it as coming from his sheep that had been stolen. The skin was traced back to Dominic and, from him, to his stepmother, who was summoned to the police station. The stepmother claimed that the sheep was hers and that she could prove it by bringing its twin from home so the skins could be compared.

Jenipher heard later that Dominic had been released the same evening and continued with his tipper business. In fact, the next time Jenipher met him, she found him underneath the dump truck trying to repair it. She managed to locate him, thanks to his mother, whom she found at the hospital caring for Dominic's sister, who had just given birth. The mother was extremely happy to see Jenipher again and expressed gratitude that she had come to see him in prison. Dominic was having money problems, she said. He had also just quarreled with his wife, because she was not helping his sick mother and his two sisters, who were in the hospital. Dominic had told his wife to go back to her parents, which she did, taking 600,000 shillings (about $235) he had been keeping at home. He needed to pay off the vehicle but could not raise the cash. He even rang Jenipher in Kampala asking for a loan (which she refused because he needed too much money). A month later, he was saying he wanted to sell the dump truck. He could not clear enough to pay it off, he said, "because they steal my money, and I have realized that I am working for nothing."

Susan joined Jenipher for the next visit. They learned that a bizarre accident had befallen Dominic. They found him lying in bed, having just been discharged from hospital. "I tell you, Jenipher, I have been here wondering whether you would come to see me and find out what is happening to me," he said. "I gave my mother your phone number, but we were waiting for someone with a phone so that we could call you and tell you." He had been selling meat at his butchery one evening when the building collapsed on him. "We were about nine people, including myself, but I was the only one who was hit by the structure," he said. "It was a whirlwind that came from the road and straight to where I was. It went into the roof and lifted everything up and then back down on me. All of the wood and bricks fell on me, and I fell down. People thought I had died. They picked everything I had in my pockets, including all the money I had made that day." (It is not uncommon to hear that the first people on scene at an accident picked the victims' pockets.)

Dominic saw a clear connection between the dump truck and the uncanny accident. He recalled that his father and wife had both advised him against going into the dump truck business with his brother. Now he wanted to sell the truck so they could share the money; if anything happened to his brother, he did not want it to be attributed to his having used witchcraft because of the conflicts over the truck. The family had agreed to hold a meeting to sort out the problem, but his brother refused to attend. It also turned out that it was the mother of that brother who had taken Dominic's TASO card; she had still not returned it, despite many requests.

Dominic asked Jenipher and Susan for a loan of 200,000 shillings (about $110) so he could start a new butcher business. That was too much money to lend, but they gave him 25,000 shillings ($14) so he could buy a goat. Jenipher noticed that the family did not even have lamp oil or soap in the home. She had brought sugar, bread, and other small things as gifts, and Dominic thanked her, but he said that next time she should give him the money instead. They went to buy the medicine that had been prescribed for him when he was admitted to the hospital after the accident but that he had not been able to afford.

A few weeks later, Jenipher received a telephone call from Dominic. He was in Iganga, undergoing treatment at the home of one of his mother's relatives who was a healer. After some searching, Jenipher and the driver of our Makerere University vehicle found the place. The healer immediately told Jenipher that Dominic had been bewitched, saying, "People are very dangerous. They wanted him dead." Dominic confirmed this, saying, "My brother and uncle wanted to kill me so they enjoy the benefits from my tipper. . . . I tell you, people are bad. Can you imagine? My own relatives." He praised the healer for saving his life, but when the man left the room, Dominic whispered to Jenipher that the healer was refusing to release him until he paid 150,000 shillings ($82), plus two goats and a white sheep, for the treatment. He had almost finished his monthly supply of ARVs and was supposed to report to his clinic for more. He did not want tell the healer that he was on ART, but he was desperate to go home. Jenipher persuaded the healer that he must send Dominic home to get the money, pointing out that he would surely do so since he was a relative. After some time, the healer called Jenipher asking for Dominic because he had not made the payments. She told him that she did not know where he was.

The last two visits found Dominic at home again. He had recovered from his accident and was engaged in farming. By this time, Jenipher had started noticing that people in the home were referring to her as *mulamu* (sister-in-law). It even happened in Dominic's presence, and he did not object to it. She realized that the family members had assumed all along that she was his wife from Kampala.

Dominic said he was planning to pay the healer but had not yet found the money and had started feeling new pain, which he feared the healer was causing. He had decided to forget about the dump truck. His brother had taken it to work in a more distant place, "where he thinks I cannot find him," Dominic said. "Let them work until they realize their mistake." Other adversities had beset the family in the meantime. A younger brother's "wife" had died after giving birth to twins. Since bridewealth had not been paid, her family fetched her corpse to bury at their home. One of the twins also died, as had one of the twins born to another brother. Dominic's father deeply regretted the losses, though he already had many grandchildren. A stepmother developed a wound on her breast and incurred a debt of 7,000 shillings ($4) for medicine. Dominic managed to make a tidy profit procuring a black sheep for someone and paid the debt. They pushed on, sharing the troubles. During Jenipher's final visit, the family was cultivating rice in a nearby swamp. A father's sister had been bitten by a big snake while working there, and Dominic's mother had gone to visit her. Dominic complained about the excessive rain that had spoiled his garden after he had spent 100,000 ($56) to prepare it. "That is the problem with farming," he said. "You can easily lose money like that without any compensation from anywhere. You can't fight with weather. You can't report it to the police. Ahhh, it's bad."

CHAPTER ELEVEN

Life

Susan Reynolds Whyte,
Hanne O. Mogensen, and
Lotte Meinert

We end our account of the first generation with the story of Dominic, for whom HIV was but one of life's many adversities. His attempts to marry were dogged by disappointment and the loss of his first child. He had been at death's door just at the time of another calamity—the madness of his mother. Initiating treatment saved his life but did not avert life's problems; the second chance was an opportunity to pursue other struggles. Overall, his story is about his efforts to establish and sustain a family, before and after he started on his "RVs." In this he is a quintessential example of life with ART. With no standard schooling, Dominic was not one of those articulate, English-speaking mobilizers who spread the message of "positive living" to others. Yet he, too, was an enlightened and conscientious client who understood "what the problem was" when he tested HIV-positive and was determined to escape from the healer so he could collect his next supply of medicine in time. He was open about his illness and treatment with his family and employer, but these were not matters on which he dwelled. Jenipher found him in the midst of other dramas—in jail accused of stealing a sheep, in a running conflict with his brother over a dump truck, in the clutches of a healer whose fee he could not pay.

In this final chapter, we reconsider the historical circumstances that characterized living with ART in Uganda in the first decade of the twenty-first century—for individuals like Dominic and for others of the first generation as we came to understand it. The disposition toward acceptance opened the way to clientship, a new pattern within Ugandan health care. Treatment brought new types of sociality, which, we argue, were facilitated by pre-existing social relations and connections. As HIV became a life sentence, not a death sentence, concerns returned to making a living and making a life with others. The certainty of death was replaced by the insecurities and uncertainties of social life.

"It Has Happened"

"When my brother told me that I was HIV-positive, I just held my heart. I took a deep breath and told him, 'Anyway, I have to accept the state I am in.'" Like Grace, the head teacher who spoke these words, many people expressed a striking sense of acceptance about their HIV infection. We heard certain turns of phrase again and again: "It has already happened"; "I am not the first to have this disease, nor will I be the last." The articulation of acceptance was less common in the time before ART became widespread, but it was a repeated theme in the accounts of the first generation.

As we discussed in chapter 1, most people had taken the initiative to be tested because they had reasons to suspect they were HIV-positive. It is thus not surprising that they were more willing to accept their status. Benjamin, a middle-aged civil servant, went for the test with his wife and explained how they prepared themselves: "our minds were already set for the outcome of the results. We said, 'Let us bear with whatever outcome.' Even when they were counseling us before giving us the result, we said to them, 'Just give us the results. We shall not fight it. We are ready for the consequences.' When the results were given, we said, 'We have nothing else to do about it. It has happened.'"

The phrases "We have nothing to do about it" and "It has happened" might seem to reflect fatalism. When Harriet, a widow in her forties, was asked whether her co-wives were bitter that their husband had infected them, she said, "They had nothing to say, apart from, 'He has killed us already. What can we say or do now?'" Hassan (case VIII) recalled the day he discovered he was HIV-positive: "I went back home and said, 'I have nothing to do since I am now infected.' With this disease, once you are infected, you have nothing else to do." "There is nothing to do" seems to mean that HIV cannot be cured. As Norah, a married woman in eastern Uganda, put it, "I was found to be HIV-positive. I took it as normal. I said, 'It has already happened, and I have no way of reversing it.'" However, our interlocutors had all found that there *was* something they could do.

Acceptance did not (only) imply fatalism. It was the positive step toward seeking help through some degree of openness, a disposition that was heavily encouraged by treatment providers. Immediately after recalling that he went home saying, "I have nothing to do since I am now infected," Hassan proceeded to tell Phoebe, "When I learned that I was sick, I decided not to hide, or else I would just die. I decided to get the drugs in order to have life. I have nothing to fear with this disease because I know that once it has come, it has come. You know with this disease, you have to be open. You die fast and so badly if you hide." Vincent, a petty trader in eastern Uganda, said the same thing: "I am open to my friends. I have counseled them because I have been counseled. I tell them, 'If you have it, be open and you will live. Those who hide have died and left me behind.'" Jackie repeated almost the same words: "there are those who died because of fear, like my brother; I tried to bring him for treatment, but he refused. Since then I learned that when you hide, you may miss someone who would have helped you. But when you are open, you can be assisted." Denial and complete secrecy are not possible for those who take treatment, even though many still wished to control the information about their serostatus. Thus, the paradox of openness and discretion came to characterize the first generation. Explicit talk was necessary, at least with health workers and a treatment companion. Moreover, the support of others in taking the test and gaining access to a treatment program meant that someone had to know in order to help you.[1]

The declarations of acceptance and openness we heard are, of course, retrospective accounts from people who have undergone counseling and who are already on ART. The acceptance of their HIV status may not have come as easily as they now remember. And everyone is not open with everyone. Still, these accounts suggest that for most people, the shock and grief they may have experienced at first are replaced by familiarization with HIV as a condition with which one can live. As Jolly (case IX) said, "I have come to realize that AIDS is not the only killer. You can die of anything. The only problem is that you live a rather uncertain life." Acceptance is not just a kind of grace; in the era of ART, it took on positive value as a pragmatic disposition that could be lifesaving. More than that, for some it was a form of enlightenment.

Enlightenment

If modernity is a sense of breaking with the past, and enlightenment is a contrast to the murk of ignorance, then many people in the first generation saw
the response to AIDS as a measure of these two qualities. Accepting your
own status and being open about it was a sign of progressiveness and virtue;
discriminating against HIV-positive people was backward. The idea that one
should not ridicule or denigrate another's debility is old and widespread in
Uganda (and is reported from other African societies). "Don't laugh because
misfortune may befall you, too," is the pith of many proverbs. Jessica's story
about the people who refused to eat in her "AIDS house" and were killed in a
car wreck shortly thereafter illustrated this maxim. There were many remarks
to the effect that those who disparaged an HIV-positive person died first, or
those who gossiped about him or her stopped after checking themselves and
finding they were also positive.

What is relatively new is that discrimination is pictured as backward. Jolly
called her neighbors primitive because they disparaged her for her sickly appearance and added, "For me, I kept quiet because it is a question of time for
everybody." Joyce (case I), one of the AIDS stars, said stigma "is an issue of
the past." Instead, HIV had made her popular and given her opportunities to
serve and represent people, including those who were HIV-negative, in various committees and projects.

People could even use their HIV-positive status to insinuate that others
were prejudiced and in need of enlightenment. Ivan said that he had once
dealt with a policewoman who demanded a bribe. "I pleaded with her and
eventually got annoyed and told her that she should be ashamed of taking a
lot of money from a patient like me," he said. "She felt embarrassed and told
me to keep my money. She would collect from [another person involved in
the matter]. You know, sometimes you need to tell these people how we feel
so they can treat us fairly."

Just as Hassan had seen a break with the past in the knowledge and organizations that had demystified AIDS, so others spoke about having learned
about the disease and its treatment. Counseling played a role for some; they
seemed to see counselors and health workers as sources of enlightenment.
Others, such as Jolly, had informed themselves by reading pamphlets provided at hospitals. Matayo, who worked for an HIV-related organization, was
pleased that he could "access information easily and be updated about current
AIDS issues." To be updated, well informed, and accepting contrasted with
being primitive, discriminating, and ignorant.

One of the clearest indications of enlightenment was to accept HIV rather than witchcraft as a diagnosis of long-standing illness. It was striking that no one said that AIDS was caused by witchcraft; either you were bewitched or you were HIV-positive, each assessment pointing to a different kind of treatment. Persistent or recurring sickness might evoke suspicion that someone had caused it maliciously, or that spirits or ghosts of the dead or some other supernatural force was at play. Like the soldier Saddam (case II), some of our interlocutors said that they had first suspected witchcraft and spent a great deal of money on specialists who claimed they could counteract the spells. In the days before ART, families often clung to such explanations in the hope that the cause could be counteracted and the discrediting shadow of AIDS denied. But once the assertion was made that the sickness was caused by HIV, then supernatural explanations were excluded.

"People said she was bewitched," said Mark, a middle-aged soldier, about a girlfriend who had died, "but I tried to find out what type of symptoms she had. The way they explained it made me suspect AIDS." People might ask themselves questions about whether they were being affected by witchcraft or HIV, and they were aware that one might very well have both in one's life. But in retrospect, many people said that they wasted time and money on witch doctors before they knew HIV was causing their symptoms. Helene, a forty-year-old farmer, described the suspicions of witchcraft that grew out of her husband's sickness. "A lot of hatred was at his place of work and among our relatives, and we were very sure that he was bewitched," she said. "However, all that was a waste of time because meanwhile my husband kept weakening due to AIDS." Jessica, a widow and food seller, said that some people called her "Slim Woman," but she did not care, "because I now know how to live positively. I tell people that it is good to disclose because sometimes people start saying that someone is bewitching you, and then they waste a lot of money trying to help you [to deal with the witchcraft]."

It was not that people denied the play of witchcraft in their lives. Both the least educated, including Dominic, and the best educated, such as the urban university graduate Cathy and the head teacher Grace, told stories about how witchcraft had brought madness and death to their closest relatives. The point is that people made a clear distinction between being HIV-positive and being bewitched. Witches did not send HIV. You could, like Dominic, be both HIV-positive and bewitched, but the bewitchment had caused a wall, not a virus, to fall on him.

Christian churches and learned Islam have long opposed beliefs and practices concerning forces of witchcraft and spirits. They consider them relics of an era before the monotheistic world religions brought truth to Uganda. Thus, the notion that these ideas were unenlightened has existed for more than a century. The success of biomedicine in discrediting such explanations—in relation to the AIDS epidemic—reinforced the contrast between modern ways and what people in Uganda call "cultural" practices.

The enlightened recognition of viral infection was facilitated, if not brought about, by the availability of ART. When HIV was a death sentence, then sorcery, witchcraft, and notions of pollution allowed a modicum of hope and a possibility of action.[2] The many herbal remedies for AIDS marketed before 2004 had the same function. But in the spirit of pragmatism, people dropped these modes of addressing misfortune when a more effective type of intervention came within reach.[3] What is remarkable is that members of the first generation not only stopped "wasting money" on treating HIV as witchcraft; they were confirmed in the view that it was unenlightened. Biomedicine was illuminating because it was mostly effective, at least for our interlocutors.

Miracles and Historical Conditions

If miracles are objects of wonder, amazing occurrences, or extraordinary events attributed to some supernatural agency, then the first generation experienced a miracle. Indeed, some saw the hand of God in the medicine. Goretti explained that when she tested HIV-positive in 2000, she realized that she and others would die because of the lack of medicine. She wished and prayed, "Let God bring drugs," and two years later her wishes were granted. People marveled at the alterations brought by treatment. Robinah (case I) reported that old friends greeted her when she returned home after some months on treatment by saying, "God is good! What a miracle! What is the magic?" Like Hassan, many spoke about having been close to death ("I was really a gone man") and said that people could hardly believe their transformation ("Are you the same Hassan, or is this another person?"). We heard many exclamations of happy disbelief: "I should have been dead. I was down. You wouldn't believe." "When people see me now, they can't believe and ask, how are these drugs of yours? What is the magic? Most people can't believe that I am the one."

Events are seen as miracles under certain conditions. They are remarkable because they go against expectations; the first generation had known AIDS as a disease of painful decline and certain death. The sudden advent of treatment that had been out of reach wrought miracles for the mortally ill. For the next generation, if funding continues, this will not necessarily be the case. Many of the first generation had been profoundly debilitated by the time they started taking ARVs; like Hassan, they experienced being snatched from the edge of the grave. Health workers in Uganda already say that people are being tested and started in treatment earlier; they no longer see many patients arriving as wasted skeletons. The World Health Organization now recommends that treatment be initiated at a higher CD4 threshold; patients do not have to be so weak to be entitled to treatment. Moreover, the widespread testing of pregnant women, together with the policy of routine testing to rule out HIV among in- and outpatients with persistent sickness, may contribute to earlier identification of people in need of treatment.

The historical conditions for the wondrous recoveries of our interlocutors were reliable supplies of ARVs. In the first years of the rollout, during the time of our study, ARVs were available, and new patients were enrolled rapidly. We heard few worries about the long-term security of drug supplies—at least, not in connection with the programs serving the people we were following. They were more preoccupied with immediate problems and uncertainties, as Steven Russell and Janet Seeley also found in their study of people on ART with the Home-Based AIDS Care (HBAC) program.[4] They developed confidence in the medicine and in the new package of care, which was quite different from what they had known before. The sensibility of assurance was a key characteristic of the shared consciousness of the first generation. This may have been a widespread tendency. In her study of an oncology ward in Botswana, Julie Livingston suggests that the ART program there evoked high expectations of biomedicine more generally. She describes how the power of ARVs contributed to an "emergent biotechnical optimism"; it firmed up hope that was focused on biotechnology and spilled over from experience with ART to the far more intractable challenges of treating cancer.[5]

What would happen to this disposition of confidence if the supply of powerful medicine failed? After the end of our study, intermittent stock-outs of ARVs were reported in several parts of the country.[6] Programs that received funding from the US President's Emergency Program for AIDS Relief (PEPFAR) had more reliable supplies and, when possible, they helped cover supply gaps for other programs. But PEPFAR itself was affected by a ceiling on funds in connection with the financial crisis. From the end of 2008 until the second quarter of 2010, a directive prohibited starting new patients in treatment unless an existing "treatment slot" became available. Peter Mugyenyi has described the effects of this ban, as crowds of very ill patients besieged clinics, pleading to be started on the lifesaving medicine. They felt cheated and betrayed. "Before PEPFAR, when the carnage was at its height most AIDS sufferers accepted their fate with gracious resignation," he writes. "All that AIDS patients were advised to do was to live positively by accepting to die peacefully. The difference this time round, was that the patients knew that death was not inevitable."[7] Many of those who were turned away had been enrolled in HIV programs for several years and were taking Septrin until the time came to start on ARVs. Now the promise was denied.

Health workers, too, who were key members of the first generation, were shaken by the return to the bad old times. Back in the 1990s, Mugyenyi writes, "health-care providers had become experts in their role as bearers of bad news. But by 2008, many had forgotten how to do it. Surely, they would look ridiculous if they once more started advising patients with the hackneyed phrases, 'Live positively, die with dignity.' We had experienced more than six years of hope when, once more, doctors could be doctors who prescribed medicine to patients—medicine that worked. Medicine that was in stock."[8]

Funding from PEPFAR to allow the enrollment of new patients was resumed in 2010, but the new expectations of biomedicine and the contingent nature of donor funding had been clearly revealed. So had the uncertain prospects for the next cohort of patients. Our interlocutors were part of a minority during the period of our study. It is estimated that coverage of those in need of ART went from 12 percent in 2004 to 33 percent in 2007 and 58 percent in 2011.[9] This means that funding must not only maintain those already in treatment; it must expand to reach others who still require it. Moreover, with new cases of HIV outstripping AIDS-related mortality, a growing number of people are going to need treatment.[10] If funding for ART does not increase, the next generation may face the situation that existed before 2004: that the miracle of ART was for the fortunate minority.

(Bio)sociality

The first generation experienced the power of biomedicine to identify a category of people through testing and to save the lives of the resourceful, willing, and fortunate among them. Two questions arise. First, to what extent did biomedicine facilitate the formation of new social ties based on diagnosis and a treatment? And second, how did these forms of biosociality relate to the sociality of households, families, and networks founded on other principles?

Clientship is the most common form taken by biosociality at this juncture in Uganda's history. This enduring, unequal relationship of dependence and obligation between treatment program and client is new in Ugandan health care. Perhaps the closest precedents are the leprosy treatment programs of the 1950s, which also registered patients and attached them to therapy sites over a period of time. But the scope of those programs and the number of people involved were limited.[11] In terms of HIV, clientship has taken several forms, as we have seen. For some, such as clients of the Joint Clinical Research Centre, the interaction was mainly with the institution that monitored them and prescribed and dispensed the next supply of medicine. Those who attended smaller rural clinics developed personal relationships with their health workers around their treatment. Jessica expounded on her relationship to the health workers at the treatment facility near the trading center where she sold cooked food: "even the health workers, they are so happy that I have been responding well. That is why the clinical officer chose me to come and talk to you." When Phoebe asked how she interacted with others in treatment, she said that she saw them at the clinic but did not know any of them: "they just sit there until they get their medicine, and then they each go home to their place."

The specific biosociality of patron-client relationships that developed in ART programs was facilitated by social technology such as "homework"—instructions to eat well, drink clean water, take medication at specific times, practice safe sex.[12] The clients could expect more complete support from their patrons if they did their homework properly. It reflected well on the health workers' job performance when their clients were "compliant."[13] But the fact that the clients' homework had to be carried out in domestic contexts meant that the biosocialities of ART projects were deeply entangled with the socialities of families and households.

The biosociality of clientship could include "expert clients" assisting in clinics or during home visits, following the GIPA (Greater Involvement of People with AIDS) Principle.[14] To assume these functions, some were given the chance to attend short training sessions on peer counseling. All of these social relations were aspects of clientship that were open only to those who tested HIV-positive and showed commitment to treatment. That is, they were biosocial because they were based on diagnostic and therapeutic criteria. But here, too, biosociality was built on pre-existing forms of sociality in that becoming and remaining a client were facilitated by support from family, friends, and acquaintances.

A minority of clients were active in Post-Test Clubs and other kinds of peer groups that some scholars have associated with biological citizenship.[15] Common identity, emotional support, advocacy, and activism were the key characteristics of such groups in the global North. Vinh-Kim Nguyen's research in Ivory Coast and Burkina Faso showed the different role they played in conditions of poverty and the absence of a strong state, where people needed material support. In his study, group leaders or facilitators attempted to foster solidarity by encouraging members to talk about ("confess") their HIV-positive status. But this kind of solidarity stood in opposition to that of the broader moral economy of kinship and community on which people depended. Announcing one's positive serostatus might lead to alienation from family members, who saw such disclosure as unnecessary, if not shaming.[16]

Members of the first generation in Uganda did not seem to feel caught between conflicting moral economies of AIDS groups and families. Many hoped that they would gain some opportunities from joining the peer groups, such as new contacts to projects and people with resources, volunteer jobs that would provide allowances, or material support. Far from alienating their families, group participation might allow them to contribute to their households and relatives. Joyce, who chaired her Post-Test Club, was clear about the advantages that she enjoyed and passed along to her sister. MamaGirl (case IV) had laid the foundation of a political career as local councilor through her involvement with a Post-Test Club and the outreach activities of the HBAC and TASO. Through TASO and, later, the Local Council 3, she brought home goats, pigs, poultry, and the prospect of orphan support for household children.

Robinah was active in the Post-Test Club that her sister Joyce led. This gave her access to other groups, including the project for which she produced her prize-winning picture. For a few years, these biosocial groups, which were organized around a shared diagnosis and therapeutic situation, were important to Robinah's transformation from being a dying AIDS victim to being an ART client. However, after the first years of learning how to be a client, she moved back to Kumi to help her children and resettle in her family. Our point is that clients joined groups not only for "self-care" and bio-fellowship, but also to (re)gain the ability to participate in family sociality. In the end, that was the most important concern for most of the people most of the time.

Ultimately, the farthest-reaching innovation in sociality for the first generation was not the support groups. Although the criterion for admission (a diagnosis) was new, the principle of groups for support and development was not. "Groupism" had been encouraged by development policy for decades; big initiatives such as the National Agricultural Advisory Services (NAADS) and Rural Water and Sanitation (RUWASA) required beneficiaries to form groups. Women's groups were widespread; there were groups for micro-credit, Anglican mothers, landmine survivors, and many more. What was more revolutionary was clientship as a form of treatment. Everyone had to join a treatment program and establish a relationship to the treatment providers, while Post-Test Clubs were optional. Clientship demanded regular contacts and should be enduring, while active participation in other groups was usually limited in duration. Clinics at health centers and hospitals that devoted a time and a space to one kind of disease were not unknown before ART. District hospitals had mental health clinics and antenatal clinics on fixed days in appointed rooms. But mental health patients were not so regular in fetching their refills as HIV patients were required to be. And pregnant women only make two to four visits in the course of nine months. The new social relations of the first generation were first and foremost to their health care providers and to the treatment programs they joined. Those relations were the basis for possible membership in support groups and HIV welfare organizations. They were, in any case, the condition for continuing life in their families. As Jessica said, "After refilling their medicine, they each go home to their place."

Chances of Problems

It was in their own places, among family, neighbors, and workmates, that people undertook their second chances. It was there the euphoria of miracles was tempered by "descent into the ordinary." With a smile, Esther talked about the wonder her recovery evoked among friends. They thought she must be taking medicine from "outside," perhaps from South Africa. Or was it herbal medicine that had transformed her? A neighbor who had just lost a son said she had money, if only Esther would tell her where to buy the medicine that might save her bereaved daughter-in-law. She could not believe that free medicine from the local hospital could be so powerful; was Esther hiding something? Yet as the discussion came to a close, Esther talked about her pain and constant sweating. She was worried about what would happen to her children if she died, and she could not sleep at night without taking a sedative. When Jenipher tried to say that it sounded as if her grown children were doing well and helping her, she fell silent. Tears ran down her cheeks.

The medicine gave people a second chance, but it was a second chance at life that was still full of problems and pain and the specter of death—a move "from certain death to uncertain survival."[17] The transition to a new life on ARVs was never a linear process, as Russell and Seeley point out.[18] Jessica, who radiated joy and amazement at her survival when Phoebe first met her, hardly smiled at all when Phoebe visited again four months later. The medicine had given her life and appetite, but she had no money to buy food; her daughter had left; her legs hurt; and the hospital had run out of ointment for the skin rash she attributed to Triomune. Physical afflictions, whether medications' side effects, opportunistic infections, or simply ordinary illnesses and injuries, plagued people time and again. Even on ART, they did not feel guaranteed of their health; many knew someone who had started on the medicine but died anyhow.

There were people for whom social hurts of the past seemed to predominate over the elation of rising from the deathbed. Cathy, a widow, denied that ARVs had changed her life. In their first long interview, Hanne and Phoebe sensed her resentment about her husband's death and her antipathy toward his relatives—perhaps a result of conflicts before or during his illness. Antiretroviral therapy may restore physical health, but it does not necessarily heal the social and emotional wounds HIV and AIDS have inflicted along the way.

In the face of loss and uncertainty, many people found support in their religious faith. We did not specifically ask people about the significance of religion in their lives, but reading through our notes we found many assertions, explicit and implicit, of the role that it played. (Like Dominic, several of our interlocutors were Muslim, and their faith was no doubt important for them, too, but they did not talk about it so emphatically, perhaps because they knew we were not Muslim.) Cathy, a widow in Kampala, had joined a Pentecostal church and asserted that nothing could change her faith. She compared her trials to those of Job, who remained steadfast. "I realize that Job could have suffered from this same disease," she said, "But he didn't change. He had sores all over, and they itched like the ones you get with AIDS. Maybe if they had had the machine, they would have found that Job had AIDS. But he didn't change. God praised him and healed him. He even had many children after that."

Faith was not only the idiom of acceptance, providing peace, self-confidence, and resolve. Many people referred to God as a social actor who intervened in practical ways in their daily lives. They spoke of God as a being with whom they communicated and who acted to help, just as living relatives did, with both small and large problems. When Phoebe brought her a gift of sugar, Dorothy, the prison officer in eastern Uganda, said, "Oh, madam, you have actually helped me so much because I specifically did not have sugar. I was going to borrow from somebody, but God is good. He has brought you at the right time. That is why I got saved after testing HIV-positive, and God has actually helped me through this period and helped me deal with my enemies." Dorothy's husband, who was also HIV-positive and saved, pointed to a calendar on the wall. "You know, God is great," he said. "You see that calendar? I bought two of them because of the words on it: 'God's power works within us. Ephesians 3.20.'" He went on to give examples of the miracles God can do—for example, God had answered his wife's prayers when he was threatened with a job transfer.

Elizabeth, a widowed midwife in middle age, said that she had to trust in God, because if the third-line medicine that she took failed, she did not know what she would do. She said that she thanked God for ensuring she had her meager salary to pay school fees and rent and to buy medicine and that God also helped her get access to free ARVs. Loyce, who had a stall in a big Kampala market, was one of several of our interlocutors who said she had been born again after an acquaintance had witnessed to her. "Being born again has helped me so much and has enabled me not to worry or be anxious," she said. "Now that I am on ARVs, I want to work for my children, to pay so that they can stay in school. It was God who helped me to complete payment of the children's school fees last year. My prayer is that they will discover drugs that cure AIDS." Loyce was fervent in her gratitude but by no means left everything to God. She knew she had to exert herself for the sake of her children. As Jessica put it, "I really thank God for these ARVs. God can give you a second chance, but you have to make an effort yourself and take the medicine."

Second chances were always chances of trouble and uncertainty. With the reprieve and relative security of ART, with the conversion to clientship, Dominic and others like him turned to the practicalities of dealing with other problems to achieve the chance and hope of relative well-being and fulfillment. They might find comfort in religion, but the examples of God's hand in paying school fees suggests that it was at least as much the challenges of everyday life as the existential uncertainties of life that preoccupied the first generation.

"A Living and a Life"

The people of the first generation were keen to emphasize that AIDS had become a normal disease. One called it "the big malaria." By "normal" they seemed to mean that it was common and could be treated; many people, all kinds of people, were HIV-positive. They were not unique in their condition. Jackie (case VI) said that gossip about her sickness had once made her angry, "But now I take it normally, because I see many people—good-looking people—who come to the clinic. Then I ask, who am I?" Dorothy remarked that others were even worse off than she was. "Although we have all those problems, I have come to realize that AIDS is with us, especially when I go to the hospital and see young girls who have not even had children," she said. "Then I relax and know that I am not alone. So I do my work, and I don't think about AIDS. That is why you see that I look like this—except having money problems."

For our interlocutors, HIV was shifting from the text to the context of their life stories. For people who had accepted their illness as a chronic disease to be treated with medicine, the "disorder was a part of the 'horizon' of their experience, rather than 'thematized' as central to their lives."[19] This impression was reinforced for us because we visited people in their homes, where they were preoccupied by domestic matters, rather than meeting them at the clinic, where their illness was in focus. The matters that *were* thematized as central to their lives were diverse, as we have shown in the case studies of this book. Basically, and too roughly, they can be summarized as "a living and a life." By "a living," we mean a sufficient livelihood; by "a life," we mean not mere survival but a social existence of reciprocity and respect.

The difference between biological survival and a living was brought home to Rosalind Morris by a young unemployed man in a South African mining town, who said, "You are saving us for dying. We want to make a living."[20] Research on the transition to living with HIV as a chronic disease among clients of the HBAC program also emphasized the overwhelming problems of livelihood: "a new life on ART had, in effect, returned participants to the *normal worries and struggles of poverty* and making a living in this resource-poor setting."[21] Our interlocutors had diverse livelihoods; some were employed. Yet "money problems" figured prominently for them all.

Lack of cash was a hindrance for everything from paying transportation costs and buying food items to covering medical expenses. The cost of education was one of the most frequently mentioned burdens. James, the university student in Kampala, was desperately searching for funds during his final semester. He had almost missed exams the previous semester because he had no money for fees. Then he was saved by a loan from a relative, to be repaid by his cousins and friends. During Godfrey's last visit to James, he was once more up against the deadline for payment, on which depended his chance to graduate. He needed money to travel to the home of a certain grandfather who might contribute. If he managed to pay his final fees (which he did, with a little help from Godfrey and more from others), he would face life after university when he would be expected to pay fees for others: his child, who should be starting nursery school, and his younger brother, who had not been able to continue to senior secondary school because of lack of money. A nurse at a military barracks hospital described the difficulties facing her clients on ART. "Soldiers are poorly paid," she said. "The salary given to them is not enough, and yet they have big families. An average soldier has four children, but many have seven—and two wives—on a salary of 140,000 shillings [about $55] a month. From this amount they have to pay school fees. So you find that although these soldiers are getting ARVs, they are strained and stressed."

The struggle to support children and pay school fees alerts us to the way livelihood was about more than staying alive. Through children, people oriented themselves toward a family future and participation in the continuing story of kinship. Jolly's urgent desire for a child was about staying alive socially. She expressed the sentiments of many people on ART when she made it clear that children make one a full person. Being childless because of failure to conceive or loss of all of one's children seemed as great a problem as being HIV-positive. In contrast, studying, as James was doing, or sending one's children or younger siblings to school was a commitment to family and future.

Livelihood was a means to achieve social participation, to care for other people, and to gain recognition as a "useful" person. That is, a living makes possible a life, with its "entailment in webs of signs, relations, and affect" and its "will to assert visibility, dignity, kinship, and attachment [that] fuels the task of everyday survival."[22] In Uganda, people wanted to be recognized as more than "HIV survivors," not so much by the state or organizations as by families, friends, and neighbors—those with whom they hoped to share future lives.

An intervention offers a solution to a particular problem, often a specific disease, and focuses the attention of policy makers and health workers on that one issue. In people's lives, problems seldom exist in the singular; either the solution to one also relieves the others or, more commonly, the tentative alleviation of one urgent problem brings others into sharper profile. Antiretroviral therapy was a reprieve and a conversion to life on chronic treatment, but in diminishing one shadow, it shed light on a great array of other problems whose resolution is still uncertain: livelihood, eating, the future of children. It brought better health but no guarantee of good health—only a tendency to worry greatly over every bout of illness. What ethnography reveals are the links between the text (the disease in focus) and the context (the other problems of health and life). Every morbidity has a "co-morbidity" in the form of other illnesses and troubles. And every medical treatment has complementary social efforts at managing the one trouble and the others.

Notes

1. S. Whyte et al., "Health Workers Entangled."
2. Mogensen, AIDS Is a Kind of Kahungu That Kills.
3. S. Whyte, Questioning Misfortune.
4. Like Russell and Seeley ("The Transition to Living with HIV as a Chronic Condition," 378), we found a few people in the HBAC's research and treatment program

who had heard it was going to close and worried about what would happen if it did. In fact, the program did end after our study finished. All of its clients were transferred to TASO, and they continued to receive medicine, although the level of service was substantially lower.

5. Livingston, *Improvising Medicine*, 170–73.

6. Park, "Stock-Outs in Global Health."

7. Mugyenyi, *A Cure Too Far*, 285.

8. Mugyenyi, *A Cure Too Far*, 286.

9. Joint United Nations Program on HIV/AIDS (UNAIDS) and World Health Organization (WHO), *Epidemiological Fact Sheet on HIV and AIDS*; Uganda AIDS Commission, *Global AIDS Response Progress Report*.

10. Uganda Government, *UNGASS Country Progress Report, Uganda*.

11. Brown, "The Uganda Leprosy Control Scheme."

12. Meinert, "Regimes of Homework."

13. Meinert, "Regimes of Homework."

14. Kyakuwa et al., "The Adopted Children of ART."

15. Rose and Novas, "Biological Citizenship."

16. Nguyen, *The Republic of Therapy*, 83–84.

17. Meinert et al., "Tests for Life Chances," 196.

18. Russell and Seeley, "The Transition to Living with HIV as a Chronic Condition in Rural Uganda," 381.

19. Good, "The Narrative Representation of Illness," 155.

20. Morris, "Rush/Panic/Rush," 205.

21. Russell and Seeley, "The Transition to Living with HIV as a Chronic Condition in Rural Uganda," 381.

22. Comaroff, "Beyond Bare Life," 209.

ACKNOWLEDGMENTS

We are grateful to the forty-eight people on antiretroviral treatment who agreed to tell us about their lives and profoundly so to the twenty-three among them who welcomed us for repeated visits. We contacted them through the generous assistance of Busolwe Hospital, the Joint Clinical Research Centre in Kampala and Mbale, the Infectious Diseases Institute at Mulago National Referral Hospital, Mukuju Health Centre, and Reach Out Mbuya. We thank the health workers Michael Mwangale and Henry Mwombekere, who took a personal interest in our study.

The research was part of a long-term collaboration funded by the Council for Development Research under the Danish Ministry of Foreign Affairs, to whom we extend deep appreciation. At Makerere University, the project's home was the Child Health and Development Centre (CHDC). The CHDC's director at the time, Jessica Jitta, and its administrator, Augustine Mutumba, were wonderfully supportive. We learned from conversations with colleagues in Uganda: Frank Kaharuza, Anne Katahoire, Edward Kirumira, Cissy Kityo, Betty Kyaddondo, Herbert Muyinda, and Janet Seeley. We are grateful to the Uganda National Council for Science and Technology for permission to carry out the study.

The Department of Anthropology was our foundation at the University of Copenhagen. We thank our good colleagues there for the stimulating academic milieu and Jørgen Pedersen for sorting out practical problems in his kind way. Thanks as well to Steen Kelså for expert help with the illustrations. Kathrin Houmoeller was our pilot reader and provided helpful suggestions, while João Biehl, Hansjörg Dilger, Paul Wenzel Geissler, Anita Hardon, Lene Diemer Jørgensen, Adriana Petryna, Ruth Prince, and Lisa Richey shared knowledge from their research and gave encouragement.

Versions of the stories of Robinah and Joyce and of Jolly appeared in Lotte Meinert, Hanne O. Mogensen, and Jenipher Twebaze, "Tests for Life Chances: CD4 Miracles and Obstacles in Uganda," *Anthropology and Medicine* 16, no. 2 (2009): 195–209. An earlier version of parts of chapters 1 and 2 appeared as Susan Reynolds Whyte, Michael A. Whyte, Lotte Meinert, and Jenipher Twebaze, "Therapeutic Clientship: Belonging in Uganda's Projectified Landscape of AIDS Care," in *When People Come First: Critical Studies in Global Health*, ed. João Biehl and Adriana Petryna (Princeton, NJ: Princeton University Press, 2013: 140–65).

BIBLIOGRAPHY

AIDS Control Program, AIDS Support Organization, United Nations Children's Fund, and World Health Organization. *Living with AIDS in the Community.* Kampala, Uganda: AIDS Control Program, 1991.

Alber, Erdmute, Sjaak van der Geest, and Susan Reynolds Whyte, eds. *Generations in Africa: Connections and Conflicts.* Münster, Germany: LIT Verlag, 2008.

Alcano, Matteo Carlo. "Living and Working in Spite of Antiretroviral Therapies: Strength in Chronicity." *Anthropology and Medicine* 16, no. 2 (2009): 119–30.

Alibhai, Arif, Walter Kipp, L. Duncan Saunders, Ambikaipakan Senthilselvan, Amy Kaler, Stan Houston, Joseph Konde-Lulu, Joa Okech-Ojony, and Tom Rubaale. "Gender-Related Mortality for HIV-Infected Patients on Highly Active Antiretroviral Therapy (HAART) in Rural Uganda." *International Journal of Women's Health* 2 (2010): 45–52.

Allen, Tim, and Suzette Heald. "The Political Environment of HIV: What Has Worked in Uganda and What Has Failed in Botswana." *Journal of International Development* 16 (2004): 1141–54.

Ankrah, E. Maxine. "The Impact of HIV/AIDS on the Family and Other Significant Relationships: The African Clan Revisited." *AIDS Care* 5, no. 1 (1993): 5–22.

Apondi, Rose, Rebecca Bunnell, Anna Awor, Nafuna Wamai, Winifred Bikaako-Kajura, Peter Solberg, Ron D. Stall, Alex Coutinho, and Jonathan Mermin. "Home-Based Antiretroviral Care Is Associated with Positive Social Outcomes in a Prospective Cohort in Uganda." *Journal of Acquired Immune Deficiency Syndrome* 44, no. 1 (2007): 71–76.

Appadurai, Arjun. "Gastro-Politics in Hindu South Asia." *American Ethnologist* 8, no. 3 (1981): 494–511.

Arendt, Hannah. *The Human Condition,* 2nd ed. Chicago: University of Chicago Press, 1998.

Barnett, Tony, and Piers Blaikie. *AIDS in Africa: Its Present and Future Impact*. New York: Guilford, 1992.

Barnett, Tony, and Alan Whiteside. *AIDS in the Twenty-First Century: Disease and Globalization*, 2nd ed. Basingstoke, UK: Palgrave Macmillan, 2006.

Baro, Mamadou, and Tara F. Deubel. "Persistent Hunger: Perspectives on Vulnerability, Famine, and Food Security in Sub-Saharan Africa." *Annual Review of Anthropology* 35 (2006): 521–38.

Beuving, J. J. "Playing Pool along the Shores of Lake Victoria: Fishermen, Careers and Capital Accumulation in the Ugandan Nile Perch Business." *Africa* 80, no. 2 (2010): 224–48.

Biehl, João. *Will to Live: AIDS Therapies and the Politics of Survival*. Princeton, NJ: Princeton University Press, 2007.

Biehl, João, and Adriana Petryna. "Critical Global Health." In *When People Come First: Critical Studies in Global Health*, ed. João Biehl and Adriana Petryna, 1–20. Princeton, NJ: Princeton University Press, 2013.

Bikaako-Kajura, Emmanuel Luyirika, David W. Purcell, Julia Downing, Frank Kaharuza, Jonathan Mermin, Samuel Malamba, and Rebecca Bunnell. "Disclosure of HIV Status and Adherence to Daily Drug Regimens among HIV-Infected Children in Uganda." *AIDS Behaviour* 10 (2006): S85–93.

Bluebond-Langner, Myra. *The Private Worlds of Dying Children*. Princeton, NJ: Princeton University Press, 1978.

Brown, J. A. Kinnear. "The Uganda Leprosy Control Scheme." *East African Medical Journal* 33, no. 7 (1956): 259–70.

Bukusuba, John, Joyce K. Kikafunda, and Roger G. Whitehead. "Nutritional Knowledge, Attitudes and Practices of Women Living with HIV in Eastern Uganda." *Journal of Health, Population and Nutrition* 28, no. 2 (2010): 182–88.

Bunnell, Rebecca, Alex Opio, Joshua Musinguzi, Wilford Kirungi, Paul Ekwaru, Vinod Mishra, Wolfgang Hladik, Jessica Kafuko, Elizabeth Madraa, and Jonathan Mermin. "HIV Transmission Risk Behavior among HIV-Infected Adults in Uganda: Results of a Nationally Representative Survey." *AIDS* 22, no. 5 (2008): 617–24.

Burnett, Judith. *Generations: The Time Machine in Theory and Practice*. Farnham, UK: Ashgate, 2010.

Byakika-Tusiime, J., J. H. Oyugi, W. A. Tumwikirize, E. T. Katabira, P. N. Mugyenyi, and D. R. Bangsberg. "Adherence to HIV Antiretroviral Therapy in HIV+ Ugandan Patients Purchasing Therapy." *International Journal of STD and AIDS* 16 (2005): 38–41.

Cammack, Diana. "The Logic of African Neopatrimonialism: What Role for Donors?" *Development Policy Review* 25, no. 5 (2007): 599–614.

Carsten, Janet. "Introduction: Cultures of Relatedness." In *Cultures of Relatedness: New Approaches to the Study of Kinship*, ed. Janet Carsten, 1–36. Cambridge: Cambridge University Press, 2000.

Carsten, Janet. "The Substance of Kinship and the Heat of the Hearth: Feeding, Personhood, and Relatedness among Malays in Pulau Langkawi." *American Ethnologist* 22, no. 2 (1995): 223–41.

Chabal, Patrick. *Africa: The Politics of Suffering and Smiling*. London: Zed, 2009.

Christiansen, Catrine. "Development by Churches, Development of Churches: Institutional Trajectories in Rural Uganda." PhD dissertation, University of Copenhagen, 2010.

Christiansen, Catrine. "The New Wives of Christ: Paradoxes and Potentials in the Remaking of Widow Lives in Uganda." In *AIDS and Religious Practice in Africa*, ed. Felicitas Becker and Paul Wenzel Geissler, 85–116. Leiden, Netherlands: Brill, 2009.

Christiansen, Catrine, Mats Utas, and Henrik Vigh, eds. *Navigating Youth, Generating Adulthood: Social Becoming in an African Context.* Uppsala, Sweden: Nordic Africa Institute, 2006.

Cohen, David W., and E. S. Atieno Odhiambo. *Burying SM: The Politics of Knowledge and the Sociology of Power in Africa*. Portsmouth, NH: Heinemann, 1992.

Cole, Jennifer, and Deborah Durham, eds. *Generations and Globalization: Youth, Age, and Family in the New World Economy*. Bloomington: Indiana University Press, 2006.

Comaroff, Jean. "Beyond Bare Life: AIDS, (Bio)Politics, and the Neoliberal Order." *Public Culture* 19, no. 1 (2007): 197–219.

Das, Veena. *Life and Words: Exploring Violence and the Descent into the Ordinary*. Berkeley: University of California Press, 2006.

deWaal, Alex, and Alan Whiteside. "New Variant Famine: AIDS and Food Crisis in Southern Africa." *The Lancet* 362, no. 9391 (2003): 1234–37.

Dilger, Hansjörg. "'My Relatives Are Running Away from Me!': Kinship and Care in the Wake of Structural Adjustment, Privatisation and HIV/AIDS in Tanzania." In *Morality, Hope and Grief: Anthropologies of AIDS in Africa*, ed. Hansjörg Dilger and Ute Luig, 102–24. New York: Berghahn, 2010.

Dilley, Roy. "The Problem of Context: An Introduction." In *The Problem of Context*, ed. Roy Dilley, 1–46. Oxford: Berghahn, 1999.

Douglas, Mary. *Natural Symbols: Explorations in Cosmology*. London: Barrie and Rockliff, 1970.

Dryden-Peterson, Sarah, and Eric Kamunvi. *Living with HIV/AIDS in Uganda and the Impact of Holistic Interventions: Clients Tell Their Stories*, ed. Reach Out Mbuya HIV/AIDS Initiative. Kampala, Uganda: Reach Out Mbuya, 2003.

Edmunds, June, and Bryan S. Turner. "Global Generations: Social Change in the Twentieth Century." *British Journal of Sociology* 56, no. 4 (2005): 559–77.

Edwards, Jeanette, and Marilyn Strathern. "Including Our Own." In *Cultures of Relatedness: New Approaches to the Study of Kinship*, ed. Janet Carsten, 149–66. Cambridge: Cambridge University Press, 2000.

Epstein, Helen. *The Invisible Cure: Why We Are Losing the Fight against AIDS in Africa*. New York: Picador, 2007.

Erdmann, Gero, and Ulf Engel. "Neopatrimonialism Reconsidered: Critical Review and Elaboration of an Elusive Concept." *Commonwealth and Comparative Politics* 45, no. 1 (2007): 95–119.

Faber, Kim. *Esthers Bog—Om at Overleve med HIV/AIDS*. Copenhagen: Politiken Bøger, 2004.

Farmer, Paul. *AIDS and Accusation: Haiti and the Geography of Blame*. Berkeley: University of California Press, 1992.

Fassin, Didier. *When Bodies Remember: Experiences and Politics of AIDS in South Africa*. Berkeley: University of California Press, 2007.

Feierman, Elizabeth Karlin. "Alternative Medical Services in Rural Tanzania: A Physician's View." *Social Science and Medicine* 15B (1981): 399–404.

Feierman, Steven. "Struggles for Control: The Social Roots of Health and Healing in Modern Africa." *African Studies Review* 28, nos. 2–3 (1985): 73–147.

Feierman, Steven, and John M. Janzen. "Introduction." In *The Social Basis of Health and Healing in Africa*, ed. Steven Feierman and John M. Janzen, 1–23. Berkeley: University of California Press, 1992.

Folmann, Birgitte. "Motherhood, Moralities and HIV: Making Lives in Northern Uganda." PhD dissertation, Aarhus University, 2012.

Fortes, Meyer. *Kinship and the Social Order*. London: Routledge and Kegan Paul, 1970 [1969].

Foucault, Michel. "Technologies of the Self." In *Technologies of the Self*, ed. Luther H. Martin, Huck Gutman, and Patrick H. Hutton, 16–49. Amherst: University of Massachusetts Press, 1998.

Geissler, Paul Wenzel. "Studying Trial Communities: Anthropological and Historical Inquiries into Ethos, Politics and Economy of Medical Research in Africa." In *Evidence, Ethos and Experiment: The Anthropology and History of Medical Research in Africa*, ed. Paul Wenzel Geissler and Catherine Molyneux, 1–28. Oxford: Berghahn, 2011.

Gluckman, Max. *Analysis of a Social Situation in Modern Zululand*. Manchester: Manchester University Press, 1958 [1940].

Goffman, Erving. *Stigma: Notes on the Management of Spoiled Identity*. Englewood Cliffs, NJ: Prentice-Hall, 1963.

Good, Byron J. "The Narrative Representation of Illness." In *Medicine, Rationality, and Experience: An Anthropological Perspective*, ed. Byron J. Good, 135–65. Cambridge: Cambridge University Press, 1994.

Green, Edward C. *Rethinking AIDS Prevention*. Westport, CT: Praeger, 2003.

Grillo, R. D. *African Railwaymen: Solidarity and Opposition in an East African Labour Force*. Cambridge: Cambridge University Press, 1973.

Guyer, Jane. "Wealth in People and Self-Realization in Equatorial Africa." *Africa Studies Review* 39, no. 3 (1993): 1–28.

Hardon, Anita, and Deborah Posel. "Secrecy as Embodied Practice: Beyond the Confessional Imperative." *Culture, Health and Sexuality* 14, supp. 1 (2012): S1–13.

Hardon, A. P., D. Akurut, C. Comoro, C. Ekezie, H. F. Irunde, T. Gerrits, J. Kglatwane, J. Kinsman, R. Kwasa, J. Maridadi, T. M. Moroka, S. Moyo, A. Nakiyemba, S. Nsimba, R. Ogenyi, T. Oyabba, F. Temu, and R. Laing. "Hunger, Waiting Time and Transport Costs: Time to Confront Challenges to ART Adherence in Africa." *AIDS Care* 19, no. 5 (2007): 658–65.

Harries, A. D., D. S. Nyangulu, N. J. Hargreaves, O. Kaluwa, and F. M. Salaniponi. "Preventing Antiretroviral Anarchy in Sub-Saharan Africa." *The Lancet* 358 (2001): 410–14.

Holtzman, Jon. "Politics and Gastropolitics: Gender and the Power of Food in Two African Pastoralist Societies." *Journal of the Royal Anthropological Institute* 8, no. 4 (2002): 259–78.

Homsy, J., R. Bunnell, D. Moore, R. King, and S. Malamba et al. "Reproductive Intentions and Outcomes among Women on Antiretroviral Therapy in Rural Uganda: A Prospective Cohort Study." *PLoS ONE* 4, no. 1 (2009): e4149.

Honwana, Alcinda, and Filip De Boeck, eds. *Makers and Breakers: Children and Youth in Postcolonial Africa*. Oxford: James Currey, 2005.

Hunter, Susan. "Orphans as a Window on the AIDS Epidemic in Sub-Saharan Africa: Initial Results and Implications of a Study in Uganda." *Social Science and Medicine* 31, no. 6 (1990): 681–90.

Iliffe, John. *The African AIDS Epidemic: A History.* Athens: Ohio University Press, 2006.

Iliffe, John. *East African Doctors: A History of the Modern Profession.* Cambridge: Cambridge University Press, 1998.

Janzen, John M. *The Quest for Therapy in Lower Zaire.* Berkeley: University of California Press, 1978.

Janzen, John M. "Therapy Management: Concept, Reality, Process." *Medical Anthropology Quarterly* 1, no. 1 (1987): 68–84.

Johnson-Hanks, Jennifer. *Uncertain Honor: Modern Motherhood in an African Crisis.* Chicago: University of Chicago Press, 2006.

Joint Clinical Research Centre, ed. "Basic Facts about Antiretroviral Therapy (ART)." Kampala, Uganda: Joint Clinical Research Centre, n.d.

Joint United Nations Program on HIV/AIDS (UNAIDS) and World Health Organization (WHO). *Epidemiological Fact Sheet on HIV and AIDS, Uganda, 2008 Update.* Geneva: UNAIDS/WHO Working Group on Global HIV/AIDS and Sexually Transmitted Infections, 2008.

Jørgensen, Line Diemer Lyng. "'We Have a Second Chance and That Chance Is Now: A Study of Conversion to Life at a Faith-Based HIV/AIDS Programme in Kampala." Paper presented at Nordic Africa Days Conference in Uppsala, Sweden, 30 September-2 October 2005.

Jørgensen, Line Diemer Lyng. "Counselling, Coping and Conversion to a New Life: A Study of the Counselling Department at Reach out Mbuya Parish HIV/AIDS Initiative in Uganda, January to April 2005, in the Light of Sociology of Religion." Masters thesis, University of Copenhagen, 2006.

Kaleeba, Noerine, with Sunanda Ray. *We Miss You All,* 2nd ed. Harare, Zimbabwe: SAf-AIDS, 2002.

Kaler, Amy, and Susan Cotts Watkins. "Disobedient Distributors: Street-Level Bureaucrats and Would-Be Patrons in Community-Based Family Planning Programs in Rural Kenya." *Studies in Family Planning* 32, no. 3 (2001): 254–69.

Kaler, Amy, Arif Alibhai, Walter Kipp, Tom Rubaale, and Joseph Konde-Lule. "'Living by the Hoe' in the Age of Treatment: Perceptions of Household Well-Being after Antiretroviral Treatment among Family Members of Persons with AIDS." *AIDS Care* 22, no. 4 (2010): 509–19.

Kalofonos, Ippolytos Andreas. "'All I Eat Is ARVs': The Paradox of AIDS Treatment Interventions in Central Mozambique." *Medical Anthropology Quarterly* 24, no. 3 (2010): 363–80.

Kapferer, Bruce. "Situations, Crisis, and the Anthropology of the Concrete: The Contribution of Max Gluckman." *Social Analysis* 49, no. 3 (2005): 85–122.

King, Rachel, David Katuntu, Julie Lifshay, Laura Packel, Richard Batamita, Sylvia Nakayiwa, Betty Abang, Frances Babirye, Pille Lindkvist, Eva Johansson, Jonathan Mermin, and Rebecca Bunnell. "Processes and Outcomes of HIV Serostatus Disclosure to Sexual Partners among People Living with HIV in Uganda." *AIDS and Behavior* 12 (2008): 232–43.

Kinsman, John. "Pragmatic Choices: Research, Politics and AIDS Control in Uganda." PhD dissertation, University of Amsterdam, 2008.

Kinsman, John. *AIDS Policy in Uganda: Evidence, Ideology, and the Making of an African Success Story.* Basingstoke, UK: Palgrave Macmillan, 2010.

Kipp, W., D. Tindyebwa, T. Rubaale, E. Karamagi, and E. Bajenja. "Family Caregivers in Rural Uganda: The Hidden Reality." *Health Care for Women International* 28, no. 12 (2007): 856–71.

Kisuule, John David. "The Social and Cultural Context of the HIV/AIDS Epidemic in Rural Areas of Jinja District." PhD dissertation, University of Oslo, 2007.

Konrad, Monica. *Narrating the New Predictive Genetics: Ethics, Ethnography and Science.* Cambridge: Cambridge University Press, 2005.

Kyakuwa, Margaret. "Ethnographic Experiences of HIV-Positive Nurses in Managing Stigma at a Clinic in Rural Uganda." *African Journal of AIDS Research* 8, no. 3 (2009): 367–78.

Kyakuwa, Margaret, and Anita Hardon. "Concealment Tactics among HIV-Positive Nurses in Uganda." *Culture, Health and Sexuality* 14, supp. 1 (2012): S123–33.

Kyakuwa, Margaret, Anita Hardon, and Zoe Goldstein. "'The Adopted Children of ART': Expert Clients and Role Tensions in ART Provision in Uganda." *Medical Anthropology* 31, no. 2 (2012): 149–61.

Leder, Drew. *The Absent Body.* Chicago: University of Chicago Press, 1990.

Leshabari, Sebalda Charles, Astrid Blystad, and Karen Marie Moland. "Difficult Choices: Infant Feeding Experiences of HIV-Positive Mothers in Northern Tanzania." *Sahara-J* 4, no. 1 (2007): 544–55.

Livingston, Julie. *Improvising Medicine: An African Oncology Ward in an Emerging Cancer Epidemic.* Durham, NC: Duke University Press, 2012.

Lock, Margaret, and Nancy Scheper-Hughes. "The Mindful Body." *Medical Anthropology Quarterly* 1, no. 1 (1987): 6–41.

Maier, Marissa, Irene Andia, Nneka Emenyonu, David Guzman, Angela Kaida, Larry Pepper, Robert Hogg, and David R. Bangsberg. "Antiretroviral Therapy Is Associated with Increased Fertility Desire, but Not Pregnancy or Live Birth, among HIV-Positive Women in an Early HIV Treatment Program in Rural Uganda." *AIDS Behavior* 13 (2009): S28–37.

Mannheim, Karl. "Essay on the Problem of Generations." In *Essays on the Sociology of Knowledge*, ed. Paul Kecskemeti. New York: Routledge and Kegan Paul, 1952 [1927].

McGrath, J. W., E. Maxine Ankrah, D. A. Schumann, S. Nkumbi, and M. Lubega. "AIDS and the Urban Family: Its Impact in Kampala, Uganda." *AIDS Care* 5, no. 1 (1993): 55–70.

Meinert, Lotte. "Sweet and Bitter Places: The Politics of Schoolchildren's Orientation in Rural Uganda." In *Children and Place: Cross-Cultural Perspectives*, ed. Karen Fog Olwig and Eva Gulløv, 179–96. London: Routledge, 2003.

Meinert, Lotte. *Hopes in Friction: Schooling, Health, and Everyday Life in Uganda.* Charlotte, NC: Information Age, 2009.

Meinert, Lotte. "Regimes of Homework: Questions of Responsibility and the Imagination of Lives in Uganda." In *Making Public Health in Africa: Ethnographic and Historical Perspectives*, ed. Ruth J. Prince and Rebecca Marsland, 119–39. Athens: Ohio University Press, 2013.

Meinert, Lotte and Susan Reynolds Whyte. "Epidemic projectification: AIDS Responses in Uganda as Event and Process." *Cambridge Anthropology* 32, no. 1 (2014): 77–94.

Meinert, Lotte, Hanne O. Mogensen, and Jenipher Twebaze. "Tests for Life Chances: CD4 Miracles and Obstacles in Uganda." *Anthropology and Medicine* 16, no. 2 (2009): 195–209.

Meinert, Lotte, Michael Whyte, Susan R. Whyte, and Betty Kyaddondo. "Faces of Globalization: AIDS and Arv Medicine in Uganda." *Folk* 45 (2004): 105–23.

Mills, C. Wright. *The Sociological Imagination*. New York: Grove, 1961 [1959].

Mitchell, J. C. "Case and Situation Analysis." In *The Manchester School. Practice and Ethnographic Praxis in Anthropology*, ed. T. M. S. Evens and D. Handelman, 23–44. New York: Berghahn, 2006.

Mogensen, Hanne O. *AIDS Is a Kind of Kahungu That Kills: The Challenge of Using Local Narratives When Exploring AIDS among the Tonga of Southern Zambia*. Copenhagen, Denmark: Scandinavian University Press, 1995.

Mogensen, Hanne O. "Finding a Path through the Health Unit: Practical Experience of Ugandan Patients." *Medical Anthropology* 24, no. 3 (2005): 209–36.

Mogensen, Hanne O. "New Hopes and New Dilemmas: Disclosure and Recognition in the Time of Antiretroviral Treatment." In *Morality, Hope and Grief: Anthropologies of AIDS in Africa*, ed. Hansjörg Dilger and Ute Luig, 61–79. New York: Berghahn, 2010.

Mogensen, Hanne O. "Ugandan Women on the Move to Stay Connected: The Concurrency of Fixation and Liberation." *Anthropologica* 53 (2011): 103–16.

Mol, Annemarie. *The Body Multiple: Ontology in Medical Practice*. Durham, NC: Duke University Press, 2002.

Moore, Henrietta L. *A Passion for Difference: Essays in Anthropology and Gender*. Cambridge: Polity, 1994.

Morris, Rosalind C. "Rush/Panic/Rush: Speculations on the Value of Life and Death in South Africa's Age of AIDS." *Public Culture* 20, no. 2 (2008): 199–231.

Mugyenyi, Peter. *Genocide by Denial: How Profiteering from HIV/AIDS Killed Millions*. Kampala, Uganda: Fountain, 2008.

Mugyenyi, Peter. "Flat-Line Funding for PEPFAR: A Recipe for Chaos." *The Lancet* 374 (2009): 292.

Mugyenyi, Peter. *A Cure Too Far: The Struggle to End HIV/AIDS*. Kampala: Fountain, 2012.

Muyinda, Herbert. "Limbs and Lives: Disability, Violent Conflict and Embodied Sociality in Northern Uganda." PhD dissertation, University of Copenhagen, 2008.

Myer, Landon, Rosalind J. Carter, Monica Katyal, Patricia Toro, Wafaa M. El-Sadr, and Elaine J. Abrams. "Impact of Antiretroviral Therapy on Incidence of Pregnancy among HIV-Infected Women in Sub-Saharan Africa: A Cohort Study." *PLoS Medicine* 7, no. 2 (2010): e1000229.

Nguyen, Vinh-Kim. "Antiretroviral Globalism, Biopolitics, and Therapeutic Citizenship." In *Global Assemblages*, ed. Aihwa Ong and Stephen Collier, 124–44. London: Blackwell, 2004.

Nguyen, Vinh-Kim. *The Republic of Therapy: Triage and Sovereignty in West Africa's Time of AIDS*. Durham, NC: Duke University Press, 2010.

Nguyen, Vinh-Kim, Cyriaque Yapo Ako, Pascal Niamba, Aliou Sylla, and Issoufou Tiendrébéogo. "Adherence as Therapeutic Citizenship: Impact of the History of Access to Antiretroviral Drugs on Adherence to Treatment." *AIDS*, supp. 5 (2007): S31–35.

Nsabagasani, Xavier, and P. Stanley Yoder. *Social Dynamics of VCT and Disclosure in Uganda*. Kampala: Uphold Project, Macro International, 2006.

Obbo, Christine. "Who Cares for the Carers? AIDS and Women in Uganda." In *Developing Uganda*, ed. Holger Bernt Hansen and Michael Twaddle, 207–14. Oxford: James Currey, 1998.

O'Neill, John. *Five Bodies: The Human Shape of Modern Society*. Ithaca, NY: Cornell University Press, 1985.

Parikh, Shanti. "Going Public: Modern Wives, Men's Infidelity, and Marriage in East-Central Uganda." In Jennifer S. Hirsch, Holly Wardlow, Daniel Jordan Smith, Harriet M. Phinney, Shanti Parikh, and Constance A. Nathanson. *The Secret: Love, Marriage and HIV*, 168–96. Nashville, TN: Vanderbilt University Press, 2009.

Park, Sung-Joon. "Stock-Outs in Global Health: Pharmaceutical Governance and Uncertainties in the Global Supply of ARVs in Uganda." In *Rethinking Biomedicine and Governance in Africa: Contributions from Anthropology*, ed. Paul Wenzel Geissler, Richard Rottenburg, and Julia Zenker, 177–94. Bielefeld: Transcript Verlag, 2012.

Parkhurst, Justin O. "The Ugandan Success Story? Evidence and Claims of HIV1 Prevention." *The Lancet* 360 (2002): 78–80.

Parkhurst, Justin O. "The Response to HIV/AIDS and the Construction of National Legitimacy: Lessons from Uganda." *Development and Change* 36, no. 3 (2005): 571–90.

Parkhurst, Justin O., and Louisiana Lush. "The Political Environment of HIV: Lessons from a Comparison of Uganda and South Africa." *Social Science and Medicine* 59 (2004): 1913–24.

Parkin, David. "The Categorization of Work: Cases from Coastal Kenya." In *Social Anthropology of Work*, ed. Sandra Wallman, 37–35. London: Academic, 1979.

Petryna, Adriana. *Life Exposed: Biological Citizens after Chernobyl*. Princeton, NJ: Princeton University Press, 2002.

Pfeiffer, James. "The Struggle for a Public Sector: PEPFAR in Mozambique." In *When People Come First: Critical Studies in Global Health*, ed. João Biehl and Adriana Petryna, 166–81. Princeton, NJ: Princeton University Press, 2013.

Pilcher, Jane. "Mannheim's Sociology of Generations: An Undervalued Legacy." *British Journal of Sociology* 45, no. 3 (1994): 481–95.

Prince, Ruth. "HIV and the Moral Economy of Survival in an East African City." *Medical Anthropology Quarterly* 26, no. 4 (2012): 534–56.

Putzel, James. "The Politics of Action on AIDS: A Case Study of Uganda." *Public Administration and Development* 24 (2004): 19–30.

Rasmussen, Louise Mubanda. "From Dying with Dignity to Living with Rules: AIDS Treatment and 'Holisitic Care' in Catholic Organisations in Uganda." PhD dissertation, University of Copenhagen, 2011.

Rasmussen, Louise Mubanda, and Lisa Ann Richey. "The Lazarus Effect of AIDS Treatment: Lessons Learned and Lives Saved." *Journal of Progressive Human Sciences* 23, no. 3 (2012): 187–207.

Redfield, Peter. *Life in Crisis: The Ethical Journey of Doctors without Borders*. Berkeley: University of California Press, 2013.

Richey, Lisa Ann. "Counselling Citizens and Producing Patronage: AIDS Treatment in South African and Ugandan Clinics." *Development and Change* 43, no. 4 (2012): 823–45.

Roby, Jini L., Stacey A. Shaw, Elinor Wanyama Chemonges, and Cole D. Hooley. "Changing Patterns of Family Care in Uganda: Father Absence and Patrilineal Neglect in the Face of HIV/AIDS." *Families in Society* 90, no. 1 (2009): 110–18.

Rose, Nikolas, and Carlos Novas. "Biological Citizenship." In *Global Assemblages: Technology, Politics, and Ethics as Anthropological Problems*, ed. Aihwa Ong and Stephen J. Collier, 439–63. Malden, MA: Blackwell, 2005.

Roth, Claudia. "'Shameful!': The Inverted Intergenerational Contract in Bobo-Dioulasso, Burkina Faso." In *Generations in Africa: Connections and Conflicts*, ed. Erdmute Alber, Sjaak van der Geest, and Susan Reynolds Whyte, 47–69. Münster, Germany: LIT Verlag, 2008.

Russell, Steven, and Janet Seeley. "The Transition to Living with HIV as a Chronic Condition in Rural Uganda: Working to Create Order and Control When on Antiretroviral Therapy." *Social Science and Medicine* 70 (2010): 375–82.

Russell, Steven, Janet Seeley, Enoch Ezati, Nafuna Wamai, Willy Were, and Rebecca Bunnell. "Coming Back from the Dead: Living with HIV as a Chronic Condition in Rural Africa." *Health Policy and Planning* 22 (2007): 344–47.

Seeley, Janet, and Steve Russell. "Social Rebirth and Social Transformation? Rebuilding Social Lives after Art in Rural Uganda." *AIDS Care* 22, supp. 1 (2010): S44–50.

Seeley, Janet, Grace Tumwekwase, and Heiner Grosskurth. "Fishing for a Living but Catching HIV: AIDS and Changing Patterns of the Organization of Work in Fisheries in Uganda." *Anthropology of Work Review* 30, no. 2 (2009): 66–76.

Seeley, Janet, E. Kajura, C. Bachengana, M. Okongo, U. Wagner, and D. Mulder. "The Extended Family and Support for People with AIDS in a Rural Population in South West Uganda: A Safety Net with Holes?" *AIDS Care* 5, no. 1 (1993): 117–22.

Seeley, Janet, Steven Russell, K. Khana, Enoch Ezati, Rachel King, and Rebecca Bunnell. "Sex after ART: The Nature of Sexual Partnerships Established by HIV-Infected Persons Taking Antiretroviral Therapy in Eastern Uganda." *Culture, Health and Sexuality* 11 (2009): 703–16.

Siu, Godfrey E., Daniel Wright, and Janet Seeley. "How a Masculine Work Ethic and Economic Circumstances Affect Uptake of HIV Treatment: Experiences of Men from an Artisanal Gold Mining Community in Rural Eastern Uganda." *Journal of the International AIDS Society* 15, supp. 1 (2012): 1/368.

Smith, Julia H., and Alan Whiteside. "The History of AIDS Exceptionalism." *Journal of the International AIDS Society* 13, no. 1 (2010): 47.

Sodemann, M., S. Biai, M.S. Jakobsen, and P. Aaby. "Knowing a Medical Doctor Is Associated with Reduced Mortality among Sick Children Consulting a Paediatric Ward in Guinea-Bissau, West Africa." *Tropical Medicine and International Health* 11, no. 12 (2006): 1868–77.

Southall, Aidan. "On Chastity in Africa." *Uganda Journal* 24, no. 2 (1960): 207–16.

Swidler, Ann. "Dialectics of Patronage: Logics of Accountability at the African AIDS-NGO Interface." In *Globalization, Philanthropy, and Civil Society*, ed. David C. Hammack and Steven Heydemann, 192–220. Bloomington: Indiana University Press, 2009.

Swidler, Ann. "Responding to AIDS in Sub-Saharan Africa: Culture, Institutions, and Health." In *Successful Societies: How Institutions and Culture Affect Health*, 128–50. Cambridge: Cambridge University Press, 2009.

Swidler, Ann, and Susan Cotts Watkins. "'Teach a Man to Fish': The Sustainability Doctrine and Its Social Consequences." *World Development* 37, no. 7 (2009): 1182–96.

Thornton, Robert J. *Unimagined Community: Sex, Networks, and AIDS in Uganda and South Africa*. Berkeley: University of California Press, 2008.

Twebaze, Jenipher. "Medicines for Life: Confidentiality and Information Control in the Lives of Clients and Providers in Ugandan ART Programs." PhD dissertation, University of Copenhagen, 2013.

Uganda AIDS Commission. *Global AIDS Response Progress Report: Country Progress Report Uganda*. Kampala, Uganda: Uganda AIDS Commission, 2012.

Uganda AIDS Commission. *National HIV/AIDS Atlas*. Kampala: Uganda AIDS Commission, 2005.

Uganda Bureau of Statistics. *The 2002 Uganda Population and Housing Census, Economic Characteristics*. Kampala, Uganda: Uganda Bureau of Statistics, 2006.

Uganda Bureau of Statistics and Macro International. *Uganda Demographic and Health Survey 2006*. Calverton, MD: Uganda Bureau of Statistics and Macro International, 2007.

Uganda Government. *UNGASS Country Progress Report Uganda, January 2008-December 2009*. http://starecuganda.jsi.com (2010).

Uganda Ministry of Health. *Uganda AIDS Indicator Survey 2011*. Kampala, Uganda: Ministry of Health, 2012.

US Department of State. *PEPFAR Blueprint: Creating an AIDS-Free Generation*. Washington, DC: Office of the Global AIDS Coordinator, 2012.

Van der Geest, Sjaak, Susan Reynolds Whyte, and Anita Hardon. "The Anthropology of Pharmaceuticals: A Biographical Approach." *Annual Review of Anthropology* 25 (1996): 153–78.

Vigh, Henrik Erdman. "Motion Squared: A Second Look at the Concept of Social Navigation." *Anthropological Theory* 9 (2009): 419–38.

Weiser, Sheri D., David M. Tuller, Edward A. Frongillo, Jude Senkungu, Nozmu Mukiibi, and David R. Bangsberg. "Food Insecurity as a Barrier to Sustained Antiretroviral Therapy Adherence in Uganda." *PLoS ONE* 5, no. 4 (2010): e10340.

Whiteside, Alan, and Julia Smith. "Exceptional Epidemics: AIDS Still Deserves a Global Response." *Globalization and Health* 5 (2009): 15.

Whyte, Michael A. "Talking about AIDS: The Biography of a Local AIDS Organization within the Church of Uganda." In *AIDS Education: Interventions in Multicultural Societies*, ed. I. Schnenker, G. Sabar-Friedman and F. Sy, 221–30. New York: Plenum, 1996.

Whyte, Michael A. "Social and Cultural Contexts of Food Production in Uganda and Kenya." In *African Families and the Crisis of Social Change*, ed. T. Weisner, C. Bradley, and P. Kilbride, 81–104. Westport, CT: Greenwood, 1997.

Whyte, Michael A. "Episodic Fieldwork, Updating, and Sociability." *Social Analysis* 57, no. 1 (2013): 110–21.

Whyte, Michael A., and David Kyaddondo. "'We Are Not Eating Our Own Food Here': Food Security and the Cash Economy in Eastern Uganda." *Land Degradation and Development* 17 (2006): 173–18.

Whyte, Susan Reynolds. "Pharmaceuticals as Folk Medicine: Transformations in the Social Relations of Health Care in Uganda." *Culture, Medicine and Psychiatry* 16, no. 2 (1992): 163–86.

Whyte, Susan Reynolds. *Questioning Misfortune: The Pragmatics of Uncertainty in Eastern Uganda*. Cambridge: Cambridge University Press, 1997.

Whyte, Susan Reynolds. "Creative Commoditization: The Social Life of Pharmaceuticals in Uganda." In *Locating Cultural Creativity*, ed. John Liep, 119–32. London: Pluto, 2001.

Whyte, Susan Reynolds. "Going Home? Burial and Belonging in the Era of AIDS." *Africa* 75, no. 2 (2005): 154–72.

Whyte, Susan Reynolds. "Discrimination: Afterthoughts on Crisis and Chronicity." *Ethnos* 73, no. 1 (2008): 97–100.

Whyte, Susan Reynolds. "Writing Knowledge and Acknowledgement: Possibilities in Medical Research. In *Evidence, Ethos and Experiment: The Anthropology and History of Medical Research in Africa*, eds. P. Wenzel Geissler and Catherine Molyneux, 29–56. Oxford: Berghahn Books, 2011.

Whyte, Susan Reynolds. "The Publics of the New Public Health: Life Conditions and 'Lifestyle Diseases' in Uganda." In *Making and Unmaking Public Health in Africa: Ethnographic and Historical Perspectives*, ed. Ruth J. Prince and Rebecca Marsland, 187–297. Athens: Ohio University Press, 2014.

Whyte, Susan Reynolds, and Harriet Birungi. "The Business of Medicines and the Politics of Knowledge in Uganda." In *Global Health Policy, Local Realities: The Fallacy of the Level Playing Field*, ed. Linda M. Whiteford and Lenore Manderson, 127–48. Boulder, CO: Lynne Rienner, 2000.

Whyte, Susan Reynolds, and Michael A. Whyte. "Children's Children: Time and Relatedness in Eastern Uganda." *Africa* 74, no. 1 (2004): 76–94.

Whyte, Susan Reynolds, Michael A. Whyte, and David Kyaddondo. "Health Workers Entangled: Confidentiality and Certification." In *Morality, Hope and Grief: Anthropologies of AIDS in Africa*, ed. Hansjörg Dilger and Ute Luig, 80–101. New York: Berghahn, 2010.

Whyte, Susan Reynolds, Michael A. Whyte, Lotte Meinert, and Betty Kyaddondo. "Treating AIDS: Dilemmas of Unequal Access in Uganda." *Journal of Social Aspects of HIV/AIDS* 1, no. 1 (2004): 14–26.

Whyte, Susan Reynolds, Michael A. Whyte, Lotte Meinert, and Jenipher Twebaze. "Therapeutic Clientship: Belonging in Uganda's Projectified Landscape of AIDS Care." In *When People Come First: Critical Studies in Global Health*, ed. João Biehl and Adriana Petryna, 140–65. Princeton, NJ: Princeton University Press, 2013.

Wilhelm-Solomon, Matthew. "Challenges for Antiretroviral Provision in Northern Uganda." *Forced Migration Review* 36 (2010): 16–18.

Wilhelm-Solomon, Matthew. "The Priest's Soldiers: HIV Therapies, Health Identities, and Forced Encampment in Northern Uganda." *Medical Anthropology* (2013): 227–46.

Wohl, Robert. *The Generation of 1914*. Cambridge, MA: Harvard University Press, 1979.

Wolf, Angelika. "Orphans' Ties: Belonging and Relatedness in Child-Headed Households in Malawi." In *Morality, Hope and Grief: Anthropologies of AIDS in Africa*, ed. Hansjörg Dilger and Ute Luig, 292–311. New York: Berghahn, 2010.

Wolf, Eric R. "Kinship, Friendship and Patron-Client Relations." In *The Social Anthropology of Complex Societies*, ed. Michael Banton, 1–22. London: Tavistock, 1966.

CONTRIBUTORS

PHOEBE KAJUBI is a doctoral student at Makerere University. Her research is on communication with children on HIV treatment in east-central Uganda and she has already published several articles from her study. She has been a guest teacher at Pomona College and a guest research student at the National University of Ireland, Maynooth.

DAVID KYADDONDO is a senior lecturer in the Department of Social Work and Social Administration, Makerere University, and has been a fellow at the Institute of Advanced Study in Berlin. He conducted his doctoral research on cash cropping and food security in eastern Uganda and has published articles on food security, children's money, and health care in Uganda.

LOTTE MEINERT is a professor in the Department of Culture and Society at Aarhus University. She is the author of *Hopes in Friction: Schooling, Health, and Everyday Life in Uganda* (2009), as well as articles on HIV based on fieldwork in eastern Uganda. She has led two collaborative research projects with Gulu University in northern Uganda and is co-director of the Center for Cultural Epidemics at Aarhus University.

HANNE O. MOGENSEN is an associate professor of anthropology at the University of Copenhagen. She is the author of *AIDS Is a Kind of Kahungu That*

Kills: The Challenge of Using Local Narratives When Exploring AIDS *among the Tonga of Southern Zambia* (1995), about the early years of the epidemic in Zambia. She has conducted fieldwork in eastern Uganda and has published articles on gender, family, child illness, and AIDS.

GODFREY ETYANG SIU is a postdoctoral researcher with the Medical Research Council in Uganda and is on the staff of Child Health and Development Centre, Makerere University. For his doctorate from the University of Glasgow he examined the relations between men's uptake of HIV treatment and their masculinity in rural eastern Uganda. He has published articles on this topic and on HIV and disclosure among adolescents living with HIV in Uganda.

JENIPHER TWEBAZE holds a master's degree in sociology from Makerere University and a doctorate in anthropology from the University of Copenhagen. Her dissertation project, "Medicines for Life," focused on health workers and clients of antiretroviral therapy in eastern and central Uganda and she has co-authored articles in this area.

MICHAEL WHYTE is an emeritus associate professor in the Department of Anthropology at the University of Copenhagen. He led the first Danish anthropological study of AIDS in Africa and is currently involved in a study of land conflict in Uganda. He has published articles on food scarcity, land conflict, and AIDS and is the co-editor (with Quentin Gausset and Torben Birch-Thomsen) of *Beyond Territory and Scarcity: Exploring Conflicts over Natural Resource Management* (2005).

SUSAN REYNOLDS WHYTE is a professor in the Department of Anthropology at the University of Copenhagen. She is the author of *Questioning Misfortune: The Pragmatics of Uncertainty in Eastern Uganda* (1997) and co-author (with Sjaak van der Geest and Anita Hardon) of *Social Lives of Medicines* (2003). She is co-editor (with Benedicte Ingstad) of *Disability and Culture* (1995) and *Disability in Local and Global Worlds* (2007), and (with Erdmute Alber and Sjaak van der Geest) of *Generations in Africa: Connections and Conflicts* (2008).

Matayo (interlocutor), 40, 134, 136, 156, 162, 225, 254, 271

Material support, 60, 65, 67, 101, 195, 211, 277. *See also* food aid

Matrifocal households, 155

Medical Access Uganda, 6

Medicine companion, 32, 239–40, 263

Medicines (other than ARVs): cost of, 75, 79, 240–41, 265–66; use practices, 52, 246, 250–51; variety of, 249–52. *See also* antiretroviral medicines, herbal medicine, nutritional supplements

Médicins sans Frontières, 6

Meinert, Lotte, 83, 106

Methodology, viii–xiv

Miracles, 3–4, 30, 31; and historical conditions, 273–75

Mobility, 80–81; accommodation and, 88–90; coordinates and, 81, 86, 87, 90, 93; fixity of programs and, 82–85, 93; homes and, 86–88; livelihood and, 90–91; topographies and, 81–82. *See also* transportation

Modernity, 271

Mogensen, Hanne O., 36, 115

Mol, Annemarie, 223

Money problems, 75, 76, 77, 183, 265, 281. *See also* school fees

Morality, 62, 135. *See also* kinship, amity of

Morris, Rosalind, 281

Moses (interlocutor), 66–67, 157, 251

Mugyenyi, Peter, 4, 13, 58, 257, 274–75

Mukuju Health Centre IV, 8, 38, 41, 49, 50, 51, 52, 53, 54, 55, 66, 83, 91

Mulago National Referral Hospital, 5, 7–8, 43, 44. *See also* Infectious Diseases Institute (IDI)

Museveni, Yoweri, 7, 11, 140

Muslims, *See* Islam

Muyinda, Herbert, 234

Mwangale Michael, 83, 84, 198

Narratives of HIV, 13–14, 64, 65

National Resistance Movement (NRM), 4–5, 6, 11–12, 140

Neopatrimonialism, 57. *See also* clientship, patron-client relations

Nevirapine, 147, 159, 243

NGOS, 5, 6, 101, 113, 162, 186–87, 209, 213, 234, 239. *See also* AIDS Information Centre, Plan International, TASO, World Vision

Nguyen, Vinh-Kim, 13, 58, 276–77

Noah, (interlocutor), 89,186

Non-governmental organizations. *See* NGOS

Norah (interlocutor), 37–38, 115, 159, 139, 225, 269–70

Nsambya Hospital, 6, 43–44, 85, 174

Nurses. *See* health workers

Nutritional supplements, 98, 251. *See also* Swissgarde

O'Neill, John, 223

Openness, 13, 16, 193, 194, 270

Orphans, 165; care of, 98, 111, 114, 115, 155, 156, 162, 164, 196, 210, 243; projects for, 101, 147

Paperwork, 59–60, 64, 69, 75, 147, 248; appointments and, 248–49; weight and, 230–31

Parikh, Shanti, 128–29, 130

Parkin, David, 177, 179

Partnership, 128–29; changes in quality of, 134–36; communication within, 131–33, 139; condoms and, 136–38; past and future of, 138–40; patterns of, 129–31; second thoughts on, 141

Patrilineality, 86, 87, 109, 130, 154

Patron-client relations, 57–58, 64, 65, 69, 276. *See also* clientship

Paul (interlocutor), 106, 116, 254

Pediatric ART, 85, 88, 240–1, 243

Pediatric Infectious Diseases Clinic, 85, 88, 241

PEPFAR, 3, 7, 8, 10–11, 58, 274–75; in Mozambique, 23n23

Personalization, 60–62, 276

Philip (interlocutor), 66, 83, 133, 139, 153, 161, 162, 255

Swissgarde, 98, 228, 251. *See also* nutritional supplements

Symptoms, 28–29, 31, 218, 224–29, 234; and CD4, 231–32, 233

TASO, 3, 60, 134; food rations provided by, 102, 198, 201, 210, 263; HBAC and, 8, 68, 99; medicines provided by, 31, 50, 67, 250; services provided by, 28, 60, 137, 195, 277

Technical Know Who (TKW), 35–37, 41, 42, 45

Technologies of the self, 234

Therapeutic citizenship, 58

Therapeutic clientship, 58–59, 80–81. *See also* clientship

Therapy managing groups, 35, 36, 38, 39–40, 42. *See also* connections

Tianshi, 251. *See also* nutritional supplements

TKW. *See* technical know who

TMG. *See* therapy managing groups

Tom (interlocutor), 41, 49, 90, 130, 139, 155, 182, 249

TORCH, ix

Tororo hospital, 49

Transfer to another ART program. *See* referral to another ART program

Transportation, 54, 196; costs of, 73, 76–77, 91–92, 172, 199, 241, 242. *See also* mobility

Travel, discomfort of, 91–92, 175

Treatment companion, 247, 254–55, 247–48, 270

Treatment seeking. *See* therapy managing group

Triomune, xi, 53, 66, 182, 203, 240, 243, 249, 250; side effects of, 256, 278

Tuberculosis, 43, 75, 146, 202, 219, 225, 228, 251, 254

Uganda AIDS Commission, 81

Uganda AIDS response history, 4–16

Uganda Cares, 6

Uganda Red Cross, 209

Uganda, AIDS history, 4–6

Ugandan Employment Act, 180

Uncertainties, 20, 62, 159, 160, 165, 176–77, 181, 188, 222, 269, 274, 278–80,

Vigh, Henrik, 82

Vincent (Interlocutor), 183

Violence against women, 97, 121–22, 138, 145, 146, 147, 150

Viral load, 147, 219, 224, 230, 248

Voluntary Counseling and Testing (VCT), 5, 37, 45, 97, 131, 133, 230

Volunteers, 65, 187–88

Vulnerability, 42, 45

Watkins, Susan Cotts, 65

Weber, Max, 57

Weight: gain, 195, 196, 199, 202, 211, 221, 222; loss as symptom, 49, 52, 99, 115, 175, 183, 201, 219, 225; monitoring, 224, 229–31, 240

WHO, 274

Widows: inheritance of, 27; pregnancy of, 156; rights of, 74, 86, 87, 98, 109, 110; support of, 104, 107, 207

William (interlocutor), 39, 114, 202, 231, 251, 255

Witchcraft, 49, 50, 99, 138, 262, 265, 266, 272–73

Wohl, Robert, 10, 16

Women's rights. *See* gender relationships

Work, 136, 176–77; contingencies of self-employment and farming, 183–4; HIV as qualification for, 186–8; kinds of, 177–79; medicine and, 240, 241–42; salary and, 193–94; second thoughts about, 188–89; security of salaried, 179–82; self-employment and, 178, 183, 197; strength and, 184–86; transfers, 41, 43, 55, 81, 90, 139, 181, 196, 279

Working class, 42, 90, 178

World Food Program, 209

World Vision, 3, 194, 209